KV-694-889

Author: Hirono I.

Date: 1987

Accn. No.:   No. 1

Location:

UDC No: 547·994 : 616-006·6

TROPICAL DEVELOPMENT AND RESEARCH
INSTITUTE LIBRARY

LIBRARY

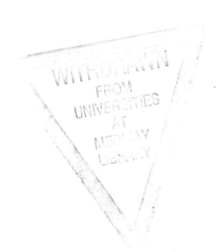

WITHDRAWN
FROM
UNIVERCITIES
AT
MEDWAY
LIBRARY

bioactive molecules

volume 2

NATURALLY OCCURRING CARCINOGENS OF PLANT ORIGIN

bioactive molecules

bioactive molecules

volume 2

4001291X

NATURALLY OCCURRING CARCINOGENS OF PLANT ORIGIN

——Toxicology, Pathology and Biochemistry

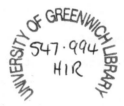

UNIVERSITY OF GREENWICH LIBRARY
547·994
HIR

Edited by

Iwao HIRONO, Professor

Fujita-Gakuen Health University School of Medicine
Toyoake, Aichi 470-11, Japan

1987

Kodansha
Tokyo

Elsevier
Amsterdam—Oxford—New York—Tokyo

Copublished by
KODANSHA LTD., Tokyo

and

ELSEVIER SCIENCE PUBLISHERS B. V., Amsterdam

exclusive sales rights in Japan
KODANSHA LTD.
12–21, Otowa 2-chome, Bunkyo-ku, Tokyo 112, Japan

for the U.S.A. and Canada
ELSEVIER SCIENCE PUBLISHING COMPANY, INC.
52 Vanderbilt Avenue, New York, NY 10017

for the rest of the world
ELSEVIER SCIENCE PUBLISHERS B. V.
25 Sara Burgerhartstraat, **P.O. Box 211, 1000 AE Amsterdam, The Netherlands**

Library of Congress Cataloging-in-Publication Data

Naturally occurring carcinogens of plant origin.

(Bioactive molecules ; v. 2)
Bibliography: p.
Includes index.
Contents: Cycasin / I. Hirono -- Pyrrolizidine
alkaloids / T. Furuya, Y. Asada, H. Mori -- Flavonoids /
S. Natori, I. Ueno -- [etc.]
1. Carcinogens. 2. Poisonous plants--Toxicology.
I. Hirono, Iwao, 1924- . II. Series.
RC268.6.N39 1987 616.99'4071 86-29338
ISBN 0-444-98972-2 (U.S. : Elsevier)

ISBN 0-444-98972-2 (Vol.2) ✓
ISBN 0-444-42633-7 (Series)

ISBN 4-06-202193-5 (Japan)

Copyright © 1987 by Kodansha Ltd.

All rights reserved.
No part of this book may be reproduced in any form, by photostat, microfilm, retrieval system, or any other means, without the written permission of Kodansha Ltd, (except in the case of brief quotation for criticism or review).

List of Contributors

Numbers in parentheses refer to the pages on which
a contributors' paper begin. Editor is asterisked.

Asada, Yoshihisa (2.1 and 2.2)   *School of Pharmaceutical Sciences, Kitasato University, Tokyo 108, Japan*

Enomoto, Makoto (7 and 8) *Biosafety Research Center, Foods, Drugs and Pesticides, Fukuda-machi, Shizuoka 477–12 & Japan Bioassay Laboratory, Hatano, Kanagawa 257, Japan*

Furuya, Tsutomu (2 1 and 2.2)   *School of Pharmacutical Sciences, Kitasato University, Tokyo 108, Japan*

Haga, Masanobu (11)   *Laboratory of Chemical Hygiene, Faculty of Pharmaceutical Sciences, Higashi Nippon Gakuen University, Tobetsu Hokkaido 061–02, Japan*

Hirata, Yoshimasa (10)   *Faculty of Pharmacy, Meijo University Nagoya 468, Japan*

*Hirono, Iwao (Introduction, 1, 4 and 5)   *Department of Pathology, Fujita-Gakuen Health University School of Medicine, Toyoake, Aichi 470–11, Japan*

Mori, Hideki (2.3–2.5 and 9)   *Department of Pathology, Gifu University School of Medicine, Gifu 500, Japan*

Natori, Shinsaku (3, 6 and 12)   *Meiji College of Pharmacy, Tanashi, Tokyo 188, Japan*

Suzuki, Eiji (10)   *Faculty of Pharmacy, Meijo University, Nagoya 468, Japan*

Ueno, Ikuko (3)   *Department of Cell Chemistry, Institute of Medical Science, University of Tokyo, Tokyo 108, Japan*

Yamada, Kiyoyuki (4.8 and 4.9)   *Department of Chemistry, Faculty of Science, Nagoya University, Nagoya 464, Japan*

Preface

This volume reviews the present state of studies of naturally occurring carcinogens of plant origin. These carcinogenic plant materials are used as human food or herbal remedies in many parts of the world. Epidemiological studies suggest that a large percentage, 80%–90%, of human cancer is of environmental origin. Thus, the chemical carcinogens in the total environment may be a major cause of human cancer. Naturally occurring carcinogens which have been so proved experimentally are relatively small in number. This does not mean that only a few natural products among the vast number of compounds are carcinogenic but rather that the number of compounds tested by adequate experimental methods is quite small compared with the number of synthetic chemicals tested. This is because feeding experiments for carcinogenicity testing require long periods of time and large amounts of materials, and in the case of natural products sufficient amounts of materials for such tests are generally not available.

The carcinogenic pyrrolizidine alkaloids and bracken carcinogen, which induce acute poisoning in livestock, are an important problem in the fields of veterinary medicine and dairy farming. This book deals with the toxicology, pathology, and biochemistry of these carcinogenic principles present in higher green plants.

It is hoped that the reviews in this book will provide a firm basis for the understanding of naturally occurring carcinogens of plant origin, and will thus make a contribution to the prevention of human cancer, in the future.

Iwao HIRONO

Contents

Introduction

It has been thirty years since the carcinogenicity of *Senecio jacobaea* L. was first discovered and a single dose of a pure pyrrolizidine alkaloid proved sufficient to induce chronic liver disease and liver tumors in rats. Since then many natural products of plant origin have been demonstrated to be carcinogenic. Very recently, ptaquiloside, a carcinogenic principle contained in bracken fern and a causative principle in bracken poisoning in cattle, was isolated. Naturally occurring carcinogens of plant origin are unique among various environmental carcinogens. They are secondary metabolites contained in certain plants used as food for human consumption and as folk (herbal) medicine since olden times. The hepatotoxic pyrrolizidine alkaloids known to occur in *Senecio jacobaea* L. are also present in honey produced from the nectar of the species. The risk of these naturally occurring carcinogens contained in food or herbal remedies for humans must not be ignored. It is probable that even a small amount of genotoxic carcinogen can induce tumors when enhancing or promoting agents act sufficiently over a long period of time. Except for occupational cancer, the cause of human cancer is still unknown. It is now clear from epidemiological data that most human cancers are induced by environmental causes. However, it is inconceivable that cancer in humans is generally caused by peculiar potent carcinogens present in daily life. A peculiar carcinogen as the causative principle of human cancer would not be detected even by epidemiological studies on environmental mutagens and carcinogens. The most probable etiological factor of human cancer is considered to be small amounts of various kinds of carcinogens and enhancing agents present in the environment.

Although it is difficult to consider these naturally occurring carcinogens of plant origin as a possible cause of human cancer from the amounts ingested as human food or herbal remedies, it is possible that even relatively small amounts can induce cancers, especially in those individuals with predisposing genetic backgrounds and/or dietary habits. A nursing infant can

1

be poisoned by mother's milk, if carcinogenic or hepatotoxic ingredients to which the adult may be resistant are present in her diet or in other products she uses. Therefore, ingestion of such plant materials should be avoided to prevent cancer and other disease. Progress in studies on the metabolism of these naturally occurring carcinogens in the human body will help elucidate the susceptibility of humans to these carcinogens and prevent cancer. Furthermore, there are still important problems to be solved in the fields of veterinary medicine and dairy farming concerning pyrrolizidine alkaloids and ptaquiloside, a bracken carcinogen, which induce acute poisoning in livestock.

1

Cycasin

Cycads are widely distributed throughout tropical and subtropical regions, and the species indigenous to Amami and Okinawa, the southwestern islands of Japan, is *Cycas revoluta* Thunb. Formerly on these islands, the seeds and trunks of cycads were invaluable food when other food supplies were destroyed by typhoons. Cycad seeds are still used as a source of starch and as a constituent of bean paste in some parts of the islands. The inhabitants of the island of Guam also use the nuts of the cycad, *Cycas circinalis* L., as a source of food starch. Accidental acute intoxication in humans caused by cycads has occasionally occurred by improper washing in the Okinawa islands. Cycasin, a toxic glycoside contained in the seeds of *Cycas revoluta*, was first isolated and identified by Nishida and his group in 1955 and later found by Riggs in *C. circinalis*.

In studies on the cause of amyotrophic lateral sclerosis, Laqueur *et al.* found that crude meal prepared from dried and ground seeds of cycad induced tumors of the liver, kidney, and intestine when fed to rats, and that the carcinogenic effect of the crude cycad material was due to its cycasin content. Spatz *et al.*, using germ-free rats, showed that cycasin is hydrolyzed to an aglycone by bacterial flora and that this aglycone is toxic and a proximate carcinogen. Studies on cycasin first demonstrated that intestinal bacterial flora may also be important in the carcinogenesis of human cancer.

1.1 Distribution of Cycads[1,2]

Cycads are ancient gymnosperms which are considered to be an intermediate in plant evolution from ferns to flowering plants. They were widely distributed throughout the world during the Mesozoic period. The cycads living today are limited to the tropical and subtropical zones around the

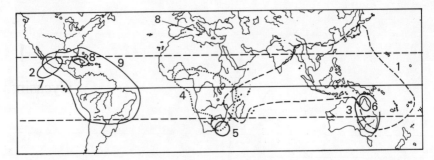

Fig. 1–1. Distribution of the genera of living cycads: 1, *Cycas*: 2, *Dioon*; 3, *Macroza-mia*: 4, *Encephalartos*; 5, *Stangeria*; 6, *Bowenia*; 7, *Ceratozamia*; 8, *Micro-cycas*; 9, *Zamia*.

globe, extending to some temperate regions such as Florida, U.S., Okinawa and Kagoshima Prefecture, Kyushu, Japan, and parts of Australia (Fig. 1–1). The cycad family, referred to as the Cycadaceae, today consits of nine living genera, each genus often having several species.

Cycas is the most widely distributed, from East Africa across the Indian Ocean and Japan to the Mariana Islands. The important species are *Cycas circinalis* L. and *C. revoluta* Thunb. The seed from *C. circinalis* is a large single round to oval body, 6 to 8 cm in diameter, whereas the seed of *C. revoluta* (Figs. 1–2, 1–3) is smaller. Both are covered by a husk, which is green and turns orange to red as the seeds mature. The masses of these seeds lie in the strobils. *Zamia* is the second most widely distributed cycad, growing on land bordering the Caribbean Sea and the northern parts of South America. It is an important genus growing in southern Florida. Two

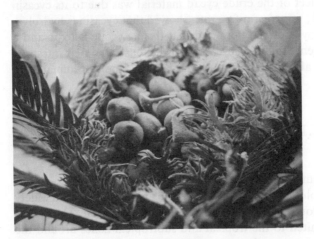

Fig. 1–2. Cycad, *Cycas revoluta* Thunb.

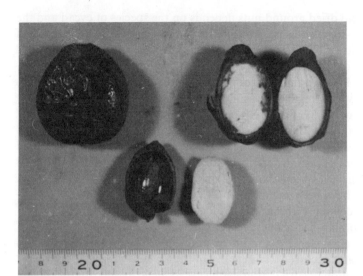

Fig. 1–3. Seed of cycad, *Cycas revoluta* Thunb.

genera, *Macrozamia* and *Bowenia,* the latter of which grows mainly in Queensland, are found in Australia. The first isolation of toxic compounds in cycads was carried out with specimens of *Macrozamia*. *Encephalartos* and *Stangeria* are the two African genera. *Microcycas* is found in Cuba and *Ceratozamia* in Mexico.

1.2 Cycad as Food

Cycas revoluta Thunb. is widely distributed in Amami and Okinawa, the southwestern islands of Japan. In these islands, the seeds and trunks of cycads were invaluable food when other food supplies were destroyed by typhoons before and during World War II. The cycad seeds are still used as a source of starch and as a constituent of the bean paste *miso* in some parts of the islands. It is also known that the inhabitants of Guam use nuts of the cycad, *C. circinalis* L., as a source of food starch. A review of the literature of the utilization and toxicity of cycads has been compiled by Whiting.[3]

Cycasin, a toxic glucoside, occurs in the seeds, trunks, and leaves of cycads. Cycad husk, which is eaten as candy by natives of Guam, also contains cycasin, and rats given diets containing 0.5 to 2% dry husk developed liver and kidney tumors.[4,5] The amount of cycasin present in cycad nuts and dried ground nuts depends on the species of cycad and the method used for drying the nuts: 0.016% cycasin was found in ground and dried nuts of *C. circinalis* prepared in Guam (leached with water and then sun-dried),[6] whereas 2.3% cycasin was found in unwashed, vacuum-dried nuts.[7] Palekar and Dastur[8] reported the cycasin content of *Cycas circinalis*. A wide range in cycasin content of seeds was observed varying from 0.55% to 3.6% in different batches. To prepare cycad starch, cycad nuts are cut into small pieces, soaked in water in a container or washed in running water, and dried. The hard dry pieces are ground and used as starch. Since cycasin is readily soluble in water, cycad starch and parts of cycads that have been thoroughly washed with water are safe to eat. Indeed, rats have been maintained on diets containing up to 10% commercial cycad flour without any evidence of a carcinogenic effect.[9]

Toxicity to man has generally been attributed to improper washing of the cycad nuts or stem. Acute intoxication in humans caused by cycads has occasionally occurred accidentally in the Okinawa islands.[10] In most cases, intoxication occurred after eating cycad *ojiya*, a kind of gruel boiled with bean paste or soy sauce. The latent time from the ingestion of cycad *ojiya* to the appearance of symptoms was 12 to 24 hr in most cases. The acute toxicity of cycasin in experimental animals also appeared at least 12 hr after oral administration of cycasin, and it is thought that the symptoms appeared only after a certain amount of aglycone had accumulated. In humans, the first sign of intoxication was the sudden development of nausea and vomiting. The victims then rapidly became unconscious, and most of them died within 20 hr after the appearance of the first sign of intoxication. In most victims, swelling of the liver was observed, and one victim who regained consciousness developed jaundice. Cycasin was carcinogenic in several kinds of test animals, and swelling of the liver and jaundice, which are symptoms of acute liver damage, were observed in the surviving victim as well as in test animals. These findings strongly suggest that cycasin is carcinogenic to man.

In 1959, the Miyako islands, Okinawa, suffered from a succession of typhoons; the inhabitants lost all their crops and had to subsist largely on cycads. A statistical survey of the mortality from cancer which was made in an attempt to assess the incidence of tumors in this community indicated no appreciable increase in cancer mortality.[10] This may have been due to the fact that the survey was made soon after the people had eaten cycads, or because the cycad foods were well prepared.

Kobayashi[11] used polarography and gas chromatography to examine the amount of cycasin in cycad materials used as food in Japan. He tested for the presence of cycasin in five samples of homemade cycad bean paste, *sotetsu miso*. Cycad bean paste is usually prepared as follows: cycad nuts are cut in half, then the kernel is washed with water and dried. The dried pieces are ground to a powder and mixed with rice or wheat to make *koji*. Beans and salt are added to the *koji* and the mixture is left to ferment. The ratio of cycad flour in the paste amounts to about one quarter to one third of the total weight of the paste. Kobayashi reported that none of the food materials containing cycad that he tested, such as cycad bean paste and starch, contained any detectable cycasin.

1.3 Discovery of the Carcinogenicity of Cycasin

An unusually high incidence of amyotrophic lateral sclerosis, a neurological disease, on the island of Guam was first reported by Kurland and Mulder.[12] It has also been reported that ingestion of cycad plant material in the tropics and subtropics where cycads are indigenous causes paralysis of the hind legs and ataxia in cattle.[3,13] Thus, studies on the cause of this disease focused on *Cycas circinalis*, which the Guamanians had long utilized as a source of food starch. In an exploratory study at the National Institutes of Health on the possible existence of neurotoxins in cycads, Laqueur *et al.*[14] found that rats fed crude cycad meal developed hepatocellular carcinomas, kidney tumors of both epithelial and mesenchymal types, and intestinal tumors, whereas nuerological disorder was not observed. Laqueur *et al.*[15,16] subsequently found that the carcinogen in cycads is cycasin (Fig. 1–4), which was first isolated from the seeds of *C. revoluta* Thunb., identified in 1955 by Nishida *et al.*,[17] and later found by Riggs[18] in *C. circinalis L.* from Guam.

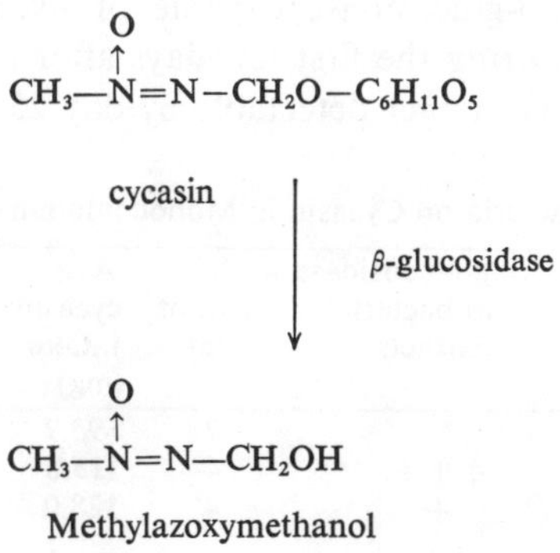

$$CH_3-\overset{\uparrow O}{N}=N-CH_2O-C_6H_{11}O_5$$

cycasin $\qquad$ β-glucosidase

$$CH_3-\overset{\uparrow O}{N}=N-CH_2OH$$

Methylazoxymethanol

Fig. 1–4. Chemical structure of cycasin and its aglycone, methylazoxymethanol.

1.4 Metabolism of Cycasin and Its Carcinogenicity

Cycasin was toxic only when given orally, and its toxicity appeared after a period of about 12 hr.[19] Thus it seemed likely that a metabolite of cycasin was the toxic compound. Since cycasin was apparently not toxic to germ-free rats, its fate in germ-free and conventional rats was compared by measuring the oral cycasin intake and its fecal and urinary excretion by these animals. Results showed that in germ-free rats excretion of cycasin was 97% of the intake, whereas in conventional rats it was only 26%.[20] These observations strongly suggested that intestinal microorganisms contained the enzyme that hydrolyzed cycasin *in vivo*. Germ-free rats were then infected with pure strains of microorganisms with or without β-glucosidase activity, as determined by *in vitro* assay. After successful colonization of the intestine, cycasin was administered by stomach intubation. Agreement was found between the enzymic activity of the microorganisms and extent of cycasin hydrolysis (Table 1–1).[21] Whereas cycasin was toxic and carcinogenic only after passage through the gastrointestinal tract, its aglycone methylazoxymethanol (MAM) (Fig. 1–4) was toxic and induced tumors in conventional and germ-free rats irrespective of the route of administration[22–27]; MAM was, therefore, the proximate carcinogen. It has also been shown that the synthetic MAM acetate induced tumors in germ-free rats.[28] MAM acetate was synthesized by oxidation of 1,2-dimethylhydrazine to azomethane, then to azoxymethane, followed by bromination and subsequent conversion of the bromoazoxymethane to the acetate by reaction with silver acetate.[29]

The skin of newborn rats and of rats during early postnatal life was found to contain a β-glucosidase capable of hydrolyzing cycasin. Its activity was highest during the first few days after birth, decreased from day 5 to 8, and was no longer detectable by day 25 after birth.[30,31] The

Table 1–1. Effects of Bacteria on Cycasin in Monocontaminated Germ-free Rats[21]

Monocontaminant	β-glucosidase in bacterial extracts	No. of rat	Avg. cycasin intake (mg)	Cycasin excreted in 48 hr	
				mg	%
None		7	95.7	88.7	92.7
Streptococcus fecalis	+++	4	115.8	34.1	29.4
Lactobacillus salivarius salicinius	+	4	128.0	93.6	73.1
Lactobacillus salivarius salivarius	−	4	97.5	93.9	96.3

demonstration of β-glucosidase activity in subcutaneous tissue of newborn and early postnatal rats provides an explanation for the toxic[32] and carcinogenic[33-37] effects of cycasin which were observed after a single sc injection of cycasin into newborn animals.

Histological types of most tumors in rats induced by cycasin or MAM were classified by Laqueur *et al.*[14,23] as follows: (1) liver—liver cell adenoma, liver cell carcinoma, bile duct adenoma, and cystadenoma; (2) kidney—adenoma, interstitial tumor, nephroblastoma, and sarcoma; (3) intestine—adenoma and adenocarcinoma.

Rats

When crude cycad meal was fed to young rats, tumors were induced in liver, kidneys and colon, in order of frequency, after long-term feeding, whereas the frequency of tumor sites was kidneys, colon and liver in short-term experiments.[14,15] Thus differences in principal tumor sites was observed depending on the length of exposure.

Rats have been the ainmals most frequently used for studies in carcinogenesis with cycad materials, and tumor induction has been successful in all strains in which it was attempted.

Hepatocellular carcinomas of the liver generally resulted after long-term feeding of crude cycad meal or of cycasin mixed with the diet. They occurred either as large often solitary carcinomas or as multiple primary hepatic carcinomas.

Although liver tumors have most readily been induced in long-term feeding experiments with cycasin or crude cycad meal, they have also developed after single intragastric instillation of cycasin or following subcutaneous injection of cycasin into newborn rats,[33] subcutaneous and intraperitoneal administration of cycasin to preweanling rats,[38] and after single or repeated doses of MAM or MAM-acetate given to conventional and germ-free rats.[28,29]

Tumors of the kidney were most frequently encountered in rats exposed for short periods of time to either cycasin or crude cycad meal as part of the diet. They were found also after administration of MAM or MAM acetate. The cycasin-induced kidney tumors usually developed multiply and bilaterally, and histologically different types were observed in the kidneys of the same rat. The tumors were derived either from epithelial cells lining the tubules, or from mesenchymal cells giving rise to adenomas and adenocarcinomas, or to mesenchymal tumors and sarcomas. Among the renal tumors, those now referred to as mesenchymal tumors have been variously interpreted as to their histogenesis. The tumors were originally designated by Laquer *et al.*[14,23] as undifferentiated proliferative lesions or interstitial tumors. Light and electron microscopic studies of cycasin-induced renal tumors have been published by Gusek *et al.*[40-43]

and Buss and Gusek.[44] Gusek et al.[40] reported that interstitial tumors have their origin in preexisting electron-microscopically demonstrable fibroblastic elements of the basal membrane and the fiber supporting framework and can be described as a special sclerosing angio-fibroblastoma because of the nature of tumor cells to differentiate into fibroblasts and angioblasts. They were readily distinguished from kidney adenomas by their location at the corticomedullary junction and by their poor delineation from the surrounding renal parenchyma. Microscopically, the interstitial tumors were composed of spindle cells lying between tubules and vessls. In larger lesions, the central part showed hyalin vascular changes. Tumors of the colon were the third most frequently observed neoplasm in the early studies in which crude cycad meal or cycasin mixed with the basal diet was fed to rats.[14,16] The tumors were situated principally in the proximal half of the colon and several in the cecum. The small intestines and lower colon and rectum were free of neoplasms.

This situation drastically changed in subsequent experiments in which the aglycone of cycasin, MAM, the synthetic MAM-acetate and MAM-glucuronide were used. The proximate carcinogen used in either its natural or synthetic form resulted in a considerable increase in the number of tumors and a much wider involvement of the intestinal tract in the neoplastic process. MAM and MAM-acetate administered either in a single or in multiple intraperitoneal doses induced tumors in the small intestine, particularly carcinomas in the duodenum in addition to large bowel tumors,[23,28] but intrarectal instillation of MAM-acetate for 2 to 26 days into Donryu rats induced a very high incidence of carcinomas extending from the cecum to the rectum.[25] The intestinal tumors were sessile or polypoid, benign or malignant.

Brain tumors occurred in rats which had been exposed to the carcinogenic activity of cycads during late fetal life.[45] The majority of the brain tumors histologically resembled oligodendrogliomas. According to Hoch-Ligeti et al.,[5] who examined ground fresh and dried cycad seed husks for oncogenic effect, malignant tumors of liver and kidneys were induced in nearly all rats. Yang et al.[4] reported similar findings. Tumor induction has also been successful with seeds of Encephalartos hildebrandtii from Kenya.[46] The azoxyglycoside in this cycad is macrozamin, according to Dossaji and Herbin.[47] The tumors induced in liver, kidney, and lung were similar to those described with cycasin.

There are many reports on the carcinogenicity of cycasin in rats.[15,16,33,42,48-50] It is noteworthy that its tumorigenic effect is not limited to rats, but has also been demonstrated in mice,[34,35,37,51] hamsters,[36] guinea pigs,[52] rabbits,[53] and aquarium fish[54] (Table 1–2). Even upon single administration, cycasin and MAM induced tumors of the kidney and large intestine in rats, tumors of the liver and lung in mice, and intrahepatic bile duct tumors in hamsters.[55]

Table 1-2. Carcinogenicity of Cycasin

Animal†	Target organs and histological findings
Rat[33]	Large intestine (Adenoma, adenocarcinoma), Kidney (Adenoma, nephroblastoma, interstitial tumor, sarcoma). Hepatocellular carcinoma also can be induced by a long-term oral administration.[14,15]
Mouse[34,35,37]	Hepatocellular carcinoma, lung adenoma
Hamster[36,55]	Cholangiocellular carcinoma
Guinea pig[57]	Hepatocellular carcinoma
Rabbit[53]	Malignant hemangioendothelioma of the liver
Monkey[58]	Hepatocellular carcinoma, renal carcinoma
Fish[54]	Hepatic tumor

† Rat, mouse and hamster received a single oral administration of cycasin. Remaining animals received long-term oral administration.

Mice

Carcinogenic effects of cycads in mice were first described by O'Gara *et al.*[51] who observed tumors in liver and kidney in male C57BL mice after repeated topical application of aqueous emulsion of seeds of *C. circinalis* to skin ulcers artificially induced with 10% croton oil. The experiment was designed to simulate situations in life where cycad juices have reportedly been used in the treatment of skin wounds and ulcers.[3] Tumors were found in 3 of 11 mice surviving the acute toxic effects. One had a hepatocellular carcinoma, kidney adenoma, and a subcutaneous hemangioma at the site of injection. A second mouse had a large kidney adenoma and multiple cystic lesions in the liver, while a third mouse had a large hemangiosarcoma of the liver. The simultaneous presence of cycasin, MAM and β-glucosidase in the seeds of cycads provides the chemicals necessary for tumor induction both at the site of application and at distant sites. Carcinogenic effects in newborn and adult mice of C57BL/6 strain by a single administration of cycasin were reported.[34] The newborn mice received single subcutaneous injections of 0.5 mg cycasin/g body weight within 24 hours after birth. Adult animals received one dose of 0.3–1.0 mg cycasin/g body weight through a stomach tube. Tumor incidence caused by cycasin was lower in mice, whether newborn or adult, than in rats. Newborn mice, however, were more susceptible to the carcinogenic effects of cycasin than the adult mice, and the newborn animals developed reticulum cell neoplasms of the liver much sooner than the control animals. Tumors of the intestine or kidney, frequently observed in cycasin-treated rats, were rarely found in mice. On the other hand, hepatomas, which were extremely rare in rats treated with a single administration of cycasin, were encountered at a high incidence in mice.

All of the newborn mice that survived for more than 280 days after the administration of cycasin developed hepatomas. It was noted that hepatomas developed and metastasized more frequently in mice treated as newborns than as adults. A subsequent study further emphasized the importance of age in the immediate postnatal period when a single subcutaneous injection of cycasin produced a 100% tumor incidence in the newborn, but only 16% in 14-day-old mice at comparable doses.[37] In another experiment on newborn mice of the dd strain, the animals received single subcutaneous injections of cycasin at two dose levels (0.5 mg or 1.0 mg cycasin/g body weight). Lung tumors were observed in 88% of mice surviving beyond 150 days and liver tumors were induced in 64% with the smaller dose, but the larger dose produced 83% lung tumors and 37% liver tumors in the mice. Early mortality was high in this group, amounting to 50% by the 16th day.[35] Many of the mice of the second group had various degrees of ataxia due to maldevelopment of the cerebellar cortex.

Hamsters

Observations on tumor induction in hamsters with cycasin have been made by our group,[36,55] and with MAM by Spatz,[56] and by Laqueur and Spatz.[57] The intrahepatic bile ducts showed the most extensive changes, and 21 intrahepatic bile duct carcinomas were recorded among 151 hamsters when cycasin was given subcutaneously to newborn hamsters or by stomach intubation to adult hamsters. Several of them were subcutaneously established as transplantable tumor lines.[36] We observed a carcinoma of the gall bladder, hepatocellular carcinomas, and hemangioendothelial sarcomas of the liver in hamsters treated as newborns, whereas such tumors were rarely seen in hamsters which had received cycasin as adults by stomach tube. A few colonic tumors, pulmonary adenomas and an occasional renal tumor, were also observed.[36] Spatz[56] reported the induction of hepatic and colonic carcinomas and of two carcinomas of the gall bladder in hamsters with MAM administered either in a single intravenous dose, or in multiple intraperitoneal injections at a dose of 20 mg/kg body weight.

Guinea Pigs

Crude cycad meal varying in concentration from 5 to 10% was fed to guinea pigs for one or two 5-day periods. The acute changes in the liver were identical to those previously seen in rats and alterations were dose-dependent. Among 27 survivors which were sacrificed between 11 and 22 months after first exposure to cycad meal, nine guinea pigs had liver tumors of which four were hepatocellular and five biliary in type. There were no metastases, but several animals had focal hyperplastic lesions in the mucosa of gall bladder and esophagus.[57] In another experiment, in which known doses of MAM or MAM-acetate instead of crude cycad meal were used, hepatocellular carcinomas were found in 30 of 45 guinea pigs surviving 6 months or longer, and 23 of them had metastasized. Bile duct carcinomas were found in two.[57]

Rabbits

Fifteen rabbits were administered cycad extract by gastric intubation, 1 ml/rabbit, once a week for 27 or 33 weeks. The extract contained 16.6 mg of cycasin/ml. Out of 9 rabbits surviving over 200 days, 7 animals developed malignant hemangioendotheliomas of the liver.[53]

Monkeys

The carcinogenic potential of cycasin and MAM acetate in monkeys was studied by Sieber *et al.*[58] Rhesus, cynomolgus, and African green monkeys received cycasin and/or MAM acetate by oral or ip routes. Hepatocellular carcinoma, intrahepatic bile duct adenoma, renal carcinoma and adenomas, and adenomatous polyps of the colon were observed in monkeys which had received cycasin and/or MAM acetate for an average of 57 months. Another group which received weekly ip injections of MAM acetate for an average of 75 months also had almost the same tumors as mentioned above. These results showed that long-term administration of cycasin and/or MAM acetate by oral and ip routes was carcinogenic in monkeys.

Fishes

Stanton[54] first described the development of tumors in the liver of aquarium fishes, *Brachydanio rerio* and *Lebistes reticulatus*, by cycasin.

Aoki and Matsudaira[59-61] reported that hepatic tumors can be initiated by treatment with MAM acetate in the small aquarium fish *medaka* (*Oryzias latipes*). A high incidence of hepatic tumors including trabecular carcinomas and cholangiomas was observed within 2–3 months after short-term exposure to high levels (0.5–10 ppm) of MAM acetate. Also, the same tumors could be detected within 5 months after long exposure to a low level (0.1 ppm) of the MAM acetate with similar incidence.[59] The same authors studied the relationship between the level of MAM acetate (0–2.0 ppm) and tumor incidence after exposure for 1 day. The incidence increased as the level of drug increased, although an apparent threshold was seen at low levels. The incorporation of [³H] thymidine into the liver greatly increased over the period of 6–20 days after treatment with 0.5 ppm for 3 days. However, only a slight increase in incorporation was found when fish were treated continuously with a low level (0.1 ppm) from days 30 through 90.[61]

Rats given cycad meal or cycasin developed intestinal tumors generally in the large intestine,[14,15,33] and consecutive administration of MAM or MAM acetate induced tumors not only in the large intestine but also in the small intestine, especially in the duodenum.[16,23] The tumorigenesis in the small intestine and cystic degeneration of intrahepatic bile ducts or the high incidence of cholangiogenic tumors induced by cycasin or MAM indicated that their metabolites might be excreted with bile.[36,62] Weisburger[63] also suggested that MAM or its conjugate was secreted into bile and by this route caused intestinal tumors in rats. The conjugate, MAM-glucosiduronic acid (MAM-GlcUA), is carried down to the colon with the bile where bacterial β-glucuronidase hydrolyzes the compound and releases free MAM, which induces neoplastic growth. This hypothesis was tested with MAM-GlcUA which was synthesized by oxidation of the primary alcohol of the glucose moiety of cycasin to a carboxylic acid.[64] The bile which was collected from male Wistar rats with cannulated bile ducts and injected with varying quantities of MAM-GlcUA (20 to 160 mg/kg body weight) was analyzed for the compound. The compound was not found in the bile. All the compound was found excreted in the urine at all levels administered. There was no indication that MAM-GlcUA was formed when MAM was injected into cannulated rats.[65] Zedeck *et al.*[66] reported that carcinogen metabolized from MAM acetate probably reaches intestinal mucosa mainly through the vascular system rather than through biliary transport. To clarify the vascular route of metabolism of MAM acetate, rats were subjected to single-barreled colostomies for the complete exclusion of the fecal stream at the proximal one third of the colon and were given consecutive intravenous injections of MAM acetate.[67] These animals developed tumors in the colon distal to the colostomy where the mucosa did not have contact with fecal stream. These results indicated that carcinogens could probably reach the intestinal mucosa via the vascular system as well as by biliary transport.

Transplacental Passage of Cycad Toxin

Transplacental passage was strongly suggested when acute liver lesions were found in pups of rats fed crude cycad meal during pregnancy. Similar observations were made with a litter of shoats, indicating transmammary passage, because the pigs had at no time access to cycad meal except through the milk from the sow.[68] Subsequent to the identification and isolation of the cycad toxins, cycasin, and its aglycone MAM,[6] it was shown that both chemicals passed through the placenta into fetal rats, and MAM was also demonstrated to be present in fetal hamster tissue when MAM was intravenously given to pregnant hamsters.[69] It was shown, in addition, that after passage through the placenta MAM reacted by methylation with constituents of rat liver,[70] with fetal rat brain after intraperitoneal administration of ^{3}H-MAM-acetate into pregnant rats,[71] as well as with nucleic acid *in vitro*.[72]

Transplacental Carcinogenesis

Transplacental tumor induction with cycad material was first accomplished with crude cycad meal containing 3% cycasin when fed to impregnated rats of the Sprague-Dawley strain during the first, second, or third week, or throughout the entire period of gestation. The concentration of the cycad meal in the diet was 1, 3, and 5%. Fifteen of 81 long-term survivors (18.5%) had tumors at various sites; most frequently gliomas and jejunal tumors.[45]

1.5 Biologic Effects of Cycasin and MAM

Acute subcellular changes in rats induced by MAM were compared with those produced by three other liver toxins, dimethylnitrosamine (DMN), carbon tetrachloride, and hydrazine sulfate. Both MAM and DMN were found to produce similar subcellular changes when compared at equivalent doses and times. The most prominent lesions were segregation of nucleolar components with depletion of granular material, hypertrophy of the smooth endoplasmic reticulum, decreases in the number of ribosomes, and formation of membrane whorls (Fig. 1–5).[73,74] Cellular necrosis was noted in nearly all of the centrilobular cells. This process of liver cell necrosis was accompanied by hemorrhage in most lobules. Rats which had died or were moribund and sacrificed at this stage frequently had free fluid in their body cavities and striking edema of the pancreas. MAM injected intravenously into golden hamsters on the eighth day of pregnancy arrested normal development, causing a variety of malformations, including hydrocephalus, microcephalus, cranioschisis, exencephaly, spina bifida, rachischisis, anophthalmia, microophthalmia, and oligodactyly.[75] Microencephaly was induced when exposure to MAM took place at the beginning of the third week of intrauterine development (on days 14, 15, and 16 of gestation) and it was found in all littermates; it was readily reproducible and inducible independent of rat strain. A single administration of 20 mg/kg body weight of MAM on day 15 of gestation was determined to be optimal. The reduction in size predominantly involved the cerebral hemispheres.[76] Histologic examination of the brain 48 hr after the administration of MAM showed extensive necrosis among the cells of the subependymal matrix zone, which provides the cells for the developing cerebral cortex under normal conditions.[76] Strong uniformity was observed within each litter in the reduction in weight of the cerebrum, although differences were noted between litters. An estimate of the cellular loss from the hemispheres of MAM-treated rats was obtained by comparing the quantitative changes with age in the DNA content of microcephalic brain with those of controls. The difference amounted to about

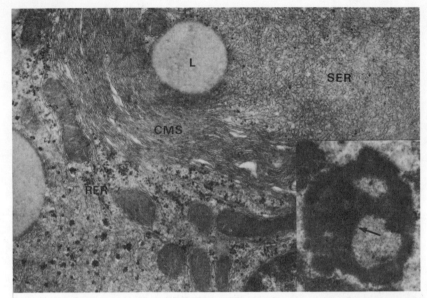

Fig. 1–5. Central portion of hepatic lobule from a rat given cycasin 250 mg/kg body weight and sacrificed at 24 hr. Deorganized rough endoplasmic reticulum forms concentric membraneous structure (CMS). The cytoplasm exhibits depletion of free ribosomes and increase of smooth endoplasmic reticulum (SER). RER; rough endoplasmic reticulum, L; lipid droplet × 21,000 A dwindled nucleolus in a hepatocyte of the central portion of the lobule from a rat given 250 mg/kg cycasin and sacrificed at 6 hr (insert). The depleted granular components (arrow) and fibrillar components have segregated into zones. × 15,000 Source: Mori, 1974.[74]

25% at birth, and persisted into maturity. The hemispheres of a 7-day-old MAM-treated rat contained about one half of the DNA content of the same parts of the brain in controls, when the hemispheres and other remaining parts of the brain were analyzed separately. There was no difference in the remaining parts of the brain.[77] These microencephalic rats showed intellectual deficits.[78] Gliomas were found in four of 44 microencephalic rats older than 1 year.[76] It has been reported also that newborn mice and hamsters that received a single administration of cycasin at 0.2 to 1.0 mg/g body weight within 24 hr after birth developed extensive necrosis of the cells of the external granular layer of the cerebellum resulting in defective development of the molecular and granule cell layers, and has ataxia and gait disturbances.[79,80] In contrast to mice and hamsters, however, a similar dosage failed to induce clinical signs of neurologic disorders in rats. The cerebellar lesions in rats were not as severe as those in mice and hamsters. The cerebellar changes in mice and hamsters persisted and were seen as late as 260 days after birth. Prerequisite for a

successful induction of the cerebellar cortical alteration was the administration of cycasin on the day of birth.[80] These observations were confirmed using MAM-acetate, which was given to newborn hamsters 2 to 4
days postnatally.[81] The necrosis of cells in the external granular layer
was more severe in the anterior than in the posterior lobes, when MAM-
acetate was administered from the 4th to 6th day of postnatal life. Haddad
et al.[82] observed dose-dependent changes in size and architecture of the
cerebellum of rats. Fine structural alterations of cerebella in mice which
were treated with cycasin within 24 hr after birth and examined 25 days
later showed marked reduction in the number of granule cells and their
processes including presynaptic terminals. Purkinje cells were present and
were essentially normal.[83,84] In addition, mice and rats which received a
single sc injection of cycasin 0.5 mg/g body weight within 24 hr after birth
produced extensive necrosis in the neuroblastic layer of the retina 72 hr
after injection. This resulted in rosette formation and abnormal structure
of the outer nuclear layer showing protrusion into the bacillary layer in
mice. In rats, the outer plexiform layer did not appear and the inner and
outer nuclear layers failed to form. Thus the retinal lesions induced by a
single administration of cycasin were much more severe in rats than in
mice.[55,85] Shimada and Langman[81] reported that severe retinal hypoplasia was noted in hamsters which received injections of MAM-acetate
between the 4th and 6th days of life and examined on the 20th postnatal
day. The thinning was most conspicuous in the prospective nuclear layer
of the retina and was accompanied by formation of rosettes.

Smith[86] showed that MAM is mutagenic in *Salmonella typhimurium*.
Observations that larvae of the arctiid moth, *Seirarctia echo*, were fed on
cycad plants without ill effects are also of interest. Extracts of larvae
feeding on cycad leaves, when analyzed, had relatively large amounts of
cycasin. The cycasin was carried over into the pupa, adult, and egg.[87] It
was also observed that all stages of *Seirarctia* except the egg contained an
emulsin-like enzyme, although free MAM was not detected in undamaged
insects or in the plant tissues. Teas,[88] in a subsequent study, reported that
larvae of *S. echo* fed MAM in an artificial diet for 24 hr had the largest
amount of cycasin in the hemolymph followed by the Malpighian tubules.
Enzymatic activity measured as β-glucosidase was strongest in the gut
and absent from the other sites. Apparently, the MAM fed to the larvae
had been glycosylated to cycasin and retained in part in the hemolymph,
and excreted in part by the Malpighian tubules, thus protecting the larvae
from the potentially hazardous effects of MAM. The acetate ester of
MAM was slightly mutagenic but preincubation with bacterial cells markedly increased the number of revertants. Pretreatment with β-glucuroni-
dase was required in the case of the gucuronide of MAM before muta-

genicity was demonstrable.[89] Gabridge, Denunzio and Legator,[90] using host-mediated assay, injected intraperitoneally histidine auxotrophs of *S. typhimurium* 2 hr after MAM and cycasin were given orally. Two hours were allowed for the hydrolysis of cycasin to proceed to its maximum. Mutation frequency was increased over control many fold more with MAM than with cycasin. Teas and Dyson[91] reported that a marked rise in sex-linked recessive lethal mutations was noted in *Drosophila melanogaster* after addition of MAM or MAM acetate to the nutrient medium. Radiomimetic effect of cycasin was also reported by Teas *et al.*[92] They found that exposure to cycasin of onion root tip cells, which show β-glucosidase activity, resulted in as many chromosomal aberrations as could be produced with 200 R of gamma rays. Then, the effect of radio-protective agents on the acute toxicity of cycasin was studied.[33] As protective agents, β-mercaptoethylamine (cysteamine) and 3-amino-1,2,4-triazole were used and given intraperitoneally once to rats at different times relative to a single gastric instillation of lethal dose of cycasin. It was found that rats could be protected from a lethal dose of cycasin by both compounds when the protective agent was given shortly before cycasin. All rats which survived beyond 6 months had tumors.

1.6 Biochemical Actions of Cycasin and MAM

The feeding of ground *Cycas circinalis* L. endosperm or cycasin produced an almost identical loss of RNA and phospholipids from rat liver cells. These changes correlated closely with loss of cytoplasmic basophilia, and with loss of ribosomes from the endoplasmic reticulum seen with the electron microscope. No effect on hepatic DNA concentration occurred.[93] Zedeck *et al.*[94] reported that a single nonlethal dose of MAM acetate inhibited thymidine incorporation into DNA of liver, small intestine, and kidney of rats. The effect was most marked in the liver, which was the only organ to show inhibition of RNA and protein synthesis. Similarities between the biochemical actions of cycasin and dimethylnitrosamine were described by Shank and Magee[70] and Miller.[95] It was speculated that cycasin and dimethylnitrosamine are metabolized to the same biochemically active compound, perhaps diazomethane[95] and methyldiazonium hydroxide.[96] Proton magnetic resonance studies on the decomposition of MAM in D_2O eliminated the possibility of formation of diazomethane.[97] Methyldiazonium hydroxide, as proposed by Druckrey,[96] is suggested as the transient methyl donor. Methyldiazonium hydroxide can arise either directly from MAM or indirectly from a cyclic intermediate through the azene and the diazo-hydroxide.[97] Schoental[98] first suggested that MAM might be activated through oxidation to methylazoxyformaldehyde by alcohol dehydrogenase (ADH). Grab and Zedeck[99] have demonstrated that MAM can serve as a substrate for ADH. They found that NAD$^+$ dependent ADH activity was present in those tissues, such as liver and colon, which are sensitive to acute and carcinogenic effects of MAM. There was no NAD$^+$-dependent ADH activity in the kidney but with NADP$^+$ ADH was more active with MAM than with ethanol. Pyrazole, an ADH inhibitor, blocked the oxidation of MAM, and when given to rats 2 hr prior to the administration of MAM reduced its lethality. Thus they suggest that ADH activity in the metabolism of MAM may be responsible for the organ-specific effects of MAM in tumor induction.[99] Matsumoto and Higa[72] and Nagata and Matsumoto[71] who studied the methylation of nucleic acids by MAM *in vitro* and in fetal rat brain, respectively, found that MAM reacted with nucleic acids and fetal proteins in rats when the compound was administered on the 14th day of gestation. Guanine methylated in the 7-position was found in both DNA and RNA. Matsumoto[65] studied the carcinogenicity of MAM-GlcUA in rats. MAM-GlcUA and cycasin have a common aglycone, MAM, and thus it would be expected that MAM-GlcUA, when administered orally, would induce tumors at the same sites as those induced by cycasin. However, the largest number of neoplasms induced by a single oral administration of MAM-GlcUA was located in the intestinal tract and predominantly in the colon. Neoplasms of the liver were few in number and consisted either of liver cell nodules or of single or multiple cystadenomas of bile duct origin. Renal tumors were also few in number. There is a reasonably high β-glucuronidase activity in both the small and large intestine, but MAM-GlcUA was not carcinogenic to germ-free rats.[100] Bacterial enzyme must hydrolyze MAM-GlcUA orally administered to rats, as is in the case with cycasin. Thus it was concluded that the conversion of the primary alcohol group of cycasin to a carboxylic acid group changed the compound from a predominantly kidney tumor inducer to an intestinal tumor inducer.[65]

REFERENCES

1. Fosberg, F.R., Résumé of the cycadaceae, *Fed. Proc.*, **23**: 1340–1342, 1964.
2. Birdsey, M.R., A brief description of the cycads, *Fed. Proc.*, **31**: 1467–1469, 1972.
3. Whiting, M.G., Toxicity of cycads, *Econ. Bot.*, **17**: 271–302, 1963.
4. Yang, M.G., Sanger, V.L., Mickelsen, O., and Laqueur, G.L., Carcinogenicity of long-term feeding of cycad husk to rats, *Proc. Soc. Exp. Biol. Med.*, **127**: 1171–1175, 1968.

5. Hoch-Ligeti, C., Stutzman, E., and Arvin, J.M., Cellular composition during tumor induction in rats by cycad husk, *J. Natl. Cancer Inst.*, **41**: 605–614, 1968.
6. Matsumoto, H., and Strong, F.M., The occurrence of methylazoxymethanol in *Cycas circinalis* L. *Arch. Biochem. Biophys.*, **101**: 299–310, 1963.
7. Campbell, M.E., Mickelsen, O., Yang M.G., Laqueur, G.L., and Keresztesy, J.C., Effects of strain, age and diet on the response of rats to the ingestion of *Cycas circinalis, J. Nutr.*, **88**: 115–124, 1966.
8. Palekar, R.S., and Dastur, D.K., Cycasin content of *Cycas circinalis, Nature* (London), **206**: 1363–1365, 1965.
9. Yang, M.G., Mickelsen, O., Campbell, M.E., Laqueur, G.L., and Keresztesy, J.C., Cycad flour used by Guamanians: Effects produced in rats by long-term feeding, *J. Nutr.*, **90**: 153–156, 1966.
10. Hirono, I., Kachi, H., and Kato, T., A survey of acute toxicity of cycads and motality rate from cancer in the Miyako islands, Okinawa, *Acta Pathol. Jpn.*, **20**: 327–337, 1970.
11. Kobayashi, A., Cycasin in cycad materials used in Japan, *Fed. Proc.*, **31**: 1476–1477, 1972.
12. Kurland, L.T., and Mulder, D.W. Epidemiologic investigations of amyotrophic lateral sclerosis, *Neurology*, **4**: 355–378, 1954.
13. Anderson, J.L., and Hall, W.T., Neurotoxic effects from cycad leaves, *Fed. Proc.*, **23**: 1349, 1964.
14. Laqueur, G.L., Mickelsen, O., Whiting, M.G., and Kurland, L.T., Carcinogenic properties of nuts from *Cycas circinalis* L. indigenous to Guam., *J. Natl. Cancer Inst.*, **31**: 919–951, 1963.
15. Laqueur, G.L., Carcinogenic effects of cycad meal and cycasin, methylazoxymethanol glycoside, in rats and effects of cycasin in germfree rats, *Fed. Proc.*, **23**: 1386–1387, 1964.
16. Laqueur, G.L., The induction of intestinal neoplasms in rats with the glycoside cycasin and its aglycone, *Virchows Arch. Path. Anat.*, **340**: 151–163, 1965.
17. Nishida, K., Kobayashi, A., and Nagahama, T., Cycasin, a new toxic glycoside of *Cycas revoluta* Thunb. 1. Isolation and structure of cycasin, *Bull. Agric. Chem. Soc. Jpn.*, **19**: 77–84, 1955.
18. Riggs, N.V., Glucosyloxyazoxymethane, a constituent of the seeds of *Cycas circinalis* L. *Chem. Ind.* (London), 926, **1956**.
19. Nishida, K., Kobayashi, A., Nagahama, T., Kojima, K., and Yamane, M., Cycasin, a new toxic glycoside of *Cycas revoluta* Thunb. IV. Pharmacology of cycasin, *Seikagaku* (J. Japan Biochem. Soc.), **28**: 218–223, 1956 (in Japanese).
20. Spatz, M., McDaniel, E.G., and Laqueur, G.L., Cycasin excretion in conventional and germfree rats, *Proc, Soc. Exp. Biol. Med.*, **121**: 417–422, 1966.
21. Spatz, M., Smith, D.W.E., McDaniel, E.G., and Laqueur, G.L., Role of intestinal microorganisms in determining cycasin toxicity, *Proc. Soc. Exp. Biol. Med.*, **124**: 691–697, 1967.
22. Kobayashi, A., and Matsumoto, H., Studies on methylazoxymethanol, the aglycone of cycasin, *Arch. Biochem. Biophys.*, **110**: 373–380, 1965.
23. Laqueur, G.L., and Matsumoto, H., Neoplasms in female Fischer rats following intraperitoneal injection of methylazoxymethanol, *J. Natl. Cancer Inst.*, **37**: 217–232, 1966.
24. Spatz, M., Laqueur, G.L., and Holmes, J.M., Carcinogenic effects of methylazoxymethanol (MAM) in hamsters, *Proc. Am. Assoc. Cancer Res.*, **10**: 86, 1969.
25. Narisawa, T., and Nakano, H., Carcinoma of the large intestine of rats induced by rectal infusion of methylazoxymethanol, *Gann*, **64**: 93–95, 1973.
26. Fushimi, K., Tumor induction in rats given consecutive injections of methylazoxymethanol acetate, *Acta. Schol. Med. Univ. Gifu*, **22**: 729–750, 1974.
27. Zedeck, M.S., and Sternberg, S.S., A model system for studies of colon carcinogenesis: Tumor induction by a single injection of methylazoxymethanol acetate, *J. Natl. Cancer Inst.*, **53**: 1419–1421, 1974.

28. Laqueur, G.L., McDaniel, E.G., and Matsumoto, H., Tumor induction in germfree rats with methylazoxymethanol (MAM) and synthetic MAM acetate, *J. Natl. Cancer Inst.*, **39**: 355–371, 1967.
29. Matsumoto, H., Nagahama, T., and Larson, H.O., Studies on methlazoxymethanol, the aglycone of cycasin: A synthesis of methylazoxymethyl acetate, *Biochem. J.*, **95**: 13c–14c, 1965.
30. Spatz, M., Hydrolysis of cycasin by β-D-glucosidase in skin of newborn rats. *Proc. Soc. Exper. Biol. Med.*, **128**: 1005–1008, 1968.
31. Spatz, M., Laqueur, G.L., and Hirono, I., Hydrolysis of cycasin by β-D-glucosidase in subcutis of newborns, *Fed. Proc.*, **27**: 722, 1968.
32. Laqueur, G.L., and Spatz, M., Toxicology of cycasin. *Cancer Res.*, **28**: 2262–2267, 1968.
33. Hirono, I., Laqueur, G.L., and Spatz, M., Tumor induction in Fischer and Osborne-Mendel rats by a single administration of cycasin, *J. Natl. Cancer Inst.*, **40**: 1003–1010, 1968.
34. Hirono, I., Shibuya, C., and Fushimi, K., Tumor induction in C57BL/6 mice by a single administration of cycasin, *Cancer Res.*, **29**: 1658–1662, 1969.
35. Hirono, I., and Shibuya, C., High incidence of pulmonary tumors in dd mice by a single injection of cycasin, *Gann*, **61**: 403–407, 1970.
36. Hirono, I., Hayashi, K., Mori, H., and Miwa, T., Carcinogenic effects of cycasin in Syrian golden hamsters and the transplantability of induced tumors, *Cancer Res.*, **31**: 283–287, 1971.
37. Shibuya, C., and Hirono, I., Relations between postnatal days of mice and carcinogenic effect of cycasin, *Gann*, **64**: 109–110, 1973.
38. Matsumoto, H., Nagata, Y., Nishimura, E.T., Bristol, R., and Haber, M., β-glucosidase modulation in preweanling rats and its association with tumor induction by cycasin, *J. Natl. Cancer Inst.*, **49**: 423–434, 1972.
39. Zedeck, M.S., and Sternberg, S.S., Tumor induction in intact and regenerating liver of adult rats by a single treatment with methylazoxymethanol acetate, *Chem. Biol. Interactions*, **17**: 291–296, 1977.
40. Gusek, W., Buss, H., and Krüger, C.H., Morphologische und histochemische Befunde an experimentellen Nierentumoren der Ratte, *Verh. Dtsch. Ges. Pathol.*, **50**: 337–343, 1966 (in German).
41. Gusek, W., Buss, H., and Laqueur, G.L. Histologische-histochemische Untersuchungen am "Interstitiellen Cycasin-Tumor" der Rattenniere, *Beitr. Path. Anat.*, **135**: 53–74, 1967(in German).
42. Gusek, W., and Mestwerdt, W. Cycasin-induzierte Nierentumoren bei der Wistar ratte unter besonderer Berücksichtigung der Adenome, *Beitr. Pathol. Anat.*, **139**: 199–218, 1969 (in German).
43. Gusek, W., Die Ultrastruktur Cycasin-induzierter Nierenadenome, *Virchows Arch. A Path. Anat. and Histol.*, **365**: 221–237, 1975 (in German).
44. Buss, H., and Gusek, W., Untersuchungen über die interstitiellen Zellen der Nierenrinde, *Virchows Arch. Abt. B Zellpath.*, **1**: 251–268, 1968 (in German).
45. Spatz, M., and Laqueur, G.L., Transplacental induction of tumors in Sprague-Dawley rats with crude cycad material, *J. Natl. Cancer Inst.*, **38**: 233–245, 1967.
46. Mugera, G.M., and Nderito, P., Tumors of the liver, kidney and lungs in rats fed *Encephalartos hildebrandtii*, *Brit. J. Cancer*, **22**: 563–568, 1968.
47. Dossaji, S.F., and Herbin, G.A., Occurrence of macrozamin in the seeds of *Encephalartos hildebrandtii*, *Fed. Proc.*, **31**: 1470–1472, 1972.
48. Hirono, I., Laqueur, G.L., and Spatz, M., Transplantability of cycasin-induced tumors in rats, with emphasis on nephroblastomas, *J. Natl. Cancer Inst.*, **40**: 1011–1025, 1968.
49. Sato, H., Yunoki, K., Hayashi, T., and Fukunishi, R., Studies on carcinogenesis of cycasin, *Igaku no Ayumi*, **65**: 525–531, 1968 (in Japanese)
50. Fukunishi, R., Terashi, S., Watanabe, K., and Kawaji, K., High yield of hepatic

tumors in rats by cycasin, *Gann*, **63**: 575–578, 1972.
51. O' Gara, R.W., Brown, J.M., and Whiting, M.G., Induction of hepatic and renal tumors by topical application of aqueous extract of cycad nut to artificial skin ulcers in mice, *Fed. Proc.*, **23**: 1383, 1964.
52. Spatz, M., Carcinogenic effect of cycad meal in guinea pigs, *Fed. Proc.*, **23**: 1384–1385, 1964.
53. Watanabe, K., Iwashita, H., Muta, K., Hamada, Y., and Hamada, K., Hepatic tumors of rabbits induced by cycad extract, *Gann*, **66**: 335–339, 1975.
54. Stanton, M.F., Hepatic neoplasms of aquarium fish exposed to *Cycas circinalis*, *Fed. Proc.*, **25**: 661, 1966.
55. Hirono, I., Carcinogenicity and neurotoxicity of cycasin with special reference to species differences, *Fed. Proc.*, **31**: 1493–1497, 1972.
56. Spatz, M., Carcinogenicity of methylazoxymethanol (MAM) in guinea pigs and hamsters, Abstr. 10th Int. Cancer Congr., Medical Arts Publ., Houston, 24–25, **1970**.
57. Laqueur, G.L., and Spatz, M., Oncogenicity of cycasin and methylazoxymethanol, *Gann Monogr. Cancer Res.*, **17**: 189–204, 1975.
58. Sieber, S.M., Correa, P., Dalgard, D.W., McIntire, K.R., and Adamson, R.H., Carcinogenicity and hepatotoxicity of cycasin and its aglycone methylazoxymethanol acetate in nonhuman primates, *J. Natl. Cancer Inst.*, **65**: 177–189, 1980.
59. Aoki, K., and Matsudaira, H., Induction of hepatic tumors in a teleost (*Oryzias latipes*) after treatment with methylazoxymethanol acetate, *J. Natl. Cancer Inst.*, **59**: 1747–1749, 1977.
60. Aoki, K., and Matsudaira, H., Factors influencing tumorigenesis in the liver after treatment with methylazoxymethanol acetate in a teleost, *Oryzias latipes*, In: *Phyletic Approaches to Cancer*, (Dawe C.J., Harshbarger, J.C. and Kondo, S., et al., eds.) Tokyo: Jpn. Sci. Soc. Press, pp. 205–216, **1981**.
61. Aoki, K., and Matsudaira, H., Factors influencing methylazoxymethanol acetate initiation of liver tumors in *Oryzias latipes*: Carcinogen dosage and time of exposure, *Natl. Cancer Inst. Monogr.*, **65**: 345–351, 1984.
62. Hirono, I., Shibuya, C. and Fushimi, K., Experimental studies on sites of tumor development in the intestine by chemical carcinogens, In: *Pathophysiology of Carcinogenesis in Digestive Organs*, (Farber, E., Kawachi, T., Nagayo, T., Sugano, H., Sugimura, T. and Weisburger, J.H., eds.), University of Tokyo Press, Tokyo, pp. 285–295, **1977**.
63. Weisburger, J.H., Colon carcinogens: Their metabolism and mode of action, *Cancer*, **28**: 60–70, 1971.
64. Matsumoto, H., Takata, R.H., and Komeiji, D.Y., Synthesis of the glucuronic acid conjugate of methylazoxymethanol, *Cancer Res.*, **39**: 3070–3073, 1979.
65. Matsumoto, H., Carcinogenicity of cycasin, its aglycone methylazoxymethanol, and methylazoxymethanol-glucosiduronic acid. In: *Naturally Occurring Carcinogens-Mutagens and Modulators of Carcinogensis*, (E.C. Miller et al., eds.) Jpn. Sci. Soc. Press, Tokyo University Park Press, Baltimore, pp.67–77, **1979**.
66. Zedeck, M.S., Grab, D.J., and Sternberg, S.S., Differences in the acute response of the various segments of rat intestine to treatment with the intestinal carcinogen, methylazoxymethanol acetate. *Cancer Res.*, **37**: 32–36, 1977.
67. Matsubara, N., Mori, H., and Hirono, I., Effect of colostomy on intestinal carcinogenesis by methylazoxymethanol acetate in rats, *J. Natl. Cancer Inst.*, **61**: 1161–1164, 1978.
68. Mickelsen, O., Campbell, E., Yang, M., Mugera, G., and Whitehair, C.K., Studies with cycad. *Fed. Proc.*, **23**: 1363–1365, 1964.
69. Spatz, M., and Laqueur, G.L., Evidence for transplacental passage of the natural carcinogen cycasin and its aglycone, *Proc. Scoc. Exp. Biol. Med.*, **127**: 281–286, 1968.
70. Shank, R.C., and Magee, P.N. Similarities between the biochemical actions of cycasin and dimethylnitrosamine, *Biochem. J.*, **105**: 521–527, 1967.

71. Nagata, Y., and Matsumoto, H., Studies on methylazoxymethanol: methylation of nucleic acids in the fetal rat brain, *Proc. Soc. Exp. Biol. Med.*, **132**: 383–385, 1969.
72. Matsumoto, H., and Higa, H.H., Studies on methylazoxymethanol, aglycone of cycasin: methylation of nucleic acids *in vitro Biochem. J.*, **98**: 20c–22c, 1966.
73. Ganote, C.E., and Rosenthal, A.S., Characteristic lesions of methylazoxymethanol-induced liver damage. A comparative ultrastructural study with dimethylnitrosamine, hydrazine sulfate, and carbon tetrachloride, *Lab. Invest.*, **19**: 382–398, 1968.
74. Mori, H., Comparative studies on liver damages induced by cycasin between rats and hamsters, *Acta Schol. Med. Univ. Gifu*, **22**: 641–677, 1974.
75. Spatz, M., Dougherty, W.J., and Smith, W.E., Teratogenic effects of Methylazoxymethanol, *Proc. Soc. Exp. Biol. Med.*, **124**: 476–478, 1967.
76. Spatz, M., and Laqueur, G.L., Transplacental chemical induction of microencephaly in two strains of rats, *Proc. Soc. Exp. Biol. Med.*, **129**: 705–710, 1968.
77. Matsumoto, H., Spatz, M., and Laqueur, G.L., Quantitative changes with age in DNA content of methylazoxymethanol-induced microcephalic rat brain, *J. Neurochem.*, **19**: 297–306, 1972.
78. Haddad, R.K., Rabe, A., Laqueur, G.L., Spatz, M., and Valsamis, M.P., Intellectual deficit associated with transplacentally induced microencephaly in the rat, *Science*, **163**: 88–90, 1969.
79. Hirono, I., and Shibuya, C., Induction of a neurological disorder by cycasin in mice. *Nature* (London), **216**: 1311–1312, 1967.
80. Hirono, I., Shibuya, C., and Hayashi, K., Induction of a cerebellar disorder with cycasin in newborn mice and hamsters. *Proc. Soc. Exp. Biol. Med.*, **131**: 593–599, 1969.
81. Shimada, M., and Langman, J., Repair of the external granular layer of the hamster cerebellum after prenatal and postnatal administration of methylazoxymethanol. *Teratology*, **3**: 119–134, 1970.
82. Haddad, R.K., Rabe, A., and Dumas, P., Comparison of effects of methylazoxymethanol acetate on brain development in different species, *Fed. Proc.*, **31**: 1520–1523, 1972.
83. Hirano, A., and Jones, M., Fine structure of cycasin-induced cerebellar alterations, *Fed. Proc.*, **31**: 1517–1519, 1972.
84. Hirano, A., Dembitzer, H.M., and Jones, M., An electron microscopic study of cycasin-induced cerebellar alterations, *J. Neuropathol. Exp. Neurology*, **31**: 113–125, 1972.
85. Fushimi, K., and Hirono, I., Induction of a retinal disorder with cycasin in newborn mice and rats, *Acta Path. Jap.*, **23**: 307–314, 1973.
86. Smith, D.W.E., Mutagenicity of cycasin aglycone (methylazoxymethanol), a naturally occurring carcinogen, *Science*, **152**: 1273–1274, 1966.
87. Teas, H.J., Dyson, J.G., and Whisenant, B.R., Cycasin metabolism in *Seirarctia echo* Abbot and Smith (Lepidoptera: Arctiidae), *J. Ga. Entomol. Soc.*, **1**: 21–22, 1966.
88. Teas, H.J., Cycasin synthesis in *Seirarctia echo* (Lepidoptera) larvae fed methylazoxymethanol, *Biochem. Biophys. Res. Commun.*, **26**: 686–690, 1967.
89. Matsushima, T., Matsumoto, H., Shirai, A., Sawamura, M., and Sugimura, T., Mutagenicity of the naturally occurring carcinogen cycasin and synthetic methylazoxymethanol conjugates in *Salmonella typhimurium*, *Cancer Res.*, **39**: 3780–3782, 1979.
90. Gabridge, M.G.A., Denunzio, A., and Legator, M.S., Cycasin: detection of associated mutagenic activity *in vivo*, *Science*, **163**: 689–691, 1969.
91. Teas, H.J., and Dyson, J.G., Mutation in *Drosophila* by methylazoxymethanol, the aglycone of cycasin, *Proc. Soc. Exp. Biol. Med.*, **125**: 988–990, 1967.
92. Teas, H.J., Sax, H.J., and Sax, K., Cycasin: Radiomimetic effect, *Science*, **149**: 541–542, 1965.
93. Williams, J.N., Jr., and Laqueur, G.L. Response of liver nucleic acids and lipids in

rats fed *Cycas circinalis* L. endosperm or cycasin, *Proc. Soc. Exp. Biol. Med.*, **118**: 1–4, 1965.

94. Zedeck, M.S., Sternberg, S.S., Poynter, R.W., and McGowan, J., Biochemical and pathological effects of methylazoxymethanol acetate, a potent carcinogen, *Cancer Res.*, **30**: 801–812, 1970.

95. Miller, J.A. Comments on chemistry of cycads, *Fed. Proc.*, **23**: 1361–1362, 1964.

96. Druckrey, H., Production of colonic carcinomas by 1,2-dialkyl-hydrazines and azoxyalkanes, In: *Carcinoma of the Colon and Antecedent Epithelium*, (Burdett, W.J., ed.) Charles C. Thomas, Springfield, Ill., pp. 267–279, **1970**.

97. Nagasawa, H.T., Shirota, F.N., and Matsumoto, H. Decomposition of methylazoxymethanol, the aglycone of cycasin, in D$_2$O., *Nature* (London), **236**: 234–235, 1972.

98. Schoental, R., The mechanisms of action of the carcinogen nitroso and related compounds, *Br. J. Cancer*, **28**: 436–439, 1973.

99. Grab, D.J., and Zedeck, M.S., Organ-specific effects of the carcinogen methylazoxymethanol related to metabolism by nicotinamide adenine dinucleotide-dependent dehydrogenases, *Cancer Res.*, **37**: 4182–4189, 1977.

100. Laqueur, G.L., Matsumoto, H., and Yamamoto, R.S., Comparison of the carcinogenicity of methylazoxymethanol-β-D-glucosiduronic acid in conventional and germfree Sprague-Dawley rats, *J. Natl. Cancer Inst.*, **67**: 1053–1055, 1981.

2

Pyrrolizidine Alkaloids

2.1 Distribution and Chemical Structure of Pyrrolizidine Alkaloids

Pyrrolizidine alkaloids were first isolated from the *Senecio* genus and found in over a hundred species of Compositae. Later, they were found to occur in many other genera, especially in *Cynoglossum*, *Lindelofia* and *Heliotropium* species of the Boraginaceae, and in the *Crotalaria* species of the Leguminosae. Pyrrolizidine alkaloids have also been found in numerous species of other families.[1] All known plant genera containing pyrrolizidine alkaloids are listed Table 2–1.[2-13] More than 200 pyrrolizidine alkaloids have been isolated from these plants.

Table 2–1. Distribution of Plants Containing Pyrrolizidine Alkaloids

Family	Genera
Apocynaceae	*Alafia, Anodendron, Parsonsia, Urechtites*
Boraginaceae	*Amsinckia, Anchusa, Asperugo, Caccinia, Cynoglossum, Echium, Ehretia, Heliotropium, Lappula, Lindelofia, Lithosperum, Macrotonia, Messerschmidia,*[2] *Myosotis, Paracaryum, Parucynoglossum, Rindera, Solenanthus, Symphytum,*[3] *Tournefortia, Trachelanthus, Trichodesma, Ulugbekia*
Celastraceae	*Bhesa*
Compositae	*Adenostyles, Brachyglottis, Cacalia,*[4] *Doronicum, Emilia, Erechtites, Eupatorium,*[5] *Farfugium,*[6] *Gynura, Kleinia, Ligularia,*[7,8] *Petasites,*[9] *Senecio,*[10,11,12] *Syneilesis,*[13] *Tussilago*
Euphorbiaceae	*Phyllanthus, Securinega*
Gramineae	*Festuca, Lolium, Thelepogon*
Leguminosae	*Adenocarpus, Crotalaria, Cytisus*
Orchidaceae	*Chysis, Doritis, Hammarbya, Kingiella, Liparis, Malaxis, Phalaenopsis, Vanda, Vandopsis*
Ranunculaceae	*Caltha*
Rhizophoraceae	*Cassipourea*
Santalaceae	*Thesium*
Sapotaceae	*Mimusops, Planchonella*
Scrophulariaceae	*Castilleja*

A diesease produced by the consumption of the plants containing toxic pyrrolizidine alkaloids affects most species of domestic livestock. This disease is known under different names, e.g., Pictow disease in Canada and Winton disease in New Zealand.[1] About 30 pyrrolizidine alkaloids have been proved to be hepatotoxic. Some of these hepatotoxic pyrrolizidine alkaloids, i.e., isatidine,[14,15] lasiocarpine,[16] monocrotaline[14] and retrosine,[15] have been demonstrated to be carcinogenic to rats. Coltsfoot (*Tussilago farfara*)[17] comfrey (*Symphytum officinale*)[3,18] and petasites (*Petasites japonicus*)[9,19] are widely used as herbal remedies or foods, and these herbs have recently been reported to contain hepatotoxic pyrrolizidine alkaloids.

The structure of pyrrolizidine alkaloids is composed of two parts, necine and necic acid (Fig. 2–1). The basic structure of necine consists of 7–hydroxy–1–methylpyrrolizidine, and necic acid represents a variety of

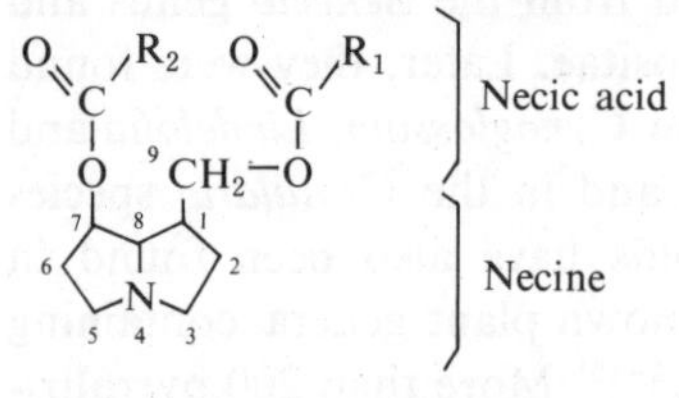

Fig. 2–1. Structure of pyrrolizidine alkaloid.

C_5–C_{10} branched chain acids. In most alkaloids, these necines and necic acids form an ester structure. By the combination of necines and necic acids, the esters can be divided into following four types: 1) nonesters, 2) monoesters, 3) acyclic diesters, and 4) macrocyclic diesters of pyrrolizidine alkaloids. Necines can be classified into four groups, i.e., a trachelanthamidine group of monohydroxylated derivatives, a retronecine group of dihydroxylated derivatives, a rosmarinecine group of trihydroxylated derivatives and an otonecine group (Fig. 2–2). The trachelanthamidine group contains trachelanthamidine, isoretronecanol, lindelofidine, laburnine and supinidine. Monoester alkaloids of the trachelanthamidine group have been found mainly in the Boraginaceae plants. The retronecine group involves retronecine, heliotridine, platynecine, hastanecine and truneforcidine. Alkaloids of the retronecine group have been found almost as acyclic and cyclic diester pyrrolizidine alkaloids. The rosmarinecine group contains rosmarinecine, crotanecine and croalbinecine. Otonecine is known as necine of otosenine and senkirkine. Otosenine and senkirkine having otonecine as necine are a transannular interaction between the carbonyl group and the tertiary nitrogen atom. Necic acids can be derived by the number of carbon atoms present in the molecule (Fig. 2–3). Angelic and

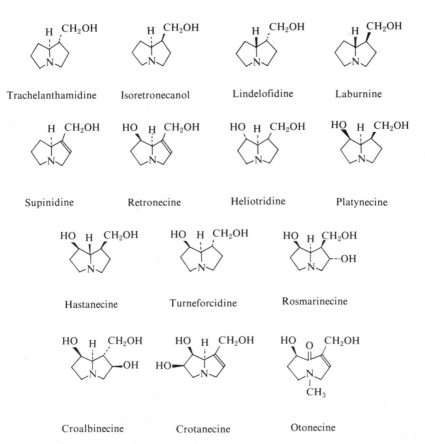

Fig. 2–2. Structures of necines.

tiglic acids have been known as C_5-acids. C_7-acids have been found almost as diester pyrrolizidine alkaloids in Boraginaceae plants. C_7-acids represent (+)-trachelanthic acids and (−)-viridifloric acid. Most C_{10}-acids have been found as macrocyclic diester pyrrolizidine alkaloids. C_{10}-acids represent senecic acid and jacobinecic acid. Representative pyrrolizidine alkaloids are shown in Fig. 2–4 in order of nonester, monoester, acyclic diester and macrocyclic diester alkaloid. The structures of the pyrrolizidine alkaloids whose pharmacological activities have been tested are shown in Fig. 2–5 (*see* sections 2.2–2.5).

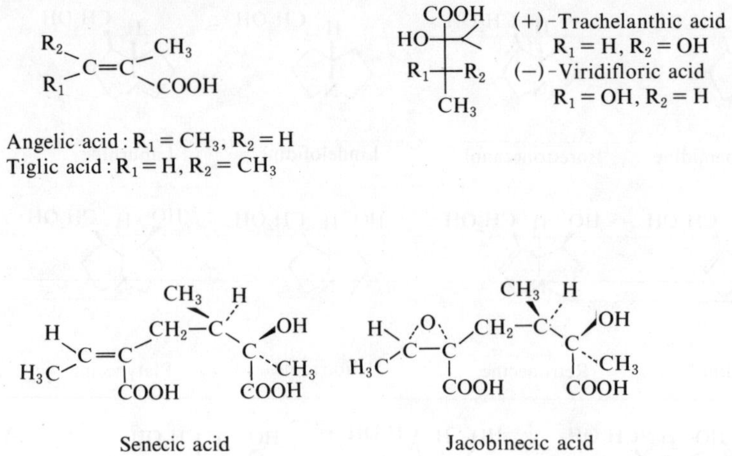

$$R_2\diagdown C=C \diagup CH_3$$
$$R_1 \diagup \qquad \diagdown COOH$$

Angelic acid : $R_1 = CH_3$, $R_2 = H$
Tiglic acid : $R_1 = H$, $R_2 = CH_3$

$$\underset{CH_3}{\overset{COOH}{HO\diagdown}} \qquad \underset{CH_3}{\overset{}{R_1 \diagdown R_2}}$$

(+)-Trachelanthic acid
$R_1 = H$, $R_2 = OH$
(−)-Viridifloric acid
$R_1 = OH$, $R_2 = H$

Senecic acid

Jacobinecic acid

Fig. 2–3. Structures of necic acids.

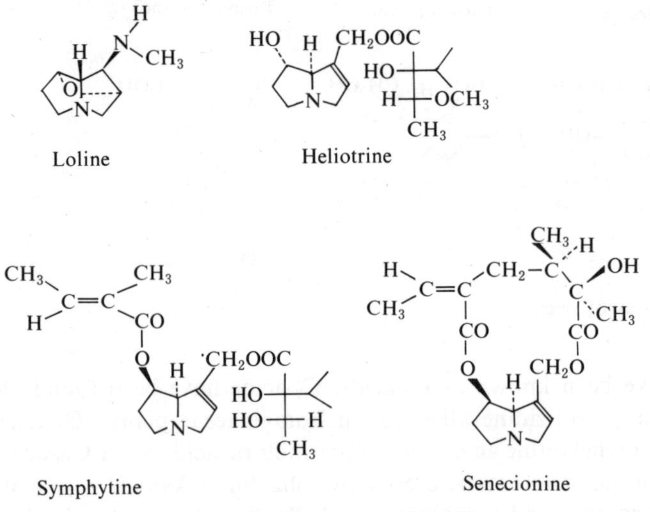

Loline

Heliotrine

Symphytine

Senecionine

Fig. 2–4. Structures of representative pyrrolizidine alkaloids.

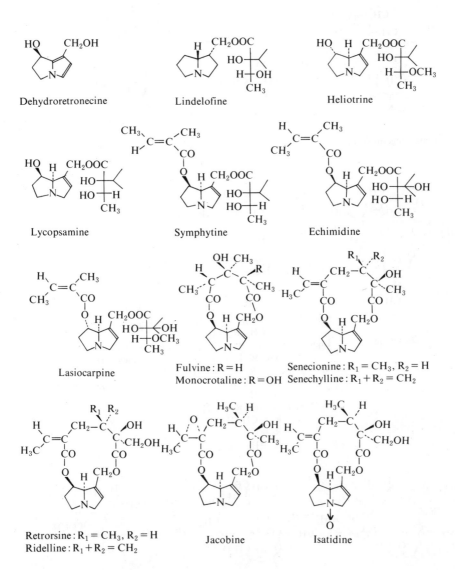

Fig. 2–5. Structures of pyrrolizidine alkaloids.

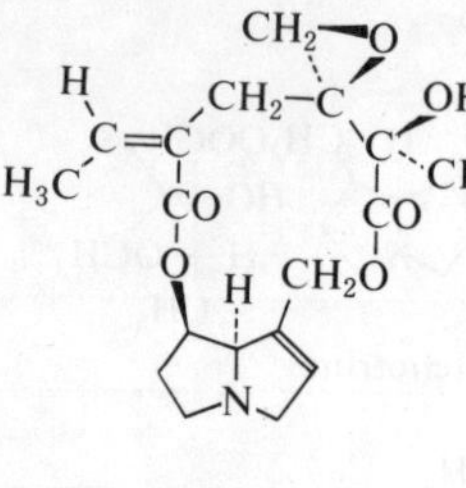

Epoxyseneciphylline 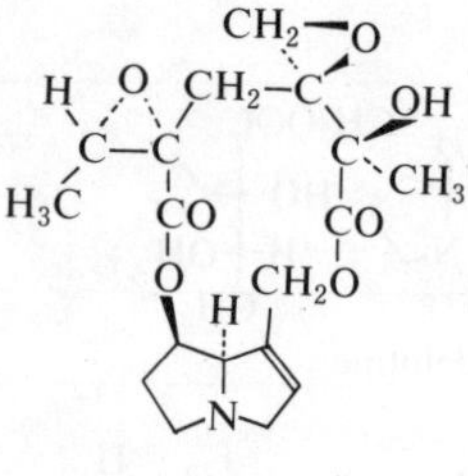   Senecicannabine 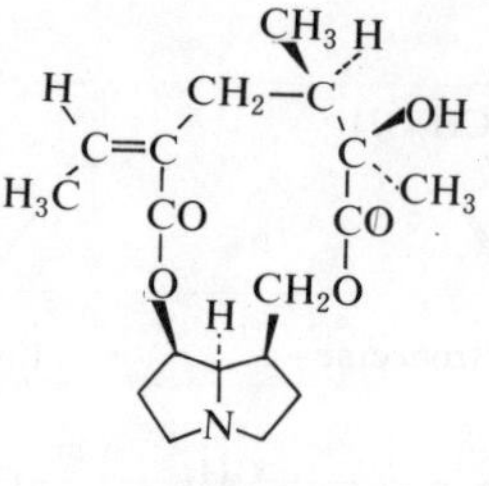   Platyphylline

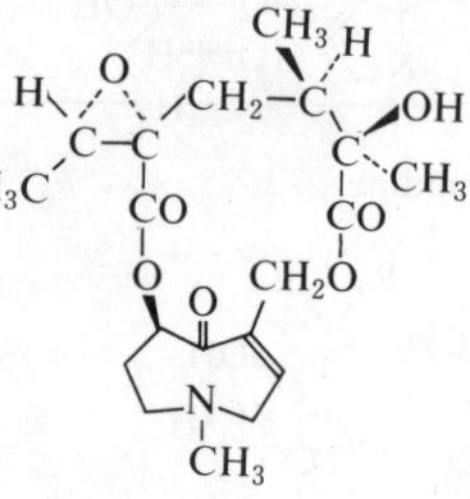

Otosenine

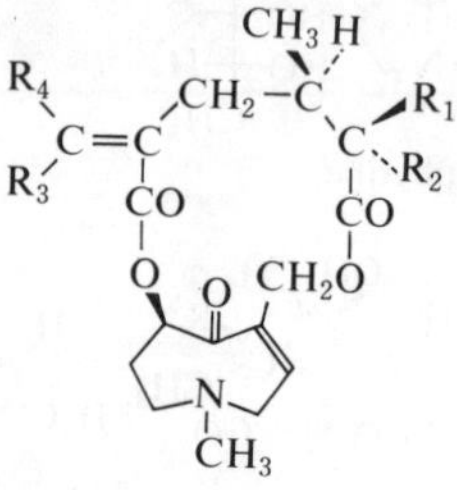

Senkirkine: $R_1 = OH$, $R_2 = R_3$
$= CH_3$, $R_4 = H$
Ligularidine: $R_1 = R_4 = CH_3$,
$R_2 = OCOCH_3$, $R_3 = H$
Neoligularidine: $R_1 = R_3 = CH_3$,
$R_2 = OCOCH_3$,
$R_4 = H$
Hydroxysenkirkine: $R_1 = OH$,
$R_2 = CH_2OH$,
$R_3 = CH_3$,
$R_4 = H$

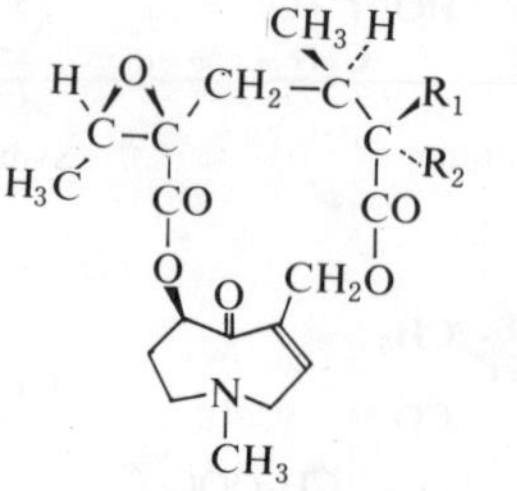

Fukinotoxin: $R_1 = OH$,
$R_2 = CH_3$
Acetylfukinotoxin:
$R_1 = OCOCH_3$, $R_2 = CH_3$
Ligularizine: $R_1 = CH_3$,
$R_2 = OCOCH_3$

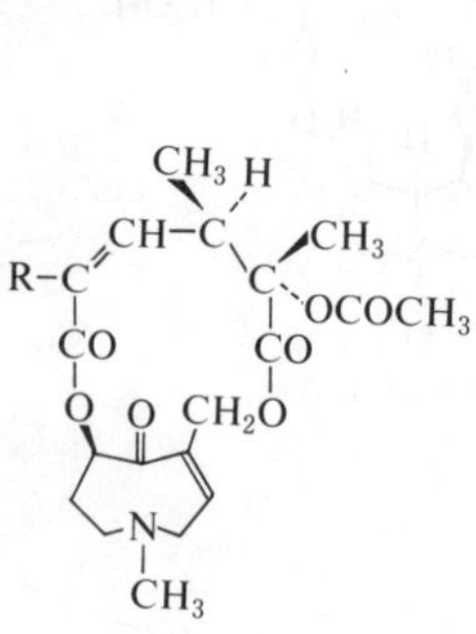

Clivorine: $R = CH = CH_2$
Dihydroclivorine: $R = C_2H_5$

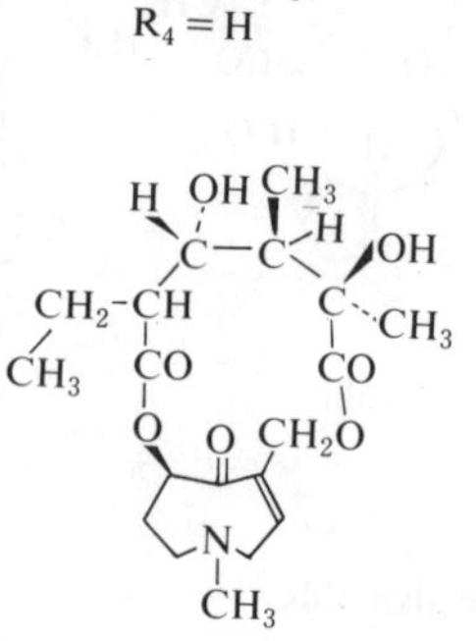

Syneilesine

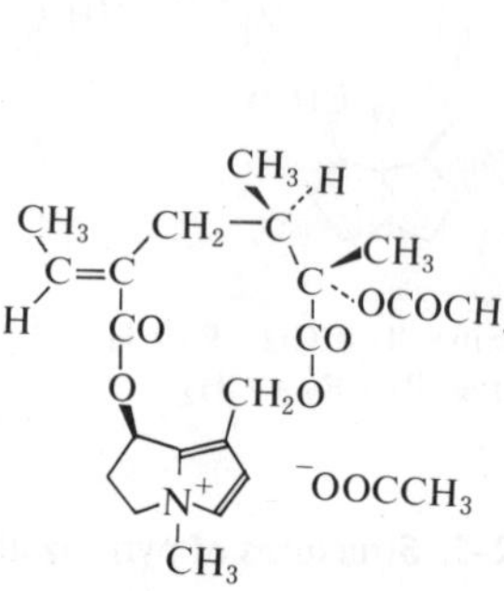

XL-201

Fig. 2–5.—*Continued*

2.2 New Macrocyclic Pyrrolizidine Alkaloids from Japanese Compositae Plants

The structure determinations of macrocyclic pyrrolizidine alkaloids isolated from Japanese Compositae plants are introduced below.

Two new alkaloids, syneilesine (Fig. 2–6) and acetylsyneilesine, together with senecionine (0.03%, 0.01% and 0.002% from dry roots) were isolated from *Syneilesis palmata* (Japanese name: *yaburegasa*),[13] young leaves of which are used for foods in various regions of Japan. Syneilesine was revealed by the mass and ^{1}H-NMR spectra to be a characteristic twelve-membered macrocyclic pyrrolizidine alkaloid of otonecine. The absolute configuration of asymmetric carbons in syneilesine was determined by hydrogenolysis and hydrolysis. Hydrogenation of syneilesine with Adam's catalyst and successive hydrolysis gave (7R)-dihydrodeoxy-otonecine. Alkaline hydrolysis of syneilesine gave three lactones designated as syneilesinolide A, B and C (Fig. 2–6). Syneilesinolide B on hydrogenation gave a dihydrosyneilesinolide B having a negative cotton effect at 238 nm in the cd spectrum. Therefore, the 5R configuration was assigned to this lactone. The formation of syneilesinolide C from A suggests that the stereochemistry at C-3 in syneilesinolide C is also R. The coupling constant $J = 5.4$ Hz between the protons on C-3 and C-4 indicated that the dihedral angle between these protons is about 36°, suggesting that the configuration at C-4 in syneilesinolide C is R. The stereochemistry at C-15 of syneilesine was not determined. The structure of acetylsyneilesine was proved by acetylation of syneilesine with acetic anhydride and sodium acetate.

A new alkaloid, yamataimine (0.004% from dry roots) (Fig. 2–7) was isolated from *Cacalia yatabei* (Japanese name: *yama-taimingasa*).[4] Mass and ^{1}H-NMR spectra of yamataimine show a typical pattern of twelve-membered macrocyclic pyrrolizidine alkaloid of retronecine and the presence of an ethyl group attached at C-15. Alkaline hydrolysis of yamataimine gave (+)-retronecine. The absolute configuration of asymmetric carbons in yamataimine was established by X-ray analysis of yamataimine hydrobromide.

A new alkaloid, fukinotoxin (0.002% semi-dry scapes), which possesses highly cytotoxic activity, was isolated from young scapes of *Petasites japonicus* (Japanese name: *fuki-no-toh*),[9] which are used for food in various parts of Japan. Mass and ^{1}H-NMR spectra of fukinotoxin show a typical pattern of twelve-membered macrocyclic pyrrolizidine alkaloid of otone-

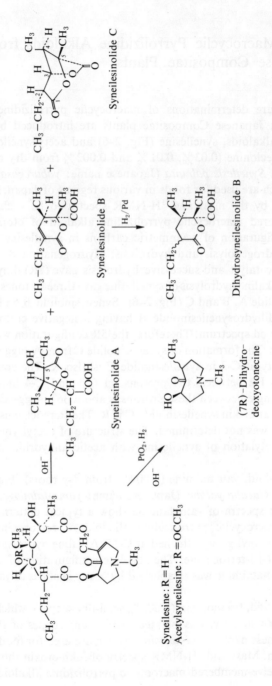

Fig. 2-6. Hydrogenolysis and hydrolysis of syneilesine.

cine and indicate that fukinotoxin is 15,20-epoxide of senkirkine. The stereochemistry of fukinotoxin, which is identical with petasitenine,[19] was established by X-ray analysis. Carcinogenicity of fukinotoxin was proved by Hirono *et al.* (Fig. 2–7).[20]

A new macrocyclic pyrrolizidine alkaloid, senecicannabine (Fig. 2–8), together with seneciphylline (Fig. 2–8) and jacozine (Fig. 2–8) (0.036%, 0.47% and 0.026%, respectively, from dry roots) was isolated from *Senecio cannabifolius* (Japanese name: *hangon-so*)[10] whose young leaves are used for food. Mass and ^{1}H-NMR spectra show a typical pattern of twelve-membered macrocyclic pyrrolizidine alkaloid of retronecine. The presence of the two epoxide groups was indicated by mass, ^{1}H and ^{13}C-NMR spectra. Alkaline hydrolysis of senecicannabine gave (+)-retronecine. The absolute configuration of asymmetric centers was established by X-ray analysis. Senecicannabine is highly oxidized in the necic acid moiety and its structure corresponds to a diepoxide of seneciphylline. Seneciphylline was transformed into senecicannabine by oxidation with performic acid. Jacozine was also oxidized with performic acid to afford senecicannabine. The epoxide structure of jacozine was thus chemically proved to be α-epoxide (Fig. 2–8).[21]

Four new macrocyclic pyrrolizidine alkaloids, ligularidine, neoligularidine, ligularizine and ligularinine, together with clivorine (0.003%, 0.0001%, 0.011%, 0.004% and 0.26%, respectively from dry roots) were isolated from *Ligularia dentata* (Japanese name: *maruba-dakebuki*).[8] The young plants are used for food in rural areas of Japan. The structures of ligularidine and neoligularidine were elucidated by mass and ^{1}H-NMR spectra to be dihydro derivatives of clivorine; these structures were confirmed by the catalytic hydrogenation of clivorine with Pd-C. Ligularizine was presumed to be 15,20-epoxide of neoligularidine by mass, ^{1}H and ^{13}C-NMR spectra. The structure of ligularizine was confirmed by the chemical transformation of neoligularidine to ligularizine, which was performed by epoxidation with performic acid (Fig. 2–9). Ligularinine was revealed by mass and ^{1}H-NMR spectra to be a typical macrocyclic pyrrolizidine alkaloid of platynecine. The structure of ligularinine was confirmed by hydrolysis which gave the same necic acid as neoligularidine (Fig. 2–10). Carcinogenicity of clivorine was proved by Kuhara *et al.*[22] The pharmacological activities of these new macrocyclic pyrrolizidine alkaloids were tested and the results are presented below.

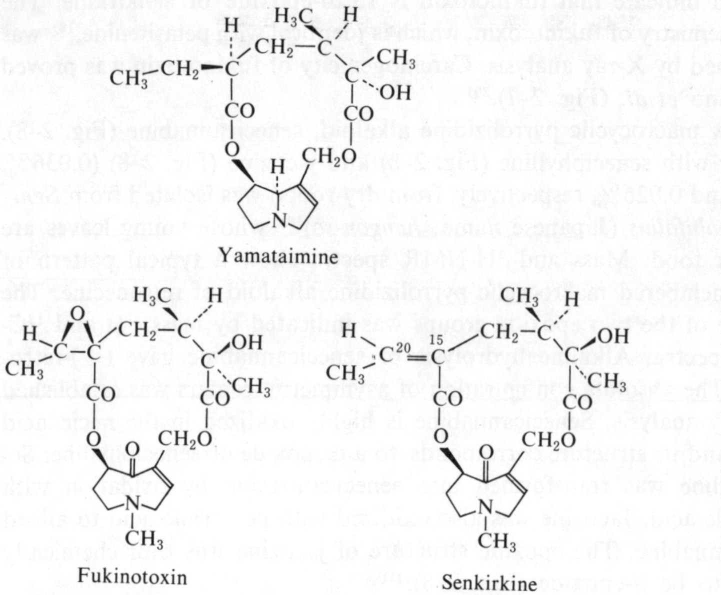

Fig. 2–7. Structure of yamataimine, fukinotoxin and senkirkine.

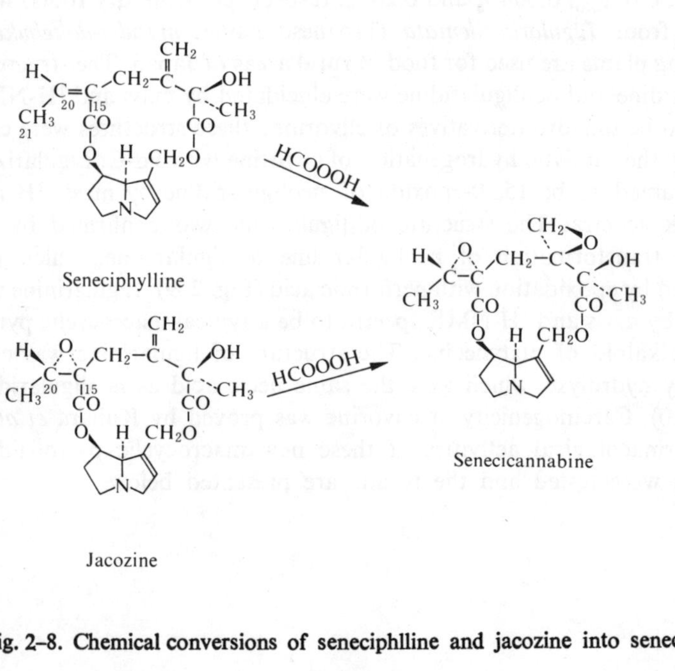

Fig. 2–8. Chemical conversions of seneciphlline and jacozine into senecicannabine.

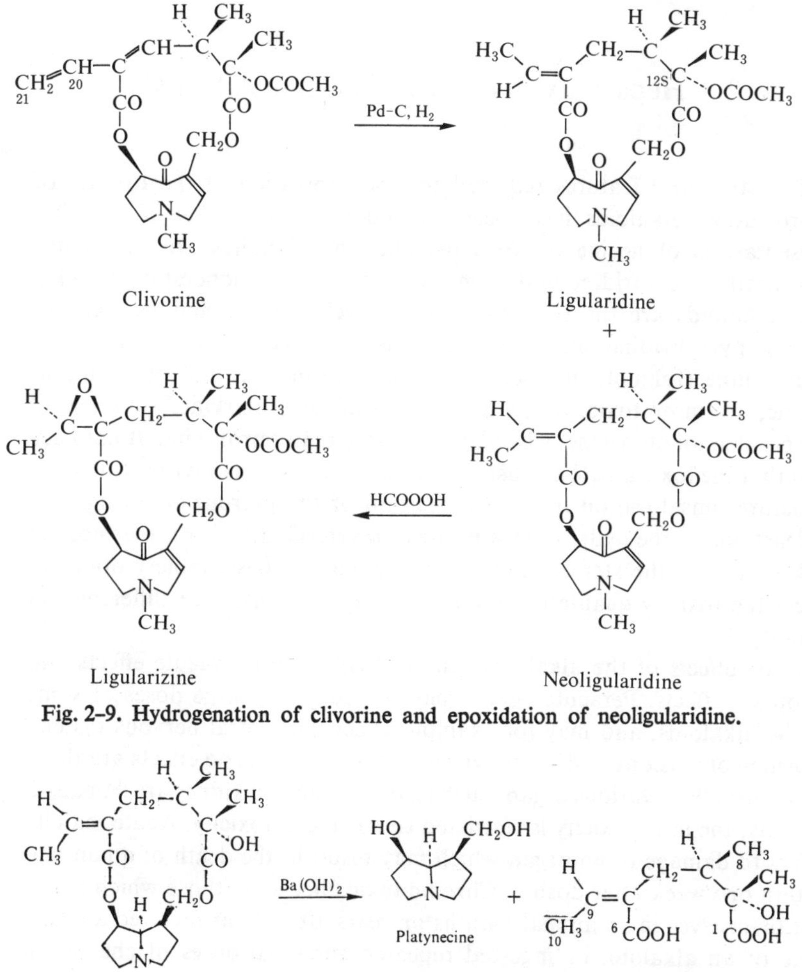

Fig. 2-9. Hydrogenation of clivorine and epoxidation of neoligularidine.

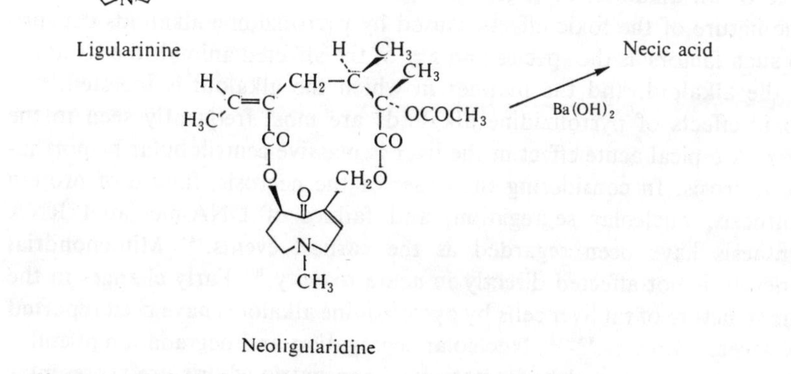

Fig. 2-10. Hydrolysis of ligularinine and neoligularidine.

2.3 Hepatotoxicity of Pyrrolizidine Alkaloids

The structural features required for the expression of the toxicity of pyrrolizidine alkaloids have been studied by Schoental *et al.*[23-25] Representatives of necine in toxic pyrrolizidine alkaloids are supinidine, retronecine, heliotridine and otonecine. In general, monoester pyrrolizidine alkaloids are the least toxic, and acyclic diester and macrocyclic diester pyrrolizidine alkaloids, such as retronecine, senecionine and petasitenine (fukinotoxin), which contain retronecine and otonecine as necine, are more toxic. A few alkaloids, such as senkirkine, are esters of amino-alcohol otonecine, which are less toxic than retronecine. It has been said that the toxic alkaloid must possess the 1-hydroxymethyl-pyrrolizidine structure, unsaturation in the 1,2-position of the pyrrolizidine ring, and at least one of the hydroxy groups must be esterified.[26,27] Furthermore, it is known that the stereochemistry of the acid or basic moiety does not affect the toxicity qualitatively, but may cause quantitative difference in toxicity.[28]

Toxic effects of the alkaloids can be divided into peracute effects and cytotoxic effects. Peracute effects may be seen after large doses of some of the alkaloids, and may for example affect the central nervous system, causing convulsions and death within minutes. Cytotoxic effects are those in which cells in various organs such as liver, lung and kidney are damaged. Usually, the term toxicity is restricted to mean cytotoxicity. Acute toxicity refers to damage to an organ which may result in the death of an animal within one week after dosing. Chronic toxic effects are those which manifest themselves in an animal months or years after it has received a single dose of an alkaloid, or ingested repeated sublethal doses of chemicals. The nature of the toxic effects caused by pyrrolizidine alkaloids depends on such factors as the species and age of the affected animal, the structure of the alkaloid, and the manner in which the alkaloid is ingested.[28,29] Toxic effects of pyrrolizidine alkaloids are most frequently seen in the liver. A typical acute effect in the liver is massive centrilobular hemorrhagic necrosis. In considering the onset of the necrosis, failure of protein synthesis, nucleolar segregation, and failure of DNA-mediated RNA synthesis have been regarded as the earliest events.[14] Mitochondrial function is not affected directly in acute toxicity.[30] Early changes in the fine structure of rat liver cells by pyrrolizidine alkaloids have been reported by several workers.[30-32] Nucleolar segregation and degradation of endoplasmic reticulum such as formation of concentric whorls are representatives of such changes (Fig. 2–11). The most characteristic chronic effect is the development of a large number of giant liver cells (megalohepatocytes[28,33,34]) (Fig. 2–12). The cells in megalocytosis appear to be too unstable to divide. A detailed description on cell division and its relation to DNA synthesis of megalocytes is provided by Maclean.[14] Megalocytes probably undergo the cell cycle without completing the M phase ("by-pass" formation[14]), and the antimitotic action of the pyrrolizidine alkaloids, as well as increased exchange of materials between the nucleus and the cytoplasm, may be the important causative factors. The electron microscopic morphology of these megalocytes has been observed by Svoboda *et al.*[32] and others.[35] Although Svoboda *et al.*[32] found no abnormality in cell nuclei, Afzelius and Schoental[35] reported increase in the number of nuclear pores and granular aggregation within the nucleus in addition to proliferation of the smooth endoplasmic reticulum and loss in the normal organization of cytoplasmic organelles. Apart from the liver, the organ most frequently affected by the pyrrolizidine alkaloids is the lung. Several alkaloids, especially fulvine and monocrotaline, cause lesions of both lung and liver.[36] In monocrotaline poisoning, lung damage is sometimes more prominent than liver damage.[37,38] Seneciphylline, one of the hepatotoxic pyrrolizidine alkaloids, also induced marked lung lesion.[39] Lung lesions in rats following a single sc injection of monocrotaline showed prominent nucleolar alterations such as disintegration of nucleolonemal structure, and segregation of granular and fibrillar components in both type I and II alveolar epithelial cells.[40]

The pyrrolizidine alkaloids are known to be metabolized in a number of different ways. Hydrolysis of the alkaloid is one.[41] The ester groups of the alkaloid are hydrolyzed by aqueous alkali.[41] Neutral alkaloids are rather resistant to hydrolysis by esterases from rat liver. Heliotrine and lasiocarpine undergo hydrolysis in rat and sheep.[28] The pyrrolizidine alkaloids are easily converted into *N*-oxides and the reaction is readily reversed by reducing agents.[36,41] The oxidation is also known to occur metabolically in rat and sheep. Mattocks has reported that *N*-oxide is reduced to the base in the rat gut, perhaps by intestinal flora, and the high toxicity of pyrrolizidine *N*-oxides ingested orally is due to metabolic reduction in the gut to alkaloid bases.[28] The hydrolysis or *N*-oxidation is considered to be a detoxication process. In the rat, toxic pyrrolizidine alkaloids are known to be metabolized to pyrrolic derivatives and the reaction is brought about by the microsomal mixed-function oxidase of rat liver. Pyrrole derivatives of the alkaloids are considered to be responsible for some or all of the toxic effects of the pyrrolizidine alkaloids. Pyrrolic derivation of the pyrrolizidine alkaloids has been studied extensively by Mattocks.[28] The derivatives of the toxic pyrrolizidine alkaloids

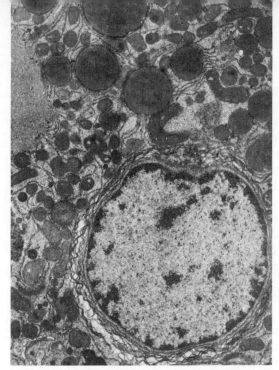

Fig. 2–11. Liver cell in the centrilobular region of a rat injected ip petasitenine 200 mg/kg and sacrificed 24 hr later. Degraded rough endoplasmic reticulum forms concentric whorls around the nucleus. Lipid droplets are increased in number. Mass of increased smooth endoplasmic reticulum is seen in the left upper portion.   × 16,500

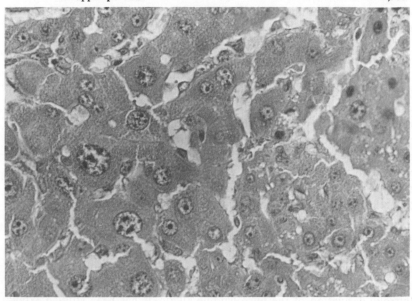

Fig. 2–12. A portion of the liver in a rat fed a diet containing *Petasites japonicus* Maxim. for 6 months. A few polyploid megalohepatocytes are seen.   × 230

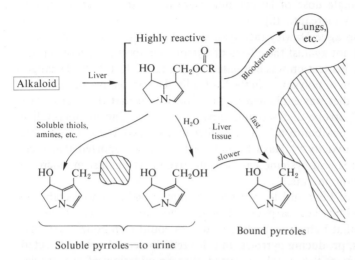

Fig. 2–13. Hypothetical fate of a reactive pyrrolic metabolite (dihydropyrrolizine ester) in the liver of a rat.

are chemically dihydro-pyrrolizidine esters, in which the ester groups are activated by conjugation with nitrogen and the ester group may readily be lost, leaving the positively charged dihydro-pyrrolizidine moiety.[27,36] Thus, the alkaloids probably act as bifunctional alkylating agents. Pyrrolic metabolites formed from pyrrolizidine alkaloid can be demonstrated when they are incubated aerobically with rat liver *in vitro*.[36] In the rat, the liver is the only organ in which the alkaloids are metabolized to pyrroles. Damage in other organs such as the pulmonary vessels appears to be due to metabolites which have escaped from the liver.[42] Thus, metabolic pyrroles are found mainly in the liver, but also in small amounts in the lung, especially after ingestion of alkaloids such as monocrotaline.[43] Fig. 2–13 shows the hypothesis proposed by Mattocks to demonstrate the fate of a reactive pyrrolic metabolite in the liver. Some of the reactive metabolites may react with structural or other macro-molecules, perhaps protein or nucleic acids within the cell, and remain for a much longer time as "bound pyrroles." Finally, some of the reactive metabolites may survive long enough to be trasported via the blood stream to other organs.[28]

Dietary effects on the toxicity of pyrrolizidine alkaloids have been studied by several workers. Newberne[44] reported that a lipotrope-deficient diet enhanced the effect of lasiocarpine on both maternal and fetal liver, when lasiocarpine was administered intra-gastrically to pregnant rats maintained on control and on lipotrope-deficient diets during gestation.

In contrast, liver damage and mortality in male Sprague-Dawley rats following a single dose of lasiocarpine were decreased by lipotrope deficiency and by mercaptoethylamine.[45] The low-lipotrope diet also protected male Sprague-Dawley rats against the acute toxic effects of monocrotaline, but not against the effects of pyrrole metabolites of monocrotaline, when the protection was evaluated by mortality, histological changes and dissociation of polysomes in the liver cells. The protective effects of the low-lipotrope diet was explained by the observation that the liver of rats fed the low-lipotrope diet was not capable of converting monocrotaline to the active metabolite at a rate sufficient to allow the characteristic expression of toxicity.[46] Hayashi and Larich[47] also reported that mercaptoethylamine and cysteine had a protective effect against monocrotaline intoxication in rats.

The ability of lung and liver tissues of human embryos to metabolize the three alkaloids lasiocarpine, retrorsine and fulvin has been tested.[48] It was found that human embryo liver tissues could metabolize pyrrolizidine alkaloids, producing pyrroles, but this reaction could not be detected with lung tissues. Schoental suggested that epoxidation of the crucial Cl,2-double bond in the dehydro-pyrrolizidine moiety rather than pyrrolic derivatives is probably an essential step in the biological action of pyrrolizidine alkaloids, this also being the reason why the cyclic diesters of retronecine are much more effectively hepatotoxic than the open-diesters.[27] However, Culvenor et al.[49] prepared both the 1α, 2α- and 1β, 2β-epoxide of monocrotaline and found that they did not cause liver damage when given as a single ip injection to 2-week-old rats in doses of up to 1,092 mg/kg for the 1α, 2α-epoxide and 546 mg/kg for the 1β, 2β-epoxide. Sex difference in the toxicity of pyrrolizidine alkaloids has been reported by many workers. Of the many pyrrolizidine alkaloids, most alkaloids such as retrosine,[50,51] isatidine,[50] ridelline,[50] monocrotaline[41] and seneciphylline[41] are more sensitive in males than in females, and some alkaloids such as lasiocarpine or pterophine (a mixture of senecionine and seneciphylline) are more toxic in females than in males.[52]

2.4 Carcinogenicity of Pyrrolizidine Alkaloids

Pyrrolizidine alkaloids were the first among natural products proved to induce tumors of the liver. Many pyrrolizidine alkaloids are present in various plants, some of which are used as food or herbal remedies. For instance, some *Senecio* plants are consumed by South African negroes from early childhood intermittently throughout life for treatment of a variety of diseases. Plants containing high levels of pyrrolizidine alkaloids have been shown to be responsible for liver damage in cattle and horses observed in chronic poisoning known under a variety of names.[14,26,53] Together with pure chemicals of pyrrolizidine alkaloids, plants with high content of pyrrolizidine alkaloids have been examined for carcinogenic activity. To date, at least six species of plants, i.e., *Senecio longilobus*,[54] *Petasites japonicus* Maxim.[55-57] *Tussilago farfara* L.,[58] *Symphytum officinale*,[59] *Farfugium japonicum*[60] and *Senecio cannabifolis*[60] have been demonstrated to have carcinogenic activities. Harris and Chen[54] studied the carcinogenic activity of prolonged administration of a diet containing dried *Senecio longilobus* in rats. The highest yield of liver cell carcinomas was obtained by alternating weekly feedings of a diet containing 0.5% *Senecio* and a *Senecio*-free diet for one year. *Petasites japonicus* Maxim., is a form of coltsfoot and herb of the tribe *Senecioneae* in the family of *Compositae*. *Petasites* is widely cultivated for use of food in Japan. The young flower stalks of wild *Petasites* are collected in early spring and used as food or herbal remedies such as cough medicine, expectorant and stomachic agent. Experiments showed that rats fed a diet containing dry powder of the fresh flower stalks of wild *Petasites* at a concentration of 4–8% developed hemangioendothelial sarcomas of the liver. Liver cell adenomas and carcinomas were also induced in a few animals.[55-57] *Tussilago farfara* L., a member of the tribe *Senecioneae*, family *Compositae*,

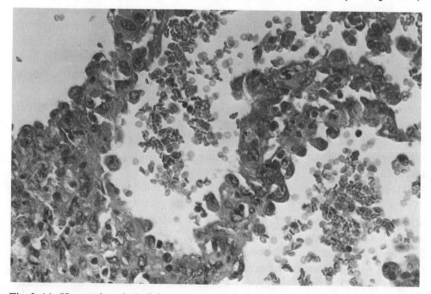

Fig. 2–14. Hemangioendothelial sarcoma of the liver in a rat fed a diet containing *Tussilago farfara* L. for 16 months. × 230

is used as a cough medicine in China and Japan. Dried and powdered buds of the coltsfoot of this plant induced hemangioendothelial sarcomas of the liver (Fig. 2-14), liver cell adenomas and carcinomas.[58] *Symphytum officinale* L., is an herb of the family *Boraginaeae*, which includes the *Heliotropium* species. This plant is called comfrey or Russian comfrey and is cultivated for use in Japan as a green vegetable or tonic. Rats fed diets containing 8 to 33% comfrey leaves or 1 to 8% roots for long periods also developed liver cell adenomas and hemangioendothelial sarcomas of the liver. The roots have much higher carcinogenicity than the leaves.[59] Carcinogenic activity of *Farfugium japonicum* and *Senecio cannabifolis* was confirmed by Hirono *et al.*[60] Both plants are herbs of the genus *Senecioneae* in the family *Compositae* and their young leaves and stalks are used in Japan as human food. 20% *Farfugium japonicum* and 1-0.2% *Senecio cannabifolis* induced hemangioendothelial sarcomas and liver cell adenomas respectively in the livers of ACI rats.[60] Although a variety of pyrrolizidine alkaloids exist in the world, very few alkaloids have so far been tested for carcinogenic activity. The major reason for the difficulty in testing carcinogenic activities of these chemicals is the limited supply of test samples. Furthermore, it has been the experience of many workers that the selection of appropriate dosage schedules which would allow the animals to survive for long periods and yet be sufficient for tumor induction is very difficult to establish. Cook *et al.*[61] examined the carcinogenicity of alkaloids of *Senecio jacobaea* and demonstrated hepatocarcinogenicity by feeding them to rats; but the alkaloids were a mixture extracted from the plant. The carcinogenicity of hydroxysenkirkine found in *Crotalaria labornifolia* L., which is used as a medical herb in Tanzania, was studied by Schoental and Cabanagh.[62] They found that after a single ip injection of the chemical, one rat developed an astrocytoma.

At least 8 pyrrolizidine alkaloids, i.e., isatidine, retrorsine, petasitenine, senkirkine, clivorine, monocrotaline, lasiocarpine and symphytine, have been demonstrated to be carcinogenic. Schoental *et al.*[15] reported that rats given isatidine, retrorsine-*N*-oxide by drinking water developed multiple hepatomas. Isatidine is not converted to pyrrol metabolites by isolated liver microsomes but is reduced to retrorsine in the intestinal tract of rats, possibly by gut flora. This explains its greater toxicity when given orally than when given intraperitoneally.[63] Rats given a solution containing 0.03 mg/ml retrorsine in drinking water 3 days weekly until death also developed hepatomas.[15] Svoboda and Reddy[16] treated male Fisher 344 rats with ip injections of lasiocarpine at a dose of 7.8 mg/kg body weight (19% of the LD_{50}) twice weekly for 4 weeks and once a week for 52 weeks. The majority of the animals were sacrificed between weeks 60 and 76. Rats developed liver cell carcinomas (61%), squamous cell carcinomas of the skin (33%), pulmonary adenomas (28%), adenocarcinomas of the small intestine, a cholangiocarcinoma and an adenomyoma of the ileum. Rao and Reddy[64] reported that among 20 male F344 rats fed a diet containing lasiocarpine at a concentration of 50 ppm for 55 weeks, malignant tumors developed in 17 animals between weeks 48 and 59. Of 20 rats, 9 (45%) developed angiosarcomas of the liver and 7 (35%) developed liver cell carcinomas. Carcinogenicity of senkirkine and symphytine was proved by Hirono *et al.*[65] All of 20 ACI rats given ip injections of freshly prepared senkirkine at a dose of 22 mg/kg body weight (10% of LD_{50}) twice weekly for 4 weeks, then once a week for 52 weeks survived more than 290 days, and 9 of them developed liver cell adenomas. Of 20 rats injected symphytine at a dose of 13 mg/kg body weight (0.1 of the LD_{50}), 4 had liver tumors (3 hemangiosarcomas and 1 liver cell adenoma). Carcinogenic activity of clivorine was demonstrated by Kuhara *et al.*[22] In their study all of the 12 ACI rats which had received a 0.005% solution of clivorine in drinking water for 340 days survived beyond 440 days. Of the 12, 8 developed liver tumors (2 hemangiosarcomas and 6 neoplastic nodules). Carcinogenicity of monocrotaline was first proved by Newberne and Rogers.[66] In this test, Sprague-Dawley rats given monocrotaline by gastric intubation once a week developed liver cell carcinomas. Hsu *et al.*[67] reported that dehydroretronecine is the major detectable pyrrole metabolite of monocrotaline in the tissues and urine of rats. Allen *et al.*,[68] and Shumaker *et al.*[69] injected either monocrotaline or dehydroretronecine sc into male Sprague-Dawley rats bi-weekly for 1 year. The rats in one experimental group were given 20 mg/kg of dehydroretronecine for 4 months and 10 mg/kg for the succeeding 8 months. The animals in another group were given 5 mg/kg of monocrotaline for 12 months. Each experimental group consisted of 60 animals. All animals were sacrificed 12 months after the cessation of the treatment. Of 60 rats that received dehydroretronecine, 39 developed rhabdomyosarcomas at the injection site, while among the monocrotaline-treated rats, 31 widely dispersed tumors of various cell types were recorded. Such a variation in tissue response may be attributable to the difference between the two alkaloids in that dehydroretronecine is a proximate carcinogen, whereas monocrotaline must first be metabolized before its carcinogenic potential is realized.[69] Recently, Robertson[70] reported that dehydroretronecine reacted with deoxyguanosine at pH 7.4 *in vitro* to yield in nearly equal quantities two major adducts with a nonexchangeable guan-8-yl proton, equimolar quantities of the pyrrole and nucleoside moieties. He emphasized that the reactive electrophile derived from protonated dehydroretronecine readily alkylates the N^2 position of deoxyguanosine at C-7 in an S_n1 reaction to yield a racemic mixture of products. Petasitenine is a stereoisomer of

otosenine and a new carcinogen isolated from *Petasites japonicus* Maxim,[9, 19)]
Carcinogenicity of petasitenine was also demonstrated by Hirono *et al.*[20)]
using ACI rats. The rats received a 0.01% solution of petasitenine and
those surviving beyond 160 days developed hemangioendothelial sarcomas of the liver and liver cell adenoma. The carcinogenic activity of
flower stalks of *Petasites jonicus* Maxim. can be attributed to petasitenine.
Seneciphylline is suspected of carcinogenicity, but nothing is known about
the carcinogenic activity of the pure chemical. However, Culvenor *et al.*[71)]
reported that rats given seneciphylline ip developed liver necrosis and
megalocytosis. Heliotrine is a monoester of heliotridine. Schoental[72)]
reported that 3 of 6 male rats surviving 22 to 27.5 months after one or
two intragastric doses of heliotrine with nicotinamide pretreatment and
one rat without nicotinamide had pancreatic tumors. Carcinogenicity of
jacobine has not yet been proved. However, rats receiving a mixture of
alkaloids from *S. jacobaea* L. in drinking water for more than 10 months
developed tumor-like masses, which were regarded as hepatomas.[61)] In
similar experiments by Schoental *et al.*[15)] using a mixture of alkaloids from
S. jacobaea, nodular hyperplasia of the liver was observed, some nodules
being described as early tarbecular hepatoma.

Species and strain differences in susceptibility to the carcinogenicity of
pyrrolizidine alkaloids are suspected. Clear data demonstrating this have
not yet been reported using pure chemicals of pyrrolizidine alkaloids.
Fushimi *et al.*[29)] conducted an experiment employing three strains of mice
and Syrian golden hamsters. Mice of ddN, Swiss and C57BL/6 strains and
Syrian golden hamsters received a 4% diet containing the flower stalks of
Petasites for 480 days. A high incidence of lung adenoma and adenocarcinoma was observed in ddN mice. No significant difference was observed
in tumor incidence between experimental groups of Swiss mice and
hamsters and their corresponding control groups. No tumors were induced in the experimental group of C57BL/6 strain mice. These results
revealed that mice and hamsters were markedly less susceptible to the
carcinogenicity of the flower stalks of *Petasites* when compared with rats
in which potent carcinogenic activity was observed. A strain difference in
susceptibility to the pyrrolizidine alkaloids was also observed.

The hazard of pyrrolizidine alkaloids regarding possible relationship to
human neoplasms, especially liver cell tumors, is not yet clear. In Africa
and other regions, plants containing carcinogenic pyrrolizidine alkaloids
are consumed as herbal remedies or foods; these plants include some
species of *Senecio* which contain isatidine, retrorsine and monocrotaline.
The consumption of foods and herbal remedies contaminated with pyrrolizidine alkaloids result in acute veno-occlusive lesions which progress
to liver cirrhosis. The Budd-Chiari syndrome, which is manifested by

hepatic vein occlusion in the native South African population is reported to be related to the consumption of bread containing *Senecio* flour.[14] Tandon *et al.*[73] reported epidemic data on veno-occlusive disease of the liver in Afganistan indicating that approximately 7,800 in a population 35,000 subjects were affected. The above authors reported that the cause was probably consumption of wheat flour heavily contaminated with the seeds of a plant of the *Heliotropium* species. Human liver cell megalocytosis due to toxic pyrrolizidine alkaloids has not yet been confirmed. However, veno-occlusive disease is a major source of cirrhosis in Jamaica.[74] The current concept of human liver disease includes the assumption that cirrhosis is an important precursor of liver malignancy.[75] Williams *et al.*[76] have reported histories of the use of herbal remedies in cases of liver cell carcinomas in infancy and childhood in western Nigeria, so far without positive correlations. Recently, Deinzer *et al.*[77] reported that hepatotoxic pyrrolizidine alkaloids which are cyclic diesters, such as senecionine, jacobine and seneciphylline, and known to occur in tansy ragwort, are also present in honey made from the nectar of this plant. It is known that the pyrrolizidine alkaloids form active metabolites and bind irreversibly to site on the liver and other organs and that their effects are accumulative.[28] Therefore, consumption of large amounts of pyrrolizidine alkaloids or the alkaloid-containing plants may be related to the occurrence of liver neoplasms and other human diseases.

2.5 Genotoxicity of Pyrrolizidine Alkaloids

Mutagenicity of pyrrolizidine alkaloids was first demonstrated in *Drosophila*. Clark[78] examined the mutagenicity of several pyrrolizidine alkaloids in *Drosophila melanogaster*, and classified the intensity of the mutagenicity in 11 alkaloids as follows: potent mutagenicity (monocrotaline, lasiocarpine and heliotrine), moderate mutagenicity (echinate, echimidine, senecionine and supinine), and weak mutagenicity (jacobine, platyphylline, heliotric acid and heliotridine).[79] Alderson and Clark[80] reported mutagenicity of two pyrrolizidine alkaloids, heliotrine and lasiocarpine, in a mutagenicity test using a methionine-dependent strain of *Aspergillus*. Chromosomal aberrations of some pyrrolizidine alkaloids in the root-tip cells of *Allium cepa* was examined by Avanzi.[81] Mutagenicity of pyrrolizidine alkaloids in bacterial systems was not proved until recently.[82] Lasiocarpine and retrorsine have been demonstrated to be mutagenic to *Salmonella typhimurium*.[83,84] In host-mediated assay, *Petasites japonicus* Maxim. was mutagenic in *his* G46 strain of *Salmonella*.[85] Yamanaka *et al.*[86] examined mutagenicity in 13 pyrrolizidine alkaloids in *Salmonella typhimurium* TA 100 in the presence of liver S9 mix. Heliotrine, lasiocarpine, fukinotoxin (petasitenine), ligularidine, senkirkine and LX201 were shown to be mutagenic, but lycopsamine, monocrotaline, retronecine, senecionine, seneciphylline and lindelofine were negative for mutagenicity. The same authors also reported that pre-incubation of the alkaloids with S9 mix and bacteria was essential for demonstration of mutagenicity in the bacterial system and that the type of ester bond does not seem to be closely related with the mutagenicity. In the same system with TA 100, symphytine was also found to be mutagenic.[57] Another systemic survey for genotoxicity of the pyrrolizidine alkaloids was performed in a hepatocyte primary culture/DNA repair test[87,88] measuring unscheduled DNA synthesis on 6 alkaloids.[89] All 6 pyrrolizidine alkaloids, i.e., monocrotaline, lasiocarpine, petasitenine, senkirkine, clivorine and LX201, elicited clear DNA repair. Very recently, further studies using this test were conducted on 17 pyrrolizidine alkaloids.[90] In the investigation, 11 pyrrolizidine alkaloids, i.e., senecionine, seneciphylline, jacobine, epoxyseneciphylline, senecicannabine, acetylfukinotoxin, syneilesine, ligularidine, neoligularidine, dihydroclivorine and ligularizine, whose carcinogenicity was not yet known, were found positive. Retronecine, an pyrrolizidine alkaloid lacking necic acid, and ligularinine, lacking the C1,2 double bond in the pyrrolizidine ring, were negative, indicating a close relationship between genotoxicity and molecular structure. This study also reported results indicating species difference in genotoxicity of pyrrolizidine alkaloids, implying species differences in their possible carcinogenic activities.[90] Chromosomal aberrations in rat lung cells related to monocrotaline was examined by Umeda and Saito.[91] The cells exposed for 48 hr to $10^{-2.5}$ M monocrotaline showed predominant chromosomal abnormalities such as breaks and fusions. Takanashi *et al.*[92] recently reported chromosomal aberration and mutagenicity by several pyrrolizidine alkaloids. Heliotrine and petasitenine induced interchromosomal exchanges, and lasiocarpine and senkirkine caused chromatid gaps. All the alkaloids tested induced an 8-azaguanine-resistant mutation in V79 cells by direct treatment for 48 hr. Mutation was also induced by treatment with the alkaloids for 1 hr in the presence of a metabolic activation system. Mutagenicity in V79 cells of 3 pyrrolizidine alkaloids, petasitenine, senkirkine and symphytine, was also proved by other investigators.[57] Transformation in hamster embryo cells was examined by Hirono *et al.*[57] Petasitenine induced transformation, while senkirkine and symphytine did not.

Teratogenic effects of a pyrrolizidine alkaloid were reported by Green and Christie.[93] They observed malformations in fetal rats following single maternal ip injections of heliotrine during the second week of gestation. Anomalies most commonly seen were general retardation of development and musculoskeletal defects involving the ribs. At high concentrations of the chemical, hypoplasia of the lower jaw, indistinguishable from that produced by irradiation, was observed.

REFERENCES

1. Bull, L.B., Culvenor, C.C.J., and Dick, A.T., *Frontiers of Biology*, Vol. 9, *The Pyrrolizidine Alkaloids*, Edited by Neuberger, A., and Tatum, E.L. Amsterdam, North-Holland Publishing Company, 1968; Klasek, A., and Weinbergora, O., *Recent Developments in the Chemistry of Natural Carbon Compounds*, Vol. VI, The Pyrrolizidine Alkaloids, Edited by Bognar, R., Bruckner, V., and Szantay, C. Budapest, Akademiai Kiado, 1975; Robins, D.J. The Pyrrolizidine Alkaloid, *Fortsch. der Chem. Org. Naturstoffe*, **41**: 115–326, 1982; Furuya, T., and Hikichi, M., Chemistry of pyrrolizidine alkaloids, *J. Synth. Org. Chem., Jpn.*, **35**: 653–668, 1977.
2. Hikichi, M., Asada, Y., and Furuya, T., Lycopsamine and O^9-Angelyl-retronecine, pyrrolizidine alkaloids from *Messerschmidia sibirica, Planta medica (Suppl)*: **1980**, 1–4.
3. Furuya, T, and Araki K, Studies on constituents of crude drugs, I. Alkaloids of *Symphytum officinale*, Chem. Pharm. Bull., **16**: 2512–2516, 1968; Furuya, T. and Hikichi, M, Alkaloids and triterpenoids of *Symphytum officinale, Phytochemistry*, **10**: 2217–2220, 1971.
4. Hikichi, M., and Furuya, T., Yamataimine, a new pyrrolizidine alkaloids from *Cacalia yatabei., Tetrahedr. Lett.*, **1978**: 767–770.
5. Furuya, T., and Hikichi, M., Lindelofine and supinine: Pyrrolizidine alkaloids from *Eupatorium stoechadosmum, Phytochemistry*, **12**: 225, 1973.
6. Furuya, T., Murakami, K., and Hikichi, M., Senkirkine, a pyrrolizidine alkaloid from *Farfugium Japonicum, Phytochemistry*, **10**: 3306–3307, 1971.
7. Asada, Y., Furuya, T., and Murakami, N., Pyrrolizidine alkaloids from *Ligularia japonica, Planta medica*, **42**: 202–203, 1981.
8. Hikichi, M., Asada, Y., and Furuya, T., Ligularidine, a new pyrrolizidine alkaloids from *Ligularia dentata, Tetrahedr. Lett.*, 1233–1236; **1979**: Asada, Y., and Furuya, T., Studies on constituents of crude drugs, XV. New pyrrolizidine alkaloids from *Ligularia dentata, Chem. Pharm. Bull.*, **32**: 475–482, 1984.
9. Furuya, T., Hikichi, M., and Iitaka, Y., Fukinotoxin, a new pyrrolizidine alkaloid from *Petasites japonicus, Chem. Pharm. Bull.*, **24**, 1120–1122, 1976.
10. Asada, Y., and Furuya, T., Shiro, M., and Nakai, H., Senecicannabine, a new pyrro lizidine Alkaloid from *Senecio cannabifolius, Tetrahedr. Lett.*, **23**: 189–192, 1982.
11. Asada, Y., Furuya, T., Neosenkirkine and senkirkine from *Senecio pierotii, Planta medica*, **44**: 182, 1982.
12. Asada, Y., Furuya, T., Takeuchi, T., and Osawa, Y., Pyrrolizidine alkaloids from *Senecio cruentus, Planta medica*, **46**: 125–126, 1982.
13. Hikichi, M., and Furuya, T., Syneilesine, a new pyrrolizidine alkaloids from *Syneilesis palmata, Tetrahedr. Lett.*, **1974**: 3657–3660; Hikichi, M., and Furuya, T., Studies on constituents of crude drugs, VII. Syneilesine and acetylsyneilesine from *Syneilesis Palmata. Chem. Pharm. Bull.*, **24**: 3178–3184, 1976.
14. Mclean, E.K., The toxic action of pyrrolizidine (*senecio*) alkaloids, *Pharmacol. Rev.*, **22**: 429–483, 1970.
15. Schoental, R., Head, M.A., and Peacock, P.R., *Senecio* alkaloids, primary liver tumours in rats as a results of treatment with (i) a mixture of alkaloids from *S. jaco-*

baea Lin.; (ii) retrorsine; (iii) isatidine, *Br. J. Cancer*, **8**: 458–465, 1954.

16. Svoboda, D.J., and Reddy, J.K. Malignant tumour in rats given lasiocarpine. *Cancer Res.*, **32**: 908–913, 1972.

17. Culvenor, C.C.J., Edgar, J.A., Smith, L.W., and Hirono, I., The occurrence of senkirkine in *Tussilago farfara. Aust. J. Chem.*, **29**: 229–230, 1976.

18. Culvenor, C.C.J., Clarke, M., Edgar, J.A., Frahn, J.L., Jago, M.V., Peterson, J.E., and Smith, L.W., Structure and toxicity of the alkaloids of Russian comfrey (*Symphytum* X *uplandicum* Nyman), a medicinal herb and item of human diet. *Experientia* **36**: 377–379, 1980.

19. Yamada, K., Tatematsu, H., Suzuki, M., Hirata, Y., Haga, M., and Hirono, I., Isolation and the structure of two new alkaloids, petasitenine and neopetasitenine from *Petasites japonicus* Maxim. *Chem. Letters*, **1976**: 461–464; Yamada, K. Tatematsu, H., Hirata, Y., Haga, M., and Hirono, I. Stereochemistry of petasitenine, the carcinogenic alkaloid from *Petasites japonicus* Maxim. and transformation of petasitenine to senkirkine. *Chem, Letters*, **1976**: 1123–1126.

20. Hirono, I., Mori, H., Yamada, K., Hirata, Y., Haga, M., Tatematsu, H., and Kanie, S., Carcinogenic activity of petasitenine, a new pyrrolizidine alkaloid isolated from *Petasites japonicus* Maxim., *J. Natl. Cancer Inst.*, **58**: 1155–1157, 1977.

21. Asada, Y., and Furuya, T., Epoxidation of Pyrrolizidine Alkaloids, (1). Chemical Conversion of Seneciphylline and Jacozine to Senecicannabine, *Chem. Pharm. Bull.*, **32**: 4616–4619, 1984.

22. Kuhara, K., Takanashi, H., Hirono, I., Furuya, T., and Asada, Y., Carcinogenic activity of clivorine, a pyrrolizidine alkaloid isolated from *Ligularia dentata, Cancer Letters*, **10**: 117–122, 1980.

23. Schoental, R., Hepatotoxic action of pyrrolidizine (senecio) alkaloids in relation to their structure, *Nature* (London), **179**: 361–363, 1957.

24. Schoental, R., Chemical structures and pathological effects of pyrrolizidine alkaloids, *Isr. J. Med. Sci.*, **4**: 1133–1145, 1968.

25. Schoental, R., Mattocks, A.R., Hepatotoxic activity of semisynthetic analogues of pyrrolizidine alkaloids, *Nature* (London), **185**: 842–843, 1960.

26. Schoental, R., Toxicology and carcinogenic action of pyrrolizidine alkaloids, *Cancer Res.*, **28**: 2237–2246, 1968.

27. Schoental, R., Hepatotoxic activity of retrorsine, senkirkine and hydroxysenkirkine in new-born rats, and the role of epoxides in carcinogenesis by pyrrolizidine alkaloids and aflatoxins, *Nature* (London) **227**: 401–402, 1970.

28. Mattocks, A.R., Toxicity and metabolism of senecio alkaloids, In: *Phytochemical Ecology* (Annual Proceeding of the Phytochemical Society No. 8). Edited by J.B. Harbone, pp. 401–402, Academic Press, London 1970.

29. Fushimi, K., Kato, K., Kato, T., and Matsubara, N., Carcinogenicity of flower stalks of *Petasites japonicus* Maxim. in mice and Syrian golden hamsters, *Toxicol. Lett.*, **1**: 201–294, 1978.

30. Mori, H., Kawai, K., Ohbayashi, F., Bunai, Y., Yamada, K., and Hirono, I., Some toxic properties of a carcinogenic pyrrolizidine alkaloid, petasitenine, *J. Toxicol. Sci.*, **9**: 143–147, 1984.

31. Svoboda, D., Racela, A., and Higginson, J., Variations in ultrastructural nucler changes in hepatocarcinogenesis, *Biochem. Pharmacol.*, **16**: 651–659, 1967.

32. Svoboda, D., and Soga, J., Early effects of pyrrolizidine alkaloids on the fine structure of rat liver cells, *Am. J. Path.*, **48**: 347–373, 1966.

33. Bull, L.B., and Dick, A.T., The chronic pathological effects on the liver of the rat of the pyrrolizidine alkaloids, heliotrine, lasiocarpine, and their *N*-oxides. *J. Pathol. Bacteriol.*, **78**: 483–502, 1959.

34. Scheuer, P., Histochemical changes in rat liver in *Senecio* and thioacetamide poisoning, *J. Pathol. Bacteriol.*, **85**: 507–512, 1963.

35. Afzelius, B.A., and Schoental, R., The ultrastructure of the enlarged hepatocytes induced in rats with a single oral dose of retrorsine, a pyrrolizidine (senecio) al-

kaloid, *J. Ultrastruct. Res.*, **20**: 328–345, 1967.

36. Mattocks, A.R., Toxicity of pyrrolizidine alkaloids, *Nature* (London), **217**: 723–728, 1968.
37. Hayashi, Y., Hussa, J.F., and Larich, J.J., Cor pulmonale in rats, *Lab. Invest.*, **16**: 875–881, 1967.
38. Schoental, R., and Head, M.A., Pathological changes in rats as a result of treatment with monocrotaline, *Br. J. Cancer*, **9**: 229–237, 1955.
39. Ohtsubo, K., Ito, Y., Saito, M., Furuya, T., and Hikichi, M., Hypertrophy of pulmonary arteries and arterioles with cor pulmonale in rats induced by seneciphylline, a pyrrolizidine alkaloid, *Experientia*, **33**: 498–499, 1977.
40. Hayashi, Y., and Hasegawa, T., Nucleolar alterations of alveolar epithelial cells in rats following a single injection of monocrotaline, *Acta Pathol. Jap.*, **19**: 315–327, 1969.
41. Bull, L.B., Culvenor, C.C.J., and Dick, A.T., *The Pyrrolizidine Alkaloids*, John Wiley & Sons, New York, **1968**.
42. Barnes, J.M., Magee, P.N., and Schoental, R., Lesions in the lungs and livers of rats posioned with the pyrrolizidine alkaloid, fulvine and its *N*-oxide. *J. Pathol. Bacteriol.*, **88**: 521–531, 1964.
43. Mattocks, A.R. and White, I.N.H., Estimation of metabolites of pyrrolizidine alkaloids in animal tissues, *Analyt. Biochem.*, **88**: 529–535, 1970.
44. Newberne, P.M. The influence of a low lipotrope diet on response of maternal and fetal rats to lasiocarpine. *Cancer Res.*, **28**: 2327–2337, 1968.
45. Rogers, A.E., and Newberne, P.M., Lasiocarpine; factors influencing its toxicity and effects on liver cell division, *Toxicol. Appl. Pharmacol.*, **18**: 356–366, 1971.
46. Newberne, P.M., Wilson, R., and Rogers, A.E., Effects of a low lipotrope diet on the response of young male rats to the pyrrolizidine alkaloid, monocrotaline, *Toxicol. Appl. Pharmacol.*, **18**: 387–397, 1971.
47. Hayashi, Y., and Larich, J., Protective effect of mercaptoethylamine and cysteine against monocrotaline intoxication in rats, *Toxical. Appl. Pharmacol.*, **12**: 36–43, 1968.
48. Armstrong, S.J., and Zuckerman, A.J., Production of pyrrolizidine alkaloids by human embryo tissue, *Nature* (London) **228**: 569–570, 1970.
49. Culvenor, C.C.J., Edgar, J.A., Smith, L.W., Jago, M.V., and Peterson, J.E., Active metabolites in the chronic hepatotoxicity of pyrrolizidine alkaloids, including otonecine esters, *Nature* (New Biol.) **229**: 255–256, 1971.
50. Schoental, R., and Head, M.A., Progression of liver lesions produced in rats by temporary treatment with pyrrolizidine (senecio). alkaloids, and the effects of betaine and high casein diets, *Br. J. Cancer*, **11**: 535–544, 1957.
51. Schoental, R., Liver lesions in young rats suckled by mothers treated with pyrrolizidine (senecio) alkaloids, lasiocarpine and retrorsine, *J. Pathol. Bacteriol.*, **77**: 485–495, 1959.
52. Jago, M.V., Factors affecting the chronic hepatotoxicity of pyrrolizidine alkaloids, *J. Pathol.*, **105**: 1–11, 1971.
53. Hirono, I., Natural carcinogenic products of plant origin, *CRC Critical Rev. Toxicol.*, **11**: 235–277, 1981.
54. Harris, P.N., and Chen, K.K., Development of hepatic tumors in rats following ingestion of *Senecio longilobus*, *Cancer Res.*, **30**: 2881–2886, 1970.
55. Hirono, I., Shimizu, M., Fushimi, K., Mori, H., and Kato, K., Carcinogenic activity of *Petasites japonicus* Maxim., a kind of coltsfoot, *Gann*, **64**: 527–528, 1973.
56. Hirono, I., Sasaoka, I., Shibuya, C., Shimizu, M., Fushimi, K., Mori, H., Kato, K., Haga, M., Natural carcinogenic products of plant origin, *Gann Monogr. Cancer Res.*, **17**: 205–217, 1975.
57. Hirono, I., Mori, H., Haga, M., Fujii, M., Yamada, K., Hirata, Y., Takanashi, H., Uchida, E., Hosaka, S., Ueno, I., Matsushima, T., Umezawa, K., and Shirai, A. Edible plants containing carcinogenic pyrrolizidine alkaloids in Japan, In: *Na-*

turally Occurring Carcinogens-Mutagens and Modulators of Carcinogenesis, Edited by E.C. Miller, J.A. Miller, I. Hirono, T. Sugimura and S. Takayama, Jap. Sci. Soc. Press & Univ. Park Press, pp. 79–87, **1979**.

58. Hirono, I. Mori, H., and Culvenor, C.C.J., Carcinogenic activity of coltsfoot, *Tussilago farfara* L. *Gann,* 67: 125–129, 1976.

59. Hirono, I., Mori, H., and Haga, M., Carcinogenic activity of *Symphytum officinale, J. Natl. Cancer Inst.,* 61: 856–869, 1978.

60. Hirono, I., Ueno, I., Aiso, S., Yamaji, T., and Haga, M., Carcinogenic activity of *Farfugium japonicum* and *Senecio cannabiofolis. Cancer Lett.,* 20: 191–198, 1983.

61. Cook, J.W., Duffy, E., and Schoental, R., Primary liver tumors in rats following feeding with alkaloids of *Senecio jacobaea. Br. J. Cancer,* 4: 405–410, 1950.

62. Schoental, R., and Cavanagh, J.B., Brain and spinal cold tumours in rats treated with pyrrolizidine alkaloids, *J. Natl. Cancer Inst.,* 49: 665–671, 1972.

63. Mattocks, A.R., Heptotoxic effects due to pyrrolizidine alkaloid N-oxides, *Xenobiotica,* 1: 563–565, 1971.

64. Rao, M.S., Reddy, J.K., Malignant neoplasms in rats fed lasiocarpine, *Br. J. Cancer,* 37: 289–293, 1978.

65. Hirono, I., Haga, M., Fujii, M., Matsuura, S., Matsubara, N., Nakayama, M., Furuya, T., Hikichi, M., Takanashi, H., Uchida, E., Hosaka, S., and Ueno, I., Induction of hepatic tumors in rats by senkirkine and symphytine, *J. Natl. Cancer Inst.,* 63: 469–472, 1979.

66. Newberne, P.M., and Rogers, A.E., Nutrition, monocrotaline and aflatoxin B_1 in liver carcinogenesis, *Plant Foods for Man,* 1: 23–31, 1973.

67. Hsu, I.C., Allen, J.R., and Chesney, C.F., Identification and toxicological effects of dehydroretrosine, a metabolite of monocrotaline, *Proc. Soc. Exp. Biol. Med.,* 144: 834–838, 1973.

68. Allen, J.R., Hsu, I.C., and Carstens, L.A., Dehydroretronecine-induced rhabdomyosarcomas in rats, *Cancer Res.,* 35: 997–1002, 1975.

69. Shumaker, R.C., Robertson, K.A., Hsu, I.C., and Allen, J.R., Neoplastic transformation in tissues of rats exposed to monocrotaline or dehydroretronecine, *J. Natl. Cancer Inst.,* 56: 787–790, 1976.

70. Robertson, K.A., Alkylation of N^2 in deoxyguanosine by dehydroretronecine, a carcinogenic metabolite of the pyrrolizidine alkaloid monocrotaline. *Cancer Res.,* 42: 8–14, 1982.

71. Culvenor, C.C.J., Edgar, J.A., Jago, M.V., Outteridge, A., Peterson, J.E., and Smith, L.W., Hepato- and pneumotoxicity of pyrrolizidine alkaloids derivatives in relation to molecular structure, *Chem. Biol. Interact.,* 12: 299–324, 1976.

72. Schoental, R., Pancreatic islet-cell and other tumors in rats given heliotrine, a monoester pyrrolizidine alkaloid, and nicotinamide, *Cancer Res.,* 35: 2020–2024, 1975.

73. Tandon, H.D., Tandon, B.N., and Mattocks, A.R., An epidemic of veno-occlusive disease of the liver in Afganistan, *Am. J. Gastroenterol.,* 70: 607–613, 1978.

74. Bras, G., Brooks, S.E.H., and Walter, D.C, Cirrhosis of the liver in Jamaica, *J. Pathol. Bacteriol.,* 82: 503–512, 1961.

75. Scheuer, P.J., Cirrhosis, In: *Pathology of the Liver,* Edited by R.N.M. Macsween, P.P. Anthony, P.J. Scheuer, Churchill Livingston Press, London & New-York, pp. 258–271, **1979**.

76. Williams, A.O., Edington, G.M., and Obakponovwe, P.C., Hepatocellular carcinoma in infancy and childhood in Ibadan, western Nigeria, *Brit. J. Cancer,* 21: 474–482, 1967.

77. Deinzer, M.L., and Thompson, P.A., Pyrrolizidine alkaloids: Their occurrence in honey from Tansy Ragwort (*Senecio jacobaea* L.), *Science,* 195: 497–499, 1977.

78. Clark, A.M. Mutagenic activity of the alkaloid heliotrine in *Drosophila, Nature* (London) 183: 731–732, 1959.

79. Clark, A.M., The mutagenic activity of some pyrrolizidine alkaloids in *Drosophila, Zeitschrift fur Vererbung,* 91: 74–80, 1960.

80. Alderson, T., and Clark, A.M., Interlocus specificity for chemical mutagens in *Aspergillus nidurans*, *Nature* (London) **210**: 593–595, 1966.
81. Avanzi, S., Chromosomal breakage by pyrrolizidine alkaloids and modification of the effects by cystein, *Caryologia*, **14**: 251–261, 1961.
82. Green, M.H.L., and Muriel, W.J., Use of repair-deficient strains of *Escherichia coli* and liver microsome to detect and characterize DNA damage caused by the pyrrolizidine alkaloids heliotrine and monocrotaline, *Mutat. Res.*, **28**: 331–336, 1975.
83. Koletsky, A., Oyasu, R., and Reddy, J.K., Mutagenicity of the pyrrolizidine (senecio) alkaloids, lasiocarpine in the *Salmonella*/microsome test, *Lab. Invest.*, **38**: 352, 1978.
84. Wehner, F.C., Thiol, P.G., and Van Rensburg, S.J. Mutagenicity of alkaloids in the *Salmonella*/microsome system, *Mutat. Res.*, **66**: 187–190, 1979.
85. Sugimura, T., Nagao, M. Kawachi, T., Honda, M., Yahagi, T., Seino, Y., Sato, S., Matsukura, N., Matsushima, T., Shirai, A., Sawamura, M., and Matsumoto, H., Mutagen-carcinogens in food, with special reference to highly mutagenic pyrolytic products in broiled foods., In: *Origin of Human Cancer* (Cold Springer Harbor Conference on Cell Proliferation 4) Edited by H.H. Hiatt, J.D. Watson, J.A. Winsten, Cold Spring Harbor Lab., pp. 1561–1577, **1977**.
86. Yamanaka, H., Nagao, M., Sugimura, T., Furuya, T., Shirai, A., and Matsushima, T., Mutagenicity of pyrrolizidine alkaloids in the *Salmonella*/mammalian-microsome test. *Mutat. Res.*, **68**: 211–216, 1979.
87. Williams, G.M., Detection of chemical-carcinogens by unscheduled DNA synthesis in rat liver primary cultures, *Cancer Res.*, **87**: 1845–1851, 1977.
88. Williams, G.M., Laspia, M.E., and Dunkel, V.C., Reliability of the hepatocyte primary culture/DNA repair test in testing of coded carcinogens and noncarcinogens, *Mutat. Res.*, **97**: 359–370, 1982.
89. Williams, G.M., Mori, H., Hirono, I., and Nagao, M., Genotoxity of pyrrolizidine alkaloids in the hepatocyte primary culture/DNA repair test, *Mutat. Res.*, **79**: 1–5, 1980.
90. Mori, H., Sugie, S., Yoshimi, N., Asada, Y., Furuya, T., and Williams, G.M., Genotoxicity of a variety of pyrrolizidine alkaloids in the hepatocycte primary culture/DNA repair test using rat, mouse and hamster hepatocytes, *Cancer Res.*, **45**: 3125–3129, 1985.
91. Umeda, M., and Saito, M., The effect of monocrotaline, a pyrrolizidine alkaloid, on Hela cells and primary culture cells from rat liver and lung, *Acta Pathol. Jap.*, **21**: 507–514, 1971.
92. Takanashi, H., Umeda, M., and Hirono, I., Chromosomal aberrations and mutation in cultured mammalian cells induced by pyrrolizidine alkaloids, *Mutat. Res.*, **78**: 67–77, 1980.
93. Green, C.R., and Christie, G.S., Malformation in foetal rats induced by pyrrolizidine alkaloid, heliotrine, *Br. J. Exp. Pathol.*, **42**: 369–378, 1961.

3

Flavonoids

3.1 Chemistry and Distribution in Plants

The flavonoids comprise one of the large groups of secondary metabolites occurring widely throughout the plant kingdom. They have a common skeleton of 1,3-diphenylpropane composed of a Ar(ring B)-C_3 subunit derived from shikimate and the other aromatic ring (ring A) of polyketide orgin (Fig. 3–1). As expected from its biosynthetic origin, oxygen functions exist usually on the 5- and 7-positions in ring A, while ring B may have a 4'-hydroxy, 3',4'-dihydroxy, or 3',4',5'-trihydroxy substitution pattern. By further oxidation, reduction, alkylation, acylation, and migration reactions, several modifications of the basic skeleton occur to produce the subgroups shown in Fig. 3–1. Further modification leads to biflavonyls, neoflavones and non-hydrolyzable tannins.

Although some occur in free form, more compounds exist in nature as the glycoside form. D-Glucose is the most frequent sugar residue but D-galactose, L-rhamnose, L-arabinose, D-xylose and D-apiose as well as some uronic acids also form the sugar part. Variation in the number of sugar residues, the binding site on the aglycones and acylation in sugar residues produce further varieties. As a result more than two thousand flavonoids have so far been characterized.[1]

The flavones give a yellow or orange color, while the anthocyanidins produce red, violet or blue colors contributing to the beauty and splendor of flowers and fruit in nature. As long as the free hydroxyl groups are retained, the flavonoids exhibit phenolic properties and show positive ferric chloride reactions. Most flavones and flavanones show characteristic red coloration with magnesium and hydrochloric acid. Spectral methods, especially UV spectra, are important in identifying this group of compounds.[2,3]

Among the subgroups shown in Fig. 3–1, chalcones are comparatively

53

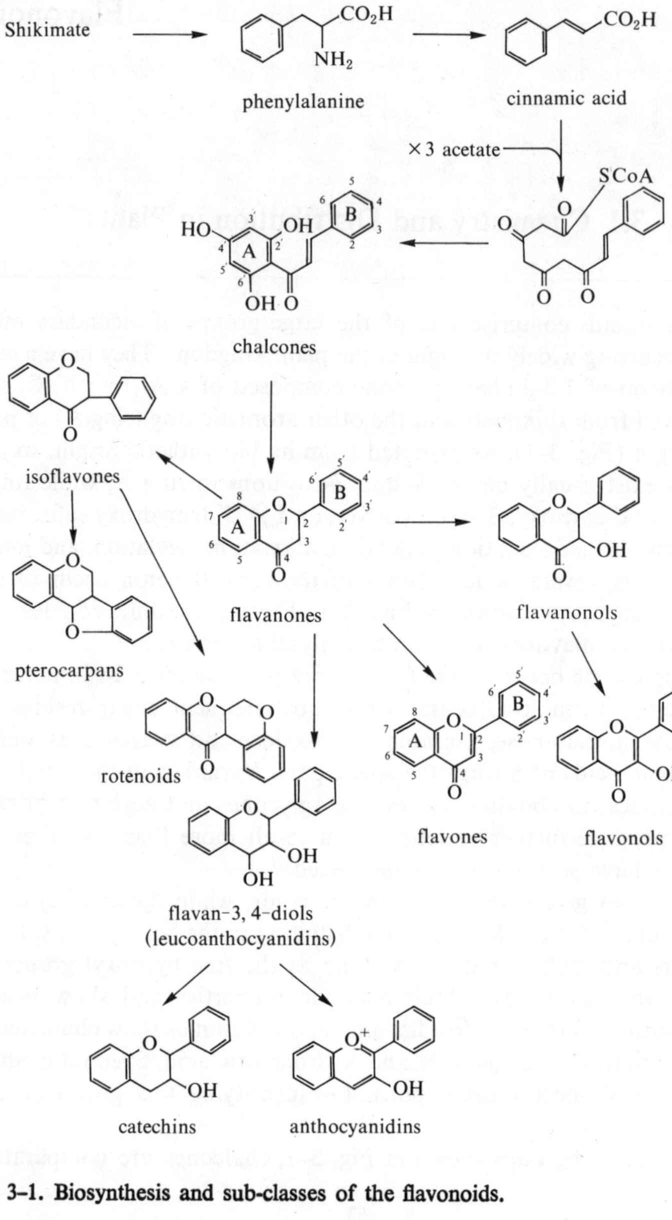

Fig. 3–1. Biosynthesis and sub-classes of the flavonoids.

rare in nature. Flavanones (2,3-dihydroflavones) and flavanonols (3-hydroxyflavanones) are also relatively uncommon, but occasionally accumulate in fruit, flowers, and wood. Both flavones and flavonols (3-hydroxyflavones) are very widely distributed. Flavonol glycosides, such as the glycosides of quercetin (3,5,7,3',4'-pentahydroxyflavone) (*e.g.* rutin (quercetin 3-rhamno-glucoside) and quercitrin (quercetin 3-rhamnoside)) and kaempherol (3,5,7,4'-tetrahydroxyflavone) (*e.g.* astragalin (kaempherol 3-glucoside)), occur most frequently. Rutin occurs at concentrations of greater than 3 % dry weight in the leaves of eucalyptus, flower buds of sophora, and buckwheat. On the contrary, the distribution of isoflavones, which occur most commonly in the family Leguminosae, is rather confined. Pterocarpans and rotenoids are the modifications. Leucoanthocyanidins produce, by polymerization, unhydrolyzable tannins (condensed tannins), one of two groups of tannins, which are widely occurring high molecular plant products. Anthocyanidins, such as pelargonidin, cyanidin, and delphinidin, occur widely in flowers in the glycoside form and produce the blue, red and violet coloration in flower petals and fruit.[4]

Flavonoids are absent in bacteria. Occurrence of the flavonoid compounds has been reported in some exceptional cases of fungi and algae. Several mosses contain flavones. In contrast, flavonoids are ubiquitous in vascular plants of a higher order than ferns. They are found particularly in the leaves and petals and have been used as markers for chemotaxonomy and chemical evolution studies.[5]

The flavonoids are widely distributed in edible parts of food plants[6] but precise quantitative analyses have not been conducted. Kaempherol and quercetin glycosides of stone and berry fruit were studied and all were proved to contain quercetin glycosides at levels of 2–240 mg/kg fresh weight. The content is lower in vegetables but the presence of flavonol glycosides was proved in potato, asparagus, carrot, onion, radish, beet and cabbage.[7] Another work on onion, lettuce, kale, chive, garlic chive, leek, horseradish, red radish and red cabbage revealed that a variety of lettuce contains 38 mg quercetin/kg fresh weight and the green portion of chive contains 55 mg kaempherol/kg fresh weight as the highest examples.[8] It is impossible to arrive at an accurate figure, but 50 mg (quercetin equivalents) per day has been estimated to be the intake of flavonol glycosides in the average diet.[6]

Many biological activities of flavonoids described in section 3.4 have been clarified recently. They are not acutely toxic to mammals and are assumed to be typical secondary metabolites with no known harmful effects on humans and animals. They play a major role in insect pollination. Some flavonoids have a bitter taste as a repelling factor. The role of flavonoids as echochemicals is quite widespread and should not be ignored.[9]

3.2 Mutagenicity

Mutagenicity of flavonoids was first reported by five groups independently in 1976–1978 using the *Salmonella typhimurium*/microsome test developed by Ames.

Pamukcu and coworkers[10] discovered mutagenicity of quercetin (1) in TA98 and TA100 strains in their course of studies of carcinogenic substances in bracken fern.

Bjeldanes and Chang[11] examined quercetin (1) and nine related compounds and found that quercetin was mutagenic against TA98 and TA100 strains without microsomal activation. With activation the mutagenic activity of quercetin was increased significantly and that of quercetin pentaacetate (2) was revealed. Since quercetin pentamethyl ether (3) and flavanones such as hesperetin (4), naringenin (5), and dihydroquercetin (6) exhibit no measurable activity, molecular planarity and free phenolic groups appeared to be a requirement for mutagenicity.

Brown *et al.*,[12] interested in genetic toxicity of food additives, examined the mutagenicity of 14 flavones and flavanones. Frameshift mutagenicity among the flavonoids tested was mainly confined to the flavonols, and quercetin (1) was found to be the most reactive. The glycosides, rutin (7) and quercitrin (8) were very weakly mutagenic but the activity increased 10–20 fold by incorporation of gut bacterial enzymic extracts. Dihydrochalcones, some of which are used as non-nutritive sweetners, were found to be non-mutagenic.

In the course of studies on the carcinogenic principles of bracken, all the compounds isolated from bracken were tested by the *Salmonella*/microsome test.[13] Unexpectedly, kaempferol (9) was found to be active to TA98 and TA100 strains of the bacteria. Thus ten flavonoids were tested by Sugimura *et al.*[14] and the flavonols quercetin (1) and galangin (10) were also found to be mutagenic.

Because of the widespread occurrence and frequent exposure to man, Hardigree and Epler[15] investigated eleven flavonoids by the same system and obtained the same results.

At that time a simple method for mutagenicity testing, the Ames test, was the focus of much attention and it was becoming increasingly evident that most chemical carcinogens are mutagens. Reports on the mutagenicity of the popular flavonols shocked many scientists, especially when the wide occurrence of flavonoids was taken into consideration.

Further work developed in four directions: i) examination of numerous

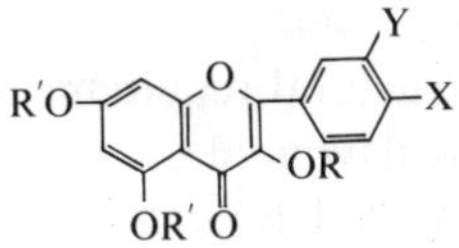

	R	R′	X	Y
quercetin (1)	H	H	OH	OH
quercetin pentaacetate (2)	Ac	Ac	OAc	OAc
quercetin pentamethyl ether (3)	Me	Me	OMe	OMe
rutin (7)	glu-rha	H	OH	OH
quercitrin (8)	rha	H	OH	OH
kaempferol (9)	H	H	OH	H
galangin (10)	H	H	H	H
myricetin (11)	H	H	OH	OH (6-OH)
rhamnetin (12)	H	H, Me	OH	OH
tamarixetin (13)	H	H	OMe	OH
morin (14)	H	H	OH	H (2′-OH)
robinin (15)	gal-rha	H, rha	OH	H
astragalin (18)	glu	H	OH	H
isorhamnetin (19)	H	H	OH	OMe
isorhamnetin 3-sulfate (20)	SO_3^-	H	OH	OMe
quercetin 3-sulfate (21)	SO_3^-	H	OH	OH

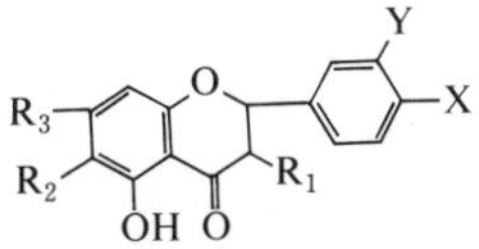

	R_1	R_2	R_3	X	Y
hesperetin (4)	H	H	OH	OMe	OH
naringenin (5)	H	OH	H	OH	H
dihydroquercetin (6)	OH	H	OH	OH	OH

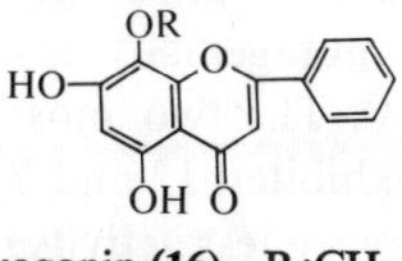

wogonin (16)   R:CH₃
norwogonin (23)   R:H

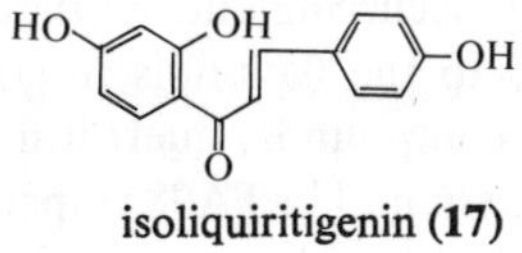

isoliquiritigenin (17)

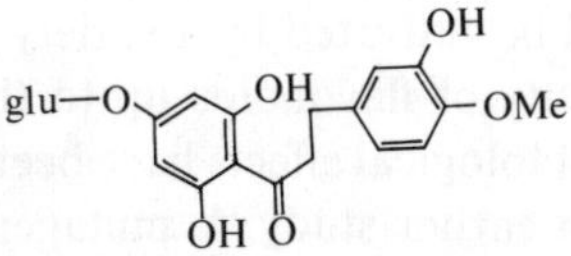

neohesperidin   dihydrocholcone (22)

Fig. 3–2. Chemical structures of mutagenic flavonoids.

flavonoid samples to clarify the structural requirements for mutagenicity,
ii) surveys on foodstuffs containing flavonoids, iii) mutagenicity testing
using systems other than bacteria, and iv) carcinogenicity testing using
experimental animals. Of the above four directions i) through iii) are
described immediately below and iv) is described in section 3.3.

Work on clarifying the structural requirements for mutagenicity was
conducted by three groups. Forty compounds related to quercetin were
tested in strain TA98 by MacGregor and Jurd.[16] Ten flavonols, quercetin
(**1**), myricetin (**11**), rhamnetin (**12**), galangin (**10**), kaempferol (**9**), tamarixe-
tin (**13**), morin (**14**), and mono- and di-methyl ethers of quercetin, exhibited
the actvity. Four compounds bearing free hydroxyl groups at the 3' and 4'
positions of the B ring were active without metabolic activation. Structural
features which appear essential for mutagenicity are a flavone ring with a
free hydroxyl group at the 3 position, a double bond at the 2,3 position, a
carbonyl group at the 4 position, and a structure which permits tautomeri-
zation of the 3-hydroxyl to a 3-keto compound. Among the sub-classes
of the flavonoids shown in Fig. 3–1, free flavonols fulfill these conditions.
Thus the ring B structures to form the quinonoid intermediates (Fig. 3–3),
by the application of the metabolic activation system, were assumed to be
essential for the activity.

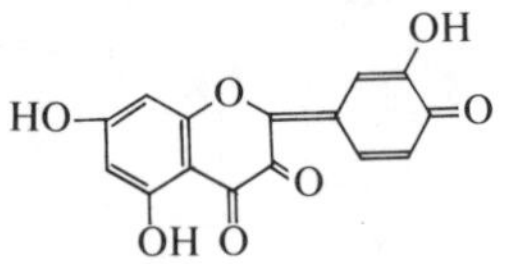

Fig. 3–3. The proposed DNA-reactive intermediate of flavonols.

Following a preliminary report,[12] Brown and Dietrich[17] using five
tester strains (TA 1535, 100, 1537, 1538 and 98) screened for over seventy
naturally occurring and synthetic flavonoids. Frameshift mutagenicity was
confined to the flavonols in strains TA98, 1537 and 100. The two most
reactive compounds, quercetin (**1**) and kaempferol (**9**), exhibited 12 and 7
revertants/n mol in TA98 respectively. Other flavonols showed less activity.
Flavonol glycosides quercitrin (**8**), rutin (**7**) and robinin (**15**) were non-
mutagenic, but they could be activated by a variety of mixed glycosidases.
The reports on mutagenicity of flavonoids up to that time together with
the general chemistry and biological effects have been reviewed by Brown.[6]

Continuing work on an earlier study,[14] mutagenicity of 61 flavonoids
was tested by Nagao *et al.*[18] using strains TA100 and 98. Among the 22
flavone derivatives tested, only wogonin (**16**) was rather strongly active.

Of the 16 flavonol derivatives, all except 3-alkoxy derivatives were mutagenic. Some flavanones and flavanonols exhibited weak mutagenicity. Among the related compounds tested only isoliquiritigenin (17), a chalcone, was weakly mutagenic. The conclusion for the structure-activity relationship was the same as above. Activation of flavonol glycosides by prenicubation with a enzyme mixture (hespridinase) obtained from *Aspergillus niger* was also reported.[18]

As for work on constituents in foodstuffs, the boiling water extract of bracken fern was fractionated using Ames' test as the monitor. Upon preincubation with hesperidinase, the fraction containing astragalin (18) was found to be mutagenic.[13] The mutagenic substance in sumac, a spice prepared from seeds of *Rhus* sp., was proved to be quercetin (1),[19] the mutagens in a Japanese pickle were proved to be kaempferol (9) with a small amount of isorhamnetin (19),[20] and those in dill weed, a spice prepared from *Anethum graveolens,* and dill seeds from *A. sawa (Umbelliferae)* were characterized as isorhamnetin 3-sulfate (20) and quercetin 3-sulfate (21) respectively.[21] Infusions of green tea and black tea were hydrolyzed and the extracts by organic solvents were examined by Ames' test. The flavonols kaempferol (9), quercetin (1) and myricetin (11) were detected in the extracts, and their combined activity was proved to represent about 70% of the total activity.[22]

Mutagenicity data on flavonoids in other microbial systems are quite limited. Quercetin exhibits activity in tester strains of *E. coli* and *Saccharomyces cerevisae*.[12,17]

Many studies have been conducted using mammalian cells and other systems. In a transformation assay with cryopreserved hamster embryo cells, kaempferol (9) did not induce transformation but quercetin (1) induced morphological transformation of cells at concentrations of 5 μg/ml and 10 μg/ml.[23] Mutagenic activity of quercetin (1) and kaempferol (9) was also tested on V79 Chinese hamster cells. Both compounds showed the activity after metabolic activation, but quercetin was also active without the activation.[24] Quercetin was found to introduce chromosomal aberrations and sister-chromatid exchanges in cultured human and Chinese hamster cells without the application of metabolic activation systems.[25] Quercetin (1), kaempferol (9), neohesperidin dihydrochalcone (22) and rutin (7) were administered to male mice for the detection of gross chromosomal anomalies by the micronucleus test. Except for rutin, the compounds were positively clastogenic in varying degrees.[26] Quercetin (1) was positive in the L5178Y mouse leukemic cell thymidine kinase locus $(TK^{+/-})$ mutation assay without metabolic activation and in DNA single-strand break assay in L5178Y cells.[27] Weak transformation of Balb/c 3T3 cells was also observed.[27] Quercetin (1) and kaempferol (9) were found to be mutagenic in *Drosophila melanogaster*.[28] The frequencies of chromosomal aberrations, gene mutation at four loci, and sister-chromatid exchange in single population of Chinese hamster ovary cells exposed to quercetin (**1**), kaempferol (**9**) and galangin (**10**) were examined; all three compounds were found to induce chromosomal aberrations and mutants at the *tk* locus, with little effect on the sister-chromatid exchange frequency or on gene mutation at three other loci (*hgprt, aprt,* and Na$^+$/ K$^+$-ATPase).[29] Induction of sister-chromatid exchange and *hgprt* mutants by quercetin (**1**) in V79 Chinese hamster cells was investigated and no induction was observed under standard conditions.[30] The induction of TK-deficient mutants in L5178Y cells with quercetin (**1**) did not result in an increase in *hgprt*-deficient mutants. These results have been discussed in relation to the negative outcome of carcinogenicity of quercetin in mammals.[30] A brief description is found in section 3.3.

Based on the oxidizability of quercetin to its quinonoid,[31,32] MacGregor and Jurd[16] proposed the quinonoid structure shown in Fig. 3–3 as an active intermediate of quercetin, but actual activation systems have not yet been demonstrated. Recently, Ochiai *et al.*[33] showed enhancement of quercetin mutagenicity in *Salmonella typhimurium* strain TA98 cells by the addition of Cu/Zn-superoxide dismutase (Cu/Zn-SOD) as well as addition of S-9 mixture (rat liver homogenate 9000 g supernatant with cofactors), and Ueno and colleagues[34] demonstrated reduction of Cu^{2+} ion of Cu/Zn-SOD by quercetin and inhibition of the direct, and Cu/Zn-, Fe- or Mn-SOD, or rat liver cytosol-stimulated mutagenicity of quercetin by diethyldithiocarbamate, a well known Cu-chelator and inhibitor of Cu/Zn-SOD. These data suggest contribution of SODs to the activation systems of quercetin.

Salmonella typhimurium strain TA98 is sensitive to frameshift type mutagens, while strain TA100 is mutated by base-pair substitutions.[11] Although certain flavonoids are mutagenic in both strains, sensitivities of some flavonoids in these two strains are not necessarily the same; in the presence of S-9 mixture, wogonin (**16**),[18] norwogonin (**23**) and several 8-hydroxyflavones,[35] most of which lack the 3-hydroxy group, were strongly mutagenic to the TA100 cells, while they showed only a minor or weak effect on the TA98 cells. Mutagenic activities of these flavones cannot be explained by the mechanism proposed by MacGregor and Jurd,[16] as pointed out by Elliger *et al.*[35]

3.3 Carcinogenicity

Ambrose and his colleagues investigated chronic toxicities and carcinogenicities of quercetin and quercitrin at 1% levels in diets of albino
rats in 1952.[36] Flavonoids were found to be neither toxic nor carcinogenic
after 410 days of feeding.

For many years Pamukcu and his colleagues[37-42] searched for the
carcinogenic principle of bracken fern, and in 1976, they discovered
mutagenicity of quercetin in *Salmonella typhimurium* strain TA98 and
TA100 cells.[10] In 1980, Pamukcu and colleagues[43] reported carcinogenicity of quercetin. They showed significantly high incidences of intestinal
neoplasms, including adenocarcinoma and bladder tumors in albino non-
inbred rats of both sexes fed grain diets containing 0.1% quercetin for
58 weeks. In their experiments, one group of rats of both sexes was fed
a diet containing 33% bracken fern for the same period as a group fed
quercetin. Both groups developed neoplasms in intestines and bladder; the
incidences of neoplasms in intestines were similar for both groups, but the
incidence of bladder neoplasms was lower in the bracken fern diet group
than in the group fed quercetin. Histopathological observations of the
neoplasms of the animals of both groups were identical. Based on these
results, Pamkcu *et al.* proposed quercetin to be the major effector of
bracken fern carcinogenesis.

Recently, however, Hirono and his colleagues[44,45] succeeded in isolating a carcinogenic principle of bracken fern, ptaquiloside, and demonstrated its carcinogenicity, casting doubt as to whether quercetin is the
carcinogenic principle of bracken fern.

Pamukcu and his colleagues[46] again exhibited significantly high incidences of hepatoma in female Sprague-Dawley rats fed a 0.5% quercetin
or 2% rutin diet for up to 139 weeks, and hepatic tumors and biliary
adenoma in female Fischer 344 rats given a 1% or 2% quercetin diet for
the same period.

As mentioned in the previous section, mutagenicity of quercetin was
confirmed by several researchers, in conjunction with new findings of
mutagenicities of other flavonoids. The problems of carcinogenicity of
these flavonoids is again the concern of many researchers. Several carcinogenic experiments have been conducted on various animals in different
laboratories mainly in Japan. However, in contrast to the results of Pamukcu *et al.,* none of these experiments demonstrated carcinogenicity of
quercetin and related flavonoids. Saito *et al.*[47] examined carcinogenicity

of quercetin at 2% levels in diets in male and female mice throughout their life span. The incidence of tumors was not significant. Hirono and his colleagues investigated carcinogenicity of quercetin, rutin and kaempferol in rats. In male and female ACI rats fed diets containing 1% or 5% quercetin, or 5% rutin for 540 days, 10% quercetin or rutin for 850 days,[48] 0.04% kaempferol for 540 days, and 0.1% quercetin for 540 days (Fischer 344 rats, both sexes[49]), no significant high incidence of tumors was observed. Hosaka and Hirono[50] examined the carcinogenicity of quercetin at a dose of 5% in diets, using pulmonary-adenoma bioassay in strain A mice. They found no significant increases in the incidence and multiplicity of lung tumors. Morino et al.[51] used non-inbred golden hamsters of both sexes. In all of the groups of hamsters fed a diet containing 10% quercetin or rutin for 735 days, 4% quercetin for 709 days and 1% quercetin for 351 days followed by either a 1% croton oil diet or control diet for 350 days, no statistically significant incidence of tumors was observed.

Related to these results, Kato et al.[52] demonstrated the suppressive effect of quercetin applied as pretreatment on the promotion effect of 12-O-tetradecanoylphorbol-13-acetate (TPA) on skin tumor formation in CD-1 mice, treated with 7,12-dimethylbenz(α) anthracene as tumor initiator. In the epidermis of the quercetin-treated mice, induction of ornithine decarboxylase (ODC) activity, but not DNA synthesis, by TPA was inhibited. Kato et al. also demonstrated potent inhibition by quercetin of lipoxygenase activity in the cytosol fraction of mouse epidermis (in vitro study). Based on these observations they assumed that the inhibitory effect of quercetin on lipoxygenase may be a major reason for the suppression of ODC activity and tumor formation in quercetin-treated mice. As described in the previous section, van der Hoeven et al.[30] found that 1) quercetin induced neither sister-chromatid exchanges nor point mutations in mammalian cells, and 2) quercetin induced TK-deficient mutants in mouse lymphoma L5178Y, with a clastogenic effect which was abolished by liver homogenate. The authors proposed that the above may be major reasons for the lack of carcinogenicity of quercetin.

3.4 Anti-inflammatory and Other Biological Effects

In 1936, Rusznyák and Szent-Györgyi published an article[53] entitled "Vitamin P: flavonols as vitamins." In a series of investigations, Szent-Györgyi and his colleagues[53-56] suggested that flavonoids present in the extracts of red pepper and lemon juice relieve increased capillary permeability and fragility of the capillary wall in scorbutic animals. They proposed the name vitamin P for the active principle. Since then, numerous studies have been conducted on the metabolism, biochemistry and pharmacology of the flavonoids. They have been comprehensively reported in reviews[57-59] and books.[1,60] This section deals with recent discoveries of pharmacological actions related to the biochemical activities and chemical structures of the flavonoids.

As can be seen in Table 3-1, many pharmacological activities of flavonoids have been demonstrated, both *in vivo* and *in vitro*. In the course of

Table 3-1. Pharmacological Activities of Flavonoids

Activities
Vitamin C sparing effect
Epinephrine sparing effect
Anti-inflammatory effect
Anti-anaphylactic effect
Anti-allergic effect
Anti-asthmatic effect
Coronary vasodilation
Anti-bacterial effect
Anti-viral effect
Anti-X-ray effect
Anti-neoplastic effect
Anti-mutagenic effect
Mutagenic effect

research conducted to elucidate the mechanisms of such pharmacological activities, a number of biochemical characteristics i.e. inhibitory actions on several enzymes (Table 3-2), have been discovered, although the exact relationships between the pharmacological and biochemical qualities are not yet known.

The chemical characteristics of flavonoids so far identified are 1) chelating actions with copper and other metal ions, and 2) potential reactivities with active oxygen species. The roles of chelation and reactions with active oxygen species have been demonstrated in several biochemical

Table 3-2. Inhibitory Actions of Flavonoids on Enzyme Activities *in vitro*.

Enzymes
Aldose reductase
Aldehyde reductase
ATPases
cAMP- and cGMP-phosphodiesterases
Prostaglandin cyclooxygenase
Prostaglandin and soybean lipoxygenases
Monooxygenase
NADPH-oxidase
Virus reverse transcriptase
RNA polymerase

phenomena described below. Present studies on the inhibitory actions of the flavonoids in certain enzyme systems suggest mimicry of adenine-nucleotide.

3.4.1 Chelating Action with Metals

In ultraviolet spectral analyses of flavonoids, Mabry et al.[2] utilised aluminum ion and correlated the positions of hydroxy groups in the flavonoid molecules and the changes in UV spectra by chelation with aluminum ion. Flavone and flavonols which possess a hydroxy group at position 3 in the pyrone ring or at position 5 of the A-ring form acid-stable complexes by chelation with aluminum ion. The flavonoids with an *o*-dihydroxy group in the A- or B-ring also chelate with aluminum ion, but the complexes formed are unstable under acidic conditions. Flavonoids also chelate with other transition metal ions.

It is known that rutin and quercetin increase the biological activities of ascorbic acid.[61] In neutral and basic solutions, L-ascorbic acid is rapidly oxidized to an unstable dehydroascorbic acid, followed by hydrolysis to diketogluconic acid of an inactive form of vitamin C. This oxidation is catalyzed by trace amounts of copper ion, or other heavy metal ions. Flavonoids such as quercetin, which possess 3-hydroxy and 4-keto groups in their pyrone ring, and a dihydroxy group at 3'- and 4'-positions of their B-ring, chelate with copper ions to prevent oxidation of ascorbic acid. Thus, the ascorbic acid sparing effects of these flavonoids are believed to be due to the chelating action with copper ion. Chelating action of flavonoids is also postulated to be responsible for their anti-viral activities.[62]

Metal ions which chelate with flavonoids prevent biological activities of the flavonoids. Middleton and Drzewiecki[63] reported prevention by Cu^{2+}, Co^{2+}, and Mn^{2+} ions of the inhibitory action of quercetin on antigen-induced basophil histamine release. Recently, Hatcher and Bryan[64] observed inhibition of quercetin mutagenicity in *Salmonella* cells by $MnCl_2$, $CuCl_2$, $FeSO_4$, and $FeCl_3$. Friedman and Smith[65] also reported inhibitory effects of heavy metals on quercetin mutagenicity in *Salmonella* cells. Interaction between flavonoids and metals may be important in biological systems.

3.4.2 Reactivity with Active Oxygen Species

Potential reactivities with active oxygen species are prominent characteristics of flavonoids. Lipid antioxidant properties of quercetin and certain flavonoids have been known for many years.[66,67] According to Letan,[68] the flavonoids structure of a conjugated chain composed of a B-ring and a 4-keto group on the pyrone ring is of primary importance, since the hydroxy groups at the 3'-and 4'-positions of the B-ring, particularly at 4'-hydroxy, play an important role in the antioxidant activities of the flavonoids.

In biological systems, phospholipids are the main constituents of cell membranes, and contain a large amount of polyunsaturated fatty acids as their components. Those polyunsaturated fatty acids are easily oxidized by active oxygen species, and lipid peroxy radicals are formed. Lipid peroxidation then proceeds as a chain reaction. Singlet oxygen and hydroxy radicals, both formed from superoxide radicals, are thought to be initiators of the peroxidation reaction. The antioxidant properties of flavonoids are believed to be due to their reactivity with free radicals participating in the peroxidation reaction.

Flavonoids react with superoxide radicals. Baumann *et al.*,[69] Salyvayre *et al.*[70] and Ueno *et al.*[71] demonstrated superoxide radical scavenging actions of flavonoids by measurements of a nitroblue tetrazolium reduction, chemiluminescence, and ESR spectrum of superoxide radical spin adduct, respectively. According to Ueno *et al.*,[71] quercetin was degraded by superoxide radicals generated in a xanthine-xanthine oxidase reaction, and the degradation of quercetin, as well as its autoxidation, was completely prevented in the presence of superoxide dismutase (SOD).

Quercetin is known to be degraded oxygenatively in a photosensitized reaction,[72] and in an enzymatic reaction catalyzed by a Cu^{2+}-containing dioxygenase, quercetinase.[73] In the former reaction, 3-hydroxyflavones are degraded to the corresponding depsides with formation of carbon monoxide and carbon dioxide.[72] Matsuura and his colleagues proposed the reaction mechanism shown in Fig. 3–4, involving singlet oxygen species. In the dioxygenase reaction, 2-protocatechuoyloxy-4, 6-dihydroxybenzoic acid and carbon monoxide are formed from quercetin, possibly through route A in the mechanism (Fig. 3–4).[72] 3-Hydroxyflavones without the 7-hydroxy group also produced depsides and carbon monoxide in a base-catalyzed reaction.[74] Thus flavonoids react with various active oxygen species. This prominent characteristic may be a major reason the diverse biological activities of flavonoids.

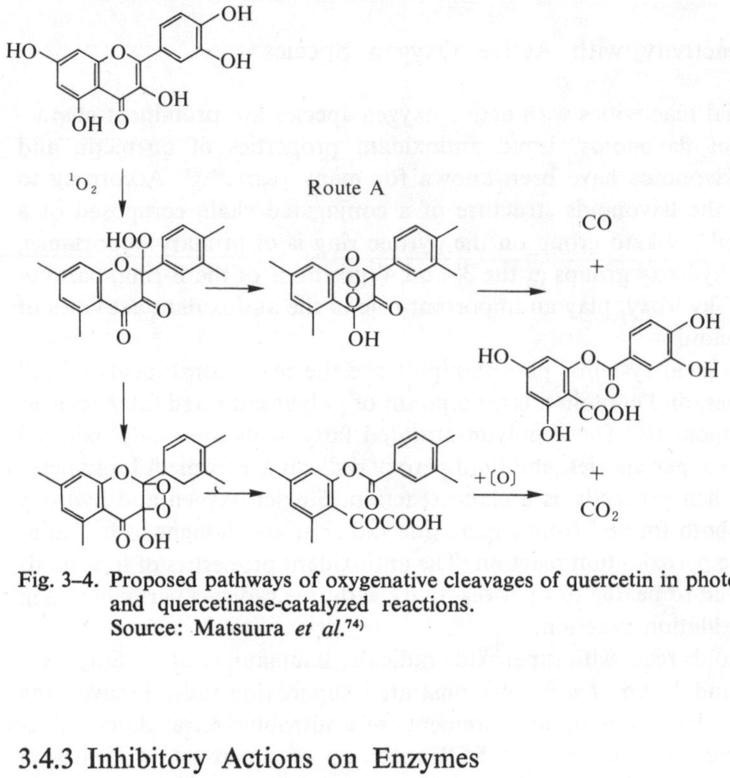

Fig. 3–4. Proposed pathways of oxygenative cleavages of quercetin in photosensitized and quercetinase-catalyzed reactions.
Source: Matsuura *et al.*[74]

3.4.3 Inhibitory Actions on Enzymes

Aldose reductase and aldehyde reductase in relation to anti-cataract reaction Lens aldose reductase is an enzyme that catalyzes the NADPH-dependent reduction of aldose to alditols. This enzyme is almost certainly involved in secondary complications of diabetes, such as cataracts,[75] neuropathy and angiopathy.[76] Certain flavonoids inhibit aldose reductase, resulting in delayed onset of cataracts in diabetic animals. According to Varma and colleagues,[76] quercitrin (8), myricetin (11), quercetin (1) and rutin (7) were strong inhibitors of aldose reductase partially purified from rat lenses. They also inhibited aldose reductase in intact rat lenses cultured in a medium with high xylose content. In *in vivo* experiments using galactosemic rodents *Octodon degus,* which develop cataracts rapidly, possibly because of high-aldose reductase activity in their lenses, Varma *et al.*[77] demonstrated that orally administered quercitrin suppresses significantly the accumulation of sorbitol and fructose; both are metabolites of the sorbitol pathway. Moreover, continuous administration of the flavonoid delayed the onset of cataracts in diabetic *O. degus.*

Flavonoids also inhibit human lens aldose reductase. Utilizing aldose reductase purified from human lenses, Chaudhry *et al.*[78] examined inhibitory actions of flavonoids, including glycosides and sulfate esters. They demonstrated that 3-*O*-acetyl-7,3',4'-trisulfate of quercetin is a potent inhibitor comparable to sorbinil. ID_{50} for the former flavonoid was 0.1 $\times$ 10^{-6} M, and that for sorbinil was 0.2 $\times$ 10^{-6} M in their test systems. They also demonstrated that glycosidation of the 3-hydroxy group with L-hexose potently intensifies the inhibitory action of aglycon, while glycosidation with glucose and galactose lowers it. The authors suggested that unsaturation of the chromone part together with a ketone group, and glycosidation with a L-sugar are necessary for greater efficiency in flavonoids. They also suggested the requirement of an electronegative group in the molecule for reaction with the center of the enzyme, which is assumed to be electrophilic.

To screen flavonoids which may be useful in the treatment of complications in diabetic patients, Okuda and colleagues[79] examined inhibitory activities of thirty-four flavonoids and thirteen coumarins on aldose reductase of rat and bovine lenses. Fourteen flavonoids showed inhibitory effects on rat and/or bovine enzymes at concentrations as low as 1 $\times 10^{-7}$ M in their test system. Axillarin (5,7,3',4'-tetrahydroxy-3,6-dimethoxyflavone) and 6,3',4'-trihydroxy-5,7,8-trimethoxyflavone were the most potent and noncompetitive inhibitors of the enzymes. For purified rat enzyme, ID_{50} of the former was 2.6 $\times$ 10^{-8} M, and that of the latter was 3.6 $\times$ 10^{-8} M. Their studies suggested that a free hydroxy group at position 7 of the A-ring is essential to the inhibitory actions, and that an *o*-dihydroxy group in the B-ring intensifies the inhibitory potency of flavonoids. Inhibitory activities of isoflavones and coumarins were at least one order of magnitude less than those of flavones. Thus, bioflavonoids showed inhibitory activity on lens aldose reductase in both humans and experimental animals; some flavonoids acted as inhibitors in diabetic cataracts.

Specific inhibitory actions by flavonoids on adenine-nucleotide-requiring enzymes have been suggested, leading Okuda *et al.*[79] to investigate inhibitory actions of axillarin and three other flavonoids on several adenine-nucleotide-requiring enzymes, including hexokinase, pyruvate kinase, lactate dehydrogenase, glucose-6-phosphate dehydrogenase, glutathione reductase, alcohol dehydrogenase and aldehyde reductase. Their results showed that only aldehyde reductase was significantly inhibited by these flavonoids, but the inhibitory activity on aldehyde reductase was one order of magnitude lower than that on aldose reductase. These results suggest the usefulness of these flavonoids as clinical drugs for treating complications in diabetes, particularly in view of their selective inhibition of aldose reductase.

To study the inhibitory actions of flavonoids on aldehyde reductase, Whittle and Thurner[80] utilized ox brain enzyme. All of the flavonoids tested (quercetin (1), morin (14), quercitrin (8), rutin (7), 7-hydroxy-ethylquercetin, and three hydroxyethyl derivatives of rutin) strongly inhibited aldehyde reductase. Quercetin, morin and quercitrin showed noncompetitive inhibition, and rutin and other flavonids showed mixed-type inhibition. Inhibitory activities of quercetin and morin were almost one hundred times greater than the activity of sodium valproate, a well-known anti-convulsant drug, and those of quercitrin and rutin and its derivatives were similar to the activity of valproate. Potency of 7-hydroxyquercetin was intermediate between quercetin and valproate. The authors suggested binding of these flavonoids to a hydrophobic region of the enzyme alongside a positively charged amino acid residue, or near or in the substrate binding site. Anti-convulsant drugs such as carbamazepine and phenacemide also inhibited aldehyde reductase. It is interesting to note that all tested flavonoids which inhibited reductase failed as anti-convulsants in the mouse maximal electro shock test. This is assumed to be due either to poor absorbability by the mucous membrane of the alimentary tract, or to inability to pass through the blood-brain barrier.

Glycolysis and ATPases   Quercetin (1), morin (14), fisetin, apigenin, but not kaempferol (9), rutin (7) and quercitrin (8), suppress the high aerobic glycolysis in Ehrlich ascites tumor cells and in rapidly growing fibroblast.[81] Flavonoids such as quercetin, also inhibit Na^+K^+-ATPase and mitochondrial ATPase,[82,83] without affecting ion transport or oxidative phosphorylation. According to Racker and his colleagues,[84] in normal cells ATPase-dependent ion pumps operate when ion flux pathways of cell membrane couple with the transport ATPase of the membranes. However, in some tumor cell lines, ion transport functions by uncoupling from the ATPases, resulting in high ATP consumption and a large concentration of ADP.[81,84] The latter support a high rate of glycolysis. Quercetin restores the efficiency of ATPase activity and suppresses glycolysis.[81] Quercetin also suppresses lactate trasnport, especially the excretion of lactate from ascites tumor cells.[85] Intracellular acidification caused by accumulated lactate is thought to be another mechanism of inhibitory action of the flavonoids on the enhanced glycolysis of tumor cells. Racker and his colleagues suggested that bioflavonoids with four or five hydroxy groups in their molecules are the most effective as inhibitors, and reduction of the 2,3-double bond and glycosidation of the 3-hydroxy group decrease their activities.

To explain the inhibitory mechanism of quercetin on Na^+K^+-ATPase, Kuriki and Racker[83] used enzymes purified from the electric organ of *Electrophorus electricus* (electric eel) and from lamb kidney. Quercetin bound reversibly to the enzyme. As a result, it interfered with the formation of ADP-insensitive phosphoenzymes from both inorganic phosphate and ADP-sensitive phosphoenzymes, and with the hydrolysis of ADP-insensitive phosphoenzymes. Lang and Racker[86] also suggested a similarity between the mechanism of the inhibitory action of quercetin and that of the mitochondrial protein inhibitor, which is assumed to block the "undesirable hydrolysis of ATP"[86] that is catalyzed by the coupling factor F_1, except inhibitory effect of quercetin on the ATP-dependent reduction of NAD^+ by succinate. Flavonoids also inhibit ATPases in *E. coli*,[87] chloroplasts,[88] and Ca^{2+}-ATPase of sarcoplasmic reticulum.[89]

Cyclic nucleotide phosphodiesterases Enhancement of cAMP level in Ehrlich ascites tumor cells by quercetin was first observed by Graziani and Chayoth in 1977.[90] Quercetin showed neither stimulatory effect on adenylate cyclase nor inhibition of hexose transport system in the cells.[91] In the following year, Beretz *et al.*[92] demonstrated inhibitory actions of quercetin and other bioflavonoids shown in Table 3–3 on beef heart cAMP phosphodiesterase, which is involved in the regulation of the cAMP level by degradation of 5'-AMP. After their findings, various kinds of flavonoid have been demonstrated as inhibitors of cAMP phosphodiesterases. Some of them are shown in Table 3–3. Although enzyme sources and experimental conditions are different in each experiment, amentoflavone, a biflavonoid, seems to be the most potent inhibitor among the flavonoids so far examined. Inhibitory potencies of amentoflavone were more than forty times greater than the potency of papaverine to beef heart phosphodiesterase, and more than five times greater to bovine lung enzyme. Inhibitory activities of biflavonoids on cAMP phosphodiesterase are greater than those of monoflavonoids.[93] However, the activities of the biflavonoids depend greatly on the nature of the bond linkage between units of the biflavonoids. For example, inhibitory potency of amentoflavone, (I-3', II-8) biapigenin, was several times greater than that of the apigenin monomer (5,7,4'-trihydroxyflavone). Biapigenins such as cupressuflavone (I-8, II-9), robstaflavone (I-3', II-6), hinokiflavone (I-4'-O, II-6) and agathiflavone (I-6, II-8) have intermediate inhibitory potency. The authors suggested the importance of the stereochemistry of the molecules in their interactions with the enzyme.

According to Nikaido *et al.*,[94] polymethoxyflavonoids were generallv more potent than the polyhydroxyflavonoids. Inhibitory activity of irisflorentin (5,3',4',5'-tetramethoxy-6,7-methylenedioxy-isoflavone, ID_{50}: 0.4 μM) was almost one order of magnitude greater than that of papaverine

Table 3-3. Inhibitory Effects of Flavonoids and Related Compounds on Prostaglandin Cyclooxygenase and Lipoxygenase and on Cyclic AMP and Cyclic GMP Phospnodiesterases

Flavonoids and related compounds		Cyclo-oxygenase[a]	Lipoxy-genase[b]	Inhibitory effects on cAMP PDE[c]				cGMP PDE[c]
Skeleton	Name			Liver fluke[d]	Rat heart[e]	Beef heart f) g)	Bovine lung[h]	Bovine lung[h]
Flavone	Flavone	88	+	80				
	Chrysin	80	+	75				
	Apigenin	63	+			9.2	53	35
	Galangin					8.6		
	Luteolin				4.3	8.7	19	19
	Fisetin			65		36		
	Kaempferol	59	20	85	5.2	2.7 206	18	23
	Morin	20	23	70			44	30
	Quercetin	97 19[i]	97 88[i]	90	5.5	3.6 317	23	15
	Robinetin			70				
	Myricetin	95 0[i]	97 68[i]	70				
	Ramnetin			80		8.3		
	Nobiletin					32	0.32	
	Cirsilineol					32		
	Pentamethyl-quercetin				7.1	129		
	Pentaacetyl-quercetin			100				
	Rutin	0	0	7.2				
	Quercitrin	19	88	75	100			
	Amentoflavone					0.12	0.66	0.54
	Sciadopitysin					42		
	Cupressflavone					4.9		
	Robstaflavone					4		
	Hinokiflavone					3.2		
	Agathisflavone					1		
	Rhusflavone					1		
Flavanone	Flavanone	66	+	55				
	Naringenin	0	0	50		45		
	Fustin			0				
	Eriodictyol						48	33

a) %Inhibition of the formation of TBX_2 from arachidonic acid of thrombin aggregated human platelets, at 50 μM of the flavonoids and related compounds. (Ref. 129)

b) %Inhibition of the formation of 12-HETE from arachidonic acid of thrombin aggregated human platelets, at 50 μM of the test compounds. (Ref. 129) +; acceleration.

c) Phosphodiesterase

d) %Inhibition at 100 μM of the test compounds. (Ref. 95)

e) ID_{50} (μM) (Ref. 96)

f) ID_{50} (μM) (Refs. 88, 92, 93)

g) ID_{50} (μM) (Ref. 94)

h) ID_{50} (μM) (Refs. 97, 98)

i) %Inhibition at 10 μM.

Table 3–3.——*Continued*

Flavonoids and related compounds		Inhibitory effects on cAMP PDE[c]						cGMP PDE[c]
Skeleton	Name	Cyclo-oxygenase[a]	Lipoxy-genase[b]	Liver fluke[d]	Rat heart[e]	Beef heart f) g)	Bovine lung[h]	Bovine lung[h]
	Hesperetin	15	+			26		
	Naringin	0	0	10				
	Hesperidin	2	0					
	(+)-Dihydro-quercetin					94	320	170
	Dihydrofisetin					320		
Isoflavone	Irisflorentin					4		
	Irigenin					11		
Catechin	(−) Catechin					300	630	300
	(+) Catechin					500	640	170
Chromone	Isoluteolin			55			42	54
	Khellin			55			125	320
	Xanthone			70			70	20
Anthraqui-none	Emodin						16	16
Others	Coumarin			5				
	Pyrone			0				
	Papaverine					5 30	5	11

(ID$_{50}$:30 μM). Nobiletin (5,6,7,8,3',4'-hexamethoxyflavone) and irigenin (5,7,3'-trihydroxy-6,4',5'-trimethoxyisoflavone) both recently isolated from peels of *Citrus reticulata* and from rhizomes of *Iris florentina* respectively, were also potent inhibitors of beef heart cAMP phosphodiesterase.[94] Inhibitory potency of irigenin was greater than the potency of papaverine and that of nobiletin was similar to that of papaverine. As for the structure-activity relationships, Beretz *et al.*[92] suggested that hydroxy groups at the 3,5,7 and 4'-positions and the 2,3-double bond are necessary for the activity. Ferrell and his colleagues[95] extensively studies correlation between chemical structures and inhibitory activities of a total of 45 compounds including flavonoids and related compounds utilizing liver fluke cyclic nucleotide phosphodiesterase. Some of the results are shown in Table 3–3. They suggested the importance of the planarity of the heterocyclic ring of the flavonoids, rather than exocyclic substituents, to the basic flavonoid skeleton for the inhibitory activities of the flavonoids. They also suggested that inhibitory action of quercetin was competitive with cAMP for the adenine-nucleotide binding site, because the pyranone ring of the flavonoid mimics the pyrimidine ring of cAMP.

Flavonoids also inhibit the activity of cGMP phosphodiesterase.[97] Ruckstuhl and Landry[98] indicated that chromone-like compounds, including flavonoids, are potent inhibitors of the cGMP and cAMP-phosphodiesterases of bovine lung, with greater activities against the former enzyme.

The highest activity was found in amentoflavone, which was five to ten times greater than that of papaverine, and more than sixty times greater than that of apigenin.

For many years, anti-anaphylactic actions of flavonoids, mainly rutin, have been reported in guinea pig.[99] The anti-anaphylactic action of rutin was thought to be due to the prevention of endogenous histamine release.[100] At present it is believed that anaphylactic reaction is initiated by the binding of polyvalent antigens to IgE antibodies which attach to the Fc receptors on the surface of the mast cells and basophils. This causes degranulation with liberation of various chemical mediators and/or modulators of anaphylactic reactions through a complex mechanism similar to that of inflammation. These sequential reactions are regulated by the intracellular levels of cAMP and cGMP. Inhibitory actions of certain flavonoids on the cyclic nucleotide phosphodiesterases and on the membrane transport-associated ATPases have been demonstrated, as described above. Therefore, it is most plausible that the inhibitory actions of the flavonoids on the phosphodiesterases and ATPases are related to the anti-anaphylactic actions of the flavonoids through enhancing the intracellular levels of cAMP and cGMP. In this regard, Rucksthul and Landry[98] suggested interactions between anti-anaphylactic properties of chromone-like compounds and their inhibition of the phosphodiesterases.

3.4.4 Anti-inflammatory Effect and Arachidonate Cascade

Inflammation is a biological process of self-defense which occurs locally at the damaged site against trauma by, for example, chemical and mechanical agents, irradiation, and heat stimulants. Pathologically, the following symptomatic sequence occurs: Congestion, that is dilatation of blood vessels of the microcirculatory system surrounding the damaged area; increase of permeability of the microcirculatory system, together with exudation of the blood plasma into intercellular spaces, leading to swelling of the inflamed area; migration of leucocytes to the damaged site, its adherence to the endothelium of the blood vessels, and invasion of the blood cells, first neutrophils and macrophages, and later lymphocytes and plasma cells, together with macrophages. Usually, secondary tissue damage occurs because of the proteolytic enzymes liberated from granules of mast cells and blood cells, and by active oxygen species produced by the phagocytic cells. Although inflammation reactions occur as defense against harmful stimuli, they occasionally have serious side effects such as severe pain and high fever. In order to relieve the pain and fever, various kinds of anti-inflammatory drugs, i.e. steroidal and non-steroidal agents, have been developed for clinical use.

For many years, anti-inflammatory actions of flavonoids, mainly rutin and its derivatives, have been demonstrated in the inhibitory actions of paw edema, changes of blood capillary endothelia, and capillary permeability, skin test, leucocyte exudation and migration, and other test systems in mice and rats. Gábor reviewed these reports,[59] and he also confirmed the anti-inflammatory effect of O-(β-hydroxyethyl) rutin by utilizing parameters of chromate ion transport of red blood cells, red paprika-induced decrease of capillary resistance and other parameters.

Inflammation proceeds through reactions induced by locally generated vasoactive agents and chemotactic factors. In recent studies on prostaglandins, the role of the arachidonate metabolites in the inflammation process has been disclosed.[101-104] Various substances that have been proposed as chemical mediators and/or modulators are thought to be produced in cells including mast cells, polymorphonuclear leucocytes (PMNL), platelets, macrophages, and endothelial cells through the following process: Inflammatory stimuli activate intracellular phospholipase A_2 which catalyzes the formation of arachidonic acid in conjunction with the initiation of the formation of PAF (platelet aggregation factor, 1-alkyl-1-acetyl-sn-glyceryl-3-phosphorylcholine),[105,106] from cell membrane phospholipid. Then, cyclooxygenase and lipoxygenase catalyze production of prostaglandins (PGs) and leukotrienes (LTs) from arachidonic acid, respectively. Thromboxanes (TXs) are produced from PG. Histamine, serotonin, bradykinin and enzymes such as proteases are also released from the stimulated cells. Among the metabolites of arachidonate cascade, PGI_2, PGE_2, LTC_4 and LTD_4 are known as potent vasoactive agents,[107-114] and hydroxyeicosatetraenoic acids (HETEs) and hydroperoxyeicosatetraenoic acid (HPETEs), LTB_4, TXA_2 and TXB_2 are known to be chemotactic agents for leucocytes.[115-118]

Based on these biochemical results, a substance that suppresses the metabolic activities of the pathways of arachidonate cascade and PAF formation would be the most suitable therapeutic anti-inflammatory agent. It stands to reason that steroidal anti-inflammatory drugs suppress the production of metabolites of the arachidonate cascade by inhibiting phospholipase A_2 through the formation of inhibitory proteins.[119-122]

Anti-inflammatory actions of flavonoids are now being researched at the cellular level, and evidence is accumulating that flavonoids inhibit enzymes which are involved in the arachidonate cascade and related reactions. Quercetin and certain other flavonoids inhibit ragweed antigen-[89] and concanavalin A (Con A)-induced[123] histamine release from rat mast cells. Quercetin also greatly affects the functions of PMNL. Quercetin inhibits the antigen-induced histamine release from human basophils,[124] and N-formylmethionylleucylphenylalanine-stimulated β-

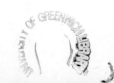

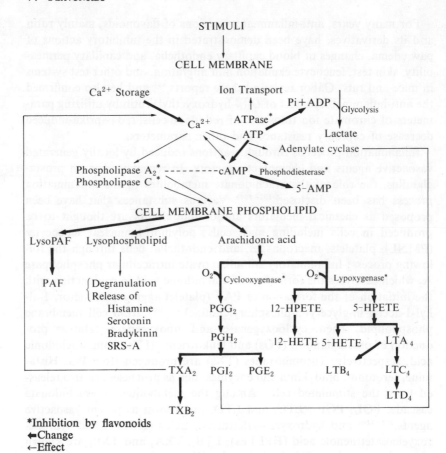

*Inhibition by flavonoids
←Change
←Effect

Fig. 3–5. Inhibitory sites of flavonoids in the pathways of energy metabolism, cyclic nucleotide metabolism and arachidonate cascade.

glucuronidase secretion from rabbit neutrophils.[123] According to Schneider et al.,[125] quercetin inhibited the con A-induced stimulation of cell respiration, lysozyme release and casein-gradient-induced chemotaxis of PMNL. Further, quercetin itself exhibited positive chemokinetic effects and chemotactic activity. Rutin showed no effect. Quercetin binding to the cells was reversible and neither viability nor oxidase activity of the cells was impaired by quercetin. They assumed that interaction between quercetin and the hydrophobic portions of the cell membrane activates cell motility, while in the presence of potential stimulants quercetin activates another reaction which suppresses the sensitivity of the cells to stimuli. For a possible explanation, they proposed participation of Ca^{2+}-dependent ion pump. However, according to Bennet *et al.*,[123] no correlation between the inhibition of secretory function and the inhibition of Ca^{2+}-ATPase, both caused by quercetin, was observed. Quercetin inhibits both the release of β-glucuronidase and arachidonic acid from human PMNL stimulated by zymosan-activated serum.[126] Activation of phospholipase A_2 is believed to be a biochemical mechanism associated with the activation of PMNL functions. Therefore, Lee *et al.*[126] proposed that the inhibitory effect of quercetin on phospholipase A_2 might be responsible for the inhibition of PMNL functions. Quercetin inhibits respiration of leucocytes activated by con A, phospholipase C, myristic acid, or antibiotic Br-X537A. However, inhibitory potency of the flavonoid was dependent on the stimulants utilized. Respiration induced by con A was highly sensitive to quercetin, while the flavonoid showed only a small effect on respiration induced by myristic acid of antibiotics. Further, quercetin added after onset of the stimulation exhibited inhibitory activity. Based on these results, Berton *et al.*[127] postulated as follows: PMNL-stimulants can be divided into two groups. Agents that belong to the first group interact with external cell surface receptors, and those of the second group interact with the hydrophobic core within the membrane. Quercetin inhibits the cell activation induced by the stimulants of the first group at the stage where the stimulants inducing morphological changes of the membrane constituents are translated into signals such as changes of ion permeability. Long *et al.*[128] observed inhibitory effect of quercetin on opsonized zymosan or phorbol myristate acetate-stimulated respiratory burst in conjunction with inhibition of Mg^{2+}-ATPase in human PMNL. Transport of non-metabolizable deoxyglucose was also inhibited. Based on their results they also proposed a generalized effect of quercetin on the membrane of PMNL. According to Middleton and Drzewiecki,[63] flavone derivatives with a 4'-hydroxy or 3'- and 4'-dihydroxy group in the B-ring, and a couplet of 4-keto and 5-hydroxy groups, are the most active inhibitors of histamine release from human basophils.

The importance of the role played by platelets in inflammatory and allergic reactions is now being recognized. According to Landolfi *et al.*[129] flavone, chrysin, apigenin, flavanone and phloretin inhibited both arachidonic acid- and collagen-induced platelet aggregation in conjunction with selective inhibition of cyclooxygenase of the platelets. Quercetin and myricetin inhibited only arachidonic acid-induced aggregation, and at a low concentration, they inhibited lipoxygenase exclusively. In the sequental study conducted by the same group, Mower *et al.*[130] concluded that inhibition of the platelet aggregation by flavone is attributable to its effect on cyclooxygenase. Both Landolfi *et al.*[129] and Beretz *et al.*[131]

assumed participation of cAMP in the inhibitory action of quercetin on platelet aggregation.

Inhibitory actions of other flavonoids on the enzyme systems that are involved in the arachidonate cascade have also been demonstrated. Baicalein inhibited activities of both lipoxygenase and cyclooxygenase of rat platelets.[132] The sensitivity of lipoxygenase to baicalein (ID_{50}: 0.12 μM) was much higher that of cyclo oxygenase (ID_{50} :0.83mM). Cirsiliol (5,3′,4′-trihydroxy-6,7-dimethoxyflavone, ID_{50}: *ca.* 0.1 μM) and pedalitin are potent inhibitors of 5-lipoxygenase of rat basophilic leukemia cells.[133] They also inhibited 12-lipoxygenase from bovine platelets and porcine leucocytes, but inhibitory activities are less than those on 5-lipoxygenase. Cirsiliol and pedalitin inhibited production of SRS-A in lung preparation obtained from passively sensitized guinea pig. Inhibitory activities of these flavonoids are much higher than those of quercetin and baicalein. Eupatilin (5,7-dihydroxy-6,3′,4′-trimethoxyflavone) and 4′-demethyleupatilin, both isolated from *Artemisia rubripes* a Chinese medicinal plant, selectively inhibited 5-lipoxygenase in cultured mastocytoma.[134] There is no significant effect on cyclooxygenase activity at the inhibitory concentration on lipoxygenase. In addition, eupatilin inhibited production of SRS-A in

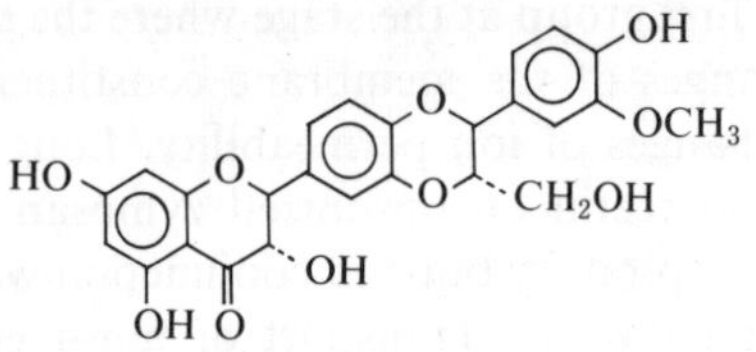

silybin

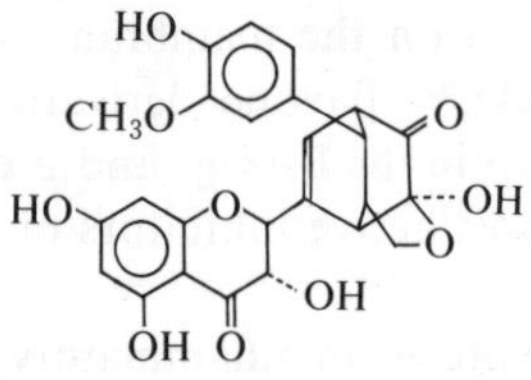

silydianin

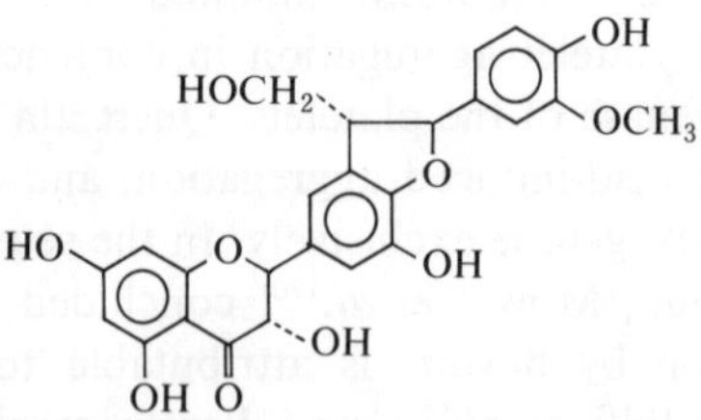

silychristin

Fig. 3–6. Structure of silybin, silydianin and silychristin.

mast tumor cells. Silymarin, an anti-hepatotoxic principle of the fruit of the milk thistle, is a complex of three flavonoids, silybin, silydianin and silychristin (Fig. 3–6). All of these flavonoids inhibit both lipoxygenase of soybean[135] and prostaglandin synthetase in the fundus of the rat stomach.[136]

Dried roots of *Scutellaria barcalensis,* a Chinese medicinal plant, is known as an effective drug for inflammatory disease. Recently, the principles of this root were identified as flavonoids: (2*S*)-5,7,2′6′-tetrahydroxy-flavanone and (2R, 3R)-3,5,7,2′,6′-pentahydroxyflavanone.[137] These flavonoids inhibited rat liver lipid peroxidation induced by ADP-NADH system, while lipid peroxidation induced by Fe^{2+}-ascorbic acid system was inhibited only by the latter flavonoid.

Recently, nepitrin (5,3′,4′-trihydroxy-6-methoxyflavone), a principle of *Nepta hindostana,* was introduced as a useful anti-inflammatory and anti-arthritic agent because it prevents various phases of inflammation with minor toxicity.[138] The anti-inflammatory action of nepitrin is assumed to be due to the anti-bradykinin and anti-angiotensin actions of the flavonoid.

As described above, quercetin and other flavonoids inhibit the activities of enzymes that play important roles in (1) energy metabolism that relates to the cell membrane transport-associated ATPase systems, (2) regulation of the cAMP and cGMP levels, and (3) arachidonate cascade, in which various kinds of chemical mediators and/or modulators of inflammation and allergy reactions are produced. Therefore, if the flavonoids truly participate in the regulation of these important reactions *in vivo* systems, their pharmacological effects such as anti-inflammation and anti-anaphylactic actions may be explained by these *in vitro* activities.

3.4.5 Anti-viral Activity

Anti-viral activities of flavonoids were first reported by Cutting *et al.*[139,140] in 1949. Quercitrin and related flavonoids were significantly prophylactic in mice, guinea pigs and rabbits infected with rabies or ectromelia viruses. For such prophylactic activities, the complete structure of the flavonoids was deemed to be necessary. It was also suggested that the nature of the sugars bound to the flavonoid aglycon is important.

Later, Apple *et al.*[141] reported that certain flavonoids with a 3-hydroxy group in their structures were potent inhibitors of viral reverse transcriptase and RNA polymerase *in vitro*. They also reported that flavonols and flavanols, which are potent inhibitors of reverse transcriptase *in vitro*, suppress incidence of RSV-induced sarcoma in chicks, while flavonols and catechins which significantly inhibited RNA polymerase *in vitro* inhibited leukemia growth in mice. According to Beladi *et al.*,[142] flavonoids such as quercetin, morin, fisetin and luteolin were anti-viral on enveloped viruses. Two hydroxy groups at the 3' and 4', and the 2' and 4' positions of the B-ring are required for anti-viral activities.

3.4.6 Miscellaneous Activities

Certain flavonoids are mutagenic in bacterial and tissue cultured mammalian cell lines, as described in section 3.2. However, flavonoids also show anti-mutagenic,[143] and anti-tumorigenic[144] activities. Biochemically, activation and inhibition of carcinogen metabolisms by flavonoids in human liver microsomes *in vitro*,[145] immediate activation of a total body metabolism of zoxazolamine by flavone in neonatal rats,[146] and induction of differentiation-associated properties such as hemoglobin synthesis in mouse leukemia B8 cells by apigenin and kaempferol[147] have recently been reported.

REFERENCES

1. Harborne, J.B., Mabry, T.J., and Mabry, H., *The Flavonoids*, Chapman & Hall, London 1975.
2. Mabry, T.J., Markham, K.R., and Thomas, M.B., *The Systematic Identification of Flavonoids*, Springer, Heidelberg 1970.
3. Harborne, J.B., and Mabry, T.J., *The Flavonoids, Advances in Research*, Chapman & Hall, London 1982.
4. Mann, J., in: *Secondary Metabolism*, pp. 252–261, Clarendon Press, Oxford 1978.
5. Swain, T., Evolution of flavonoid compounds. in: *The Flavonoids* (eds. Harborne, J.B., Mabry, T.J., and Mabry, H.), pp. 1096–11209, Chapman & Hall, London 1975.
6. Brown, J.P., A review of the genetic effects of naturally occurring flavonoids, anthraquinones and related compounds, *Mut. Res.*, 75: 243–277, 1980.
7. Herrmann, K., Flavonols and Flavones in Food Plants: A Review. *J. Fd. Technol.*, 11: 433–448, 1976.
8. Bilyk, A., and Sapers, G.M., Distribution of quercetin and kaempferol in lettuce, kale, chive, garlic chive, leek, horseradish, red radish, and red cabbage tissues, *J. Agric. Food Chem.*, 33: 226–228, 1985.
9. Torsell, K.B.G., in: *Natural Product Chemistry*, pp. 138–145, John Wiley & Sons, Chichester, 1983.
10. Wang, C.Y., Pamukcu, A.M., and Bryan, G.T., Bracken fern as naturally occurring carinogens, in: *Ecological Perspectives on Carcinogens and Cancer Control. Medicine Biologie Environment*, 4: 565–572, 1976.

11. Bjeldanes, L.F., and Chang, G.W., Mutagenic activity of quercetin and related compounds, *Science*, **197**: 577–578, 1977.
12. Brown, J.P., Dietrich, P.S., and Brown, R.J., Frameshift mutagenicity of certain naturally occurring phenolic compounds in the '*Salmonella*/microsome' test: activation of anthraquinone and flavonol glycosides by gut bacterial enzymes, *Biochem. Soc. Trans.*, 1489–1492, **1977**.
13. Fukuoka, M., Kuroyanagi, M., Yoshihira, K., Natori, S., Nagao, M., Takahashi, Y., and Sugimura, T., Chemical and toxicological studies on bracken fern, *Pteridium Aquilinum* var. *latiusculum*. IV. Surveys on bracken constituents by mutagen test, *J. Pharmacobio-Dyn.*, **1**: 324–331, 1978.
14. Sugimura, T., Nagao, M., Matsushima, T., Yahagi, T., Seino, Y. Shirai, A., Sawamura, M., Natori, S., Yoshihira, K., Fukuoka, M., and Kuroyanagi, M., Mutagenicity of flavone derivatives, *Proc. Japan Acad.*, **53**: Ser. B 194–197, 1977.
15. Hardigree, A.A., and Epler, J.L., Comparative mutagenesis of plant flavonoids in microbial systems, *Mut. Res.*, **58**: 231–239, 1978.
16. MacGregor, J.T., and Jurd, L., Mutagenicity of plant flavonoids: structural requirements for mutagenic activity in *Salmonella typhimurium*. *Mut. Res.*, **54**: 297–309, 1978.
17. Brown, J., and Dietrich, P.S., Mutagenicity of plant flavonols in the *Salmonella*/mammalian microsome test, activation of flavonol glycosides by mixed glycosidases from rat cecal bacteria and other sources, *Mut. Res.*, **66**: 223–240, 1979.
18. Nagao, M., Morita, N., Yahagi, T., Shimizu, M., Kuroyanagi, M., Fukuoka, M., Yoshihira, K., Natori, S., Fujino, T., and Sugimura, T., Mutagenicities of 61 flavonoids and 11 related compounds, *Environmental Mutagenesis*, **3**: 401–419, 1981.
19. Seino, Y., Nagao, M., Yahagi, T., Sugimura, T., Yasuda, T., and Nishimura, S., Identification of a mutagenic substance in a spice, sumac, as quercetin. *Mut. Res.*, **58**: 225–229, 1978.
20. Takahashi, Y., Nagao, M., Fujino, T., Yamaizumi, Z., and Sugimura, T., Mutagens in Japanese pickle identified as flavonoids, *Mut. Res.*, **68**: 117–123, 1979.
21. Fukuoka, M., Yoshihira, K., Natori, S., Sakamoto, K., Iwahara, S., Hosaka, S., and Hirono, I., Characterization of mutagenic principles and carcinogenicity test of dill weed and seeds, *J. Pharm. Dyn.*, **3**: 236–244, 1980.
22. Uyeta, M., Taue, S., and Mazaki, M., Mutagenicity of hydrolysates of tea infusions, *Mut. Res.*, **88**: 233–240, 1981.
23. Umezawa, K., Matsushima, T., Sugimura, T., Hirakawa, T., Tanaka, M., Katoh, Y., and Takayama, S., *In vitro* transformation of hamster embryo cells by quercetin, *Toxicol. Lett.*, **1**: 175–178, 1977.
24. Maruta, A., Enaka, K., and Umeda, M., Mutagenicity of quercetin and kaempferol on cultured mammalian cells, *Gann*, **70**: 273–276, 1979.
25. Yoshida, M., Sasaki, M., Sugimura, K., and Kawachi, T., Cytogenetic effects of quercetin on cultured mammalian cells, *Pro. Japan Acad.*, **56**: Ser B 433–447, 1980.
26. Sahu, R.K., Basu, R., and Sharma, A., Genetic toxicological testing of some plant flavonoids by the micronucleus test, *Mut. Res.*, **89**: 69–74, 1981.
27. Meltz, M.L., and MacGregor, J.T., Activity of the plant flavonol quercetin in the mouse lymphoma L5178Y TK$^{+/-}$ mutation, DNA single-strand break, and Balb/c 3T3 chemical transformation assays, *Mut. Res.*, **88**: 317–324, 1981.
28. Watson, W.A.F., The mutagenic activity of quercetin and kaempferol in *Drosophila melanogaster*. *Mut. Res.*, **103**: 145–147, 1982.
29. Carver, J.H., Carrano, A.V., and MacGregor, J.T., Genetic effects of the flavonols quercetin, kaempferol, and galangin on Chinese hamster ovary cells *in vitro*. *Mut. Res.*, **113**: 45–60, 1983.
30. Hoeven, J.C.M., Bruggeman, I.M., and Debets, F.M.H., Genotoxicity of quercetin in cultured mammalian cells, *Mut. Res.*, **136**: 9–21, 1984.
31. Gottlieb, O.R., Flavonols, in: *The Flavonoids* (eds. Harborne, J.B., Mabry, T.J., and Mabry, H., pp. 296–375, Chapman & Hall, London; **1975**.
32. Loth, H., and Diedrich, H., Chinone von Flavon und Flavonolderivaten, *Tetrahedr*

on Lett., 715–718, **1968** (in German).

33. Ochiai M., Nagao, M., Wakabayashi, K., and Sugimura, T., Superoxide dismutase acts as an enhancing factor for quercetin mutagenesis in rat-liver cytosol by preventing its decomposition, *Mut. Res.*, **129**: 19–24, 1984.

34. Ueno. I., Haraikama, K., Kohno, M. Hinomoto, T., Ohya-Nishiguchi, H., Tomatsuri, T., and Yoshihira, K., Possible involvement of superoxide dismutase in the mutagencity of quercetin in Salmonella typhimurim strain TA98. in: Plant flanonoids in biology and medicine. (eds. V. Cody, E. Middleton, Fr. and J.B. Harborne) pp. 425–428, Alan R. Liss, Inc. New York. 1986.

35. Elliger, C.A., Henika, P.R., and MacGregor, J.T., Mutagenicity of flavones, chromones and acetophenones in *Salmonella typhimurium*: New structure-activity relationships, *Mut. Res.*, **135**: 77–86, 1984.

36. Ambrose, A.M., Robbins, D.J., and DeEds, F., Comparative toxicities of quercetin and quercitrin, *J. Am. Pharm. Assoc.*, **41**: 119–122, 1952.

37. Pamukcu, A.M., Göksoy, S.K., and Price, J.M., Urinary bladder neoplasms induced by feeding bracken fern (*Pteris aquilina*) to cows, Cancer Res., **27**: 917–924, 1967.

38. Price, J.M., and Pamukcu, A.M., The induction of neoplasms of the urinary bladder of the cow and the small intestine of the rat by feeding bracken fern (*Pteris aquilina*). *Cancer Res.*, **28**: 2247–2251, 1968.

39. Pamukcu, A.M., Price, J.M., Induction of intestinal and urinary bladder cancer in rats by feeding bracken fern (*Pteris aquilina*). *J. Natl. Cancer Inst.*, **43**: 275–281, 1969.

40. Wang, C.Y., Pamukcu, A.M., and Bryan, G.T., Isolation of fumaric acid, succinic acid, astragalin, isoquercitrin and tiliroside from *Pteridium aquilinum*. *Phytochemistry*, **12**: 2298–2299, 1973.

41. Wang, C.Y., Chiu, C.W., Pamukcu, A.M., and Bryan, G.T., Identification of carcinogenic tannin isolated from bracken fern (*Pteridium aquilinum*). *J. Natl. Cancer Inst.*, **56**: 33–36, 1976.

42. Pamukcu, A.M., Wang, C.Y., Hatcher, J., and Bryan, G.T., Carcinogenicity of tannin and tannin-free extracts of bracken fern (*Pteridium aquilinum*) in rats. *J. Natl. Cancer. Inst.*, **65**: 131–136, 1980.

43. Pamukcu, A.M., Yalciner, S., Hatcher, J.H., and Bryan, G.T., Quercetin, a rat intestinal and bladder carcinogen present in bracken fern (*Pteridium aquilinum*). *Cancer Res.*, **40**: 3468–3472, 1980.

44. Hirono, I., Yamada, K., Niwa, H., Shizuri, Y., Ojika, M., Hosaka, S., Yamaji, T., Wakamatsu, K., Kigoshi, H., Niiyama, K., and Uosaki, Y., Separation of carcinogenic fraction of bracken fern. *Cancer Lett.*, **21**: 239–246, 1984.

45. Hirono, I., Aiso, S., Yamaji, T., Mori, H., Yamada, K., Niwa, H., Ojika, M., Wakamatsu, K., Kigoshi, H., Niiyama, K., and Uosaki, Y., Carcinogenicity in rats of ptaquiloside isolated from bracken. *Gann*, **75**: 833–836, 1984.

46. Erturk, E., Hatcher, J.F., Nunoya, T., Pamukcu, A.M., and Bryan, G.T., Hepatic tumors in Sprague-Dawley (SD) and Fischer 344 (F) female rats chronically exposed to quercetin or its glycoside rutin (R). *Proc. Am. Assoc. Cancer Res.*, **25**: 95, 1984.

47. Saito, D., Shirai, A., Matsushima, T., Sugimura, T., and Hirono, I., Test of carcinogenicity of quercetin, a widely distributed mutagen in food. *Teratogenesis, Carcinogenesis, and Mutagenesis*, **1**: 213–221, 1980.

48. Hirono, I., Ueno, I., Hosaka, S., Takanashi, H., Matsushima, T., Sugimura, T., and Natori, S., Carcinogenicity examination of quercetin and rutin in ACI rats. *Cancer Lett.*, **13**: 15–21, 1981.

49. Takanashi, H., Aiso, O., and Hirono, I., Carcinogenicity test of quercetin and kaempferol in rats by oral administration. *J. Food Safety*, **5**: 55–60, 1983.

50. Hosaka, S., Hirono, I., Carcinogenicity test of quercetin by pulmonary-adenoma bioassay in strain A mice. *Gann*, **72**: 327–328, 1981.

51. Morino, K., Matsukura, N., Kawachi, T., Ohgaki, H., Sugimura, T., and Hirono,

I., Carcinogenicity test of quercetin and rutin in golden hamsters by oral administration. *Carcinogenesis*, **3**: 93–97, 1982.

52. Kato, R., Nakadate, T., Yamamtoto, S., and Sugimura, T., Inhibition of 12-*O*-tetradecanoylphorbol-13-acetate-induced tumor promotion and ornithine decarboxylase activity by quercetin: Possible involvement of lipoxygenase inhibition. *Carcinogenesis*, **4**: 1301–1305, 1983.

53. Rusznyák, S., Szent-Györgyi, A., Vitamin P: Flavonols as vitamins. *Nature*, **138**: 27, 1936.

54. Almentano, von, L., Bentasáth, A., Béres, T., Rusznyák, S., and Szent-Györgyi, A., Über den Einfluss von Substanzen der Flavongruppe auf die Permeabilität der Kapilláren. Vitamin P. *Deutsche Medizinische Wochenshrift*, **62**: 1325–1328, 1936 (in German).

55. Bentsáth, A., Rusznyák, S., and Szent-Györgyi, A., Vitamin nature of flavones. *Nature*, **138**: 798, 1936.

56. Bruckner, V., and Szent-Györgyi, A., Chemical nature of citrin. *Nature*, **138**: 1057, 1936.

57. Willaman, J.J., Some biological effects of the flavonoids. *J. Am. Pharmac. Assoc.*, **44**: 404–408, 1955.

58. DeEds, F., Flavonoid metabolism. *Comp. Biochem.*, **20**: 127–170, 1968.

59. Gábor, M., The anti-inflammatory action of flavonoids. *Akademiai Kiado. Budapest*, **1972**.

60. Scheline, R.R., *Mammalian Metabolism of Plant Xenobiotics*. Academic Press, London, **1978**.

61. Clementson, C.A.B., and Andersen, L., Plant polyphenols as antioxidants for ascorbic acid. *Ann. N.Y. Acad. Sci.*, **136**: 339–376, 1966.

62. Perrin, D.D., and Stünzi, H., Viral chemotherapy: Antiviral actions of metal ions and metal-chelating agents. *Pharmacol. Ther.*, **12**: 255–297, 1981.

63. Middleton, E. Jr., and Drzewiecki, G. Effects of flavonoids and transitional metal cations on antigen-induced histamine release from human basophils. *Biochem. Pharmacol.*, **31**: 1449–1453, 1982.

64. Hatcher, J.F., and Bryan, G.T., Factors affecting the mutagenic activity of quercetin for *Salmonella typhimurium* TA98: Metal ions, antioxidants and pH. *Mut. Res.*, **148**: 13–23, 1985.

65. Friedman, M., and Smith, G.A., Inactivation of quercetin mutagenicity. *Fd. Chem. Toxicol.*, **22**: 535–539, 1984.

66. Pratt, D.E., and Watts, B.M., The antioxidant activity of vegetable extracts. I. Flavone aglycones. *J. Food Sci.*, **29**: 27–33, 1964.

67. Pratt, D.E., Lipid antioxidants in plant tissue. *J. Food Sci.*, **30**: 737–741, 1965.

68. Letan, A., The relation of structure to antioxidant activity of quercetin and some of its derivatives. I. Primary activity. *J. Food Sci.*, **31**: 518–523, 1966.

69. Baumann, J., Wurm, G., and Bruchhausen, F.V., Hemmung der Prostaglandin-synthetase durch Flavonoide und Phenolderivate im Vergleich mit deren O_2^--Radikalfängereigenschaften. *Arch. Pharm.*, **313**: 330–337, 1980 (in German).

70. Salvayre, R., Braquet, P., Perruchot, T. and Douste-Blazy, L., Comparison of the scavenger effect of bilberry anthocyanosides with various flavonoids. in: *Flavonoids and Bioflavonoids*. (eds. L. Farkas, F. Kallay, M. Gábor and H. Wagner) *Studies in Organic Chemistry*, **11**. pp. 437–446, Elsevier, Amsterdam, **1981**.

71. Ueno, I., Kohno, M., Haraikawa, K., and Hirono, I., Interaction between quercetin and superoxide radicals. Reduction of the quercetin mutagenicity. *J. Pharm. Dyn.* **7**: 798–803, 1984.

72. Matsuura, T., Matsushima, H., and Nakadate, R., Photoinduced reactions. —XXXVI. Photosensitized oxygenation of 3-hydroxyflavones as a non-enzymatic model for quercetinase. *Tetrahedron*, **26**: 435–443, 1970.

73. Oka, T., Simpson, F.J., and Krishnamurty, H.G., Degradation of rutin by *Aspergillus flavus*. Studies on specificity, inhibition and possible reaction mechanism of quercetinase. *Can. J. Microbiol.*, **18**: 493–508, 1972.

74. Nishinaga, A., Tojo, T., Tomita, H., and Matsuura, T., Base-catalysed oxygenolysis of 3-hydroxyflavones. *J. Chem. Soc.*, Perkin Trans. 1: 2511–2516, **1979**.
75. Heyningen, R., Formation of polyols by the lens of the rat with 'sugar' cataract., *Nature*, **18**: 194–195, 1959.
76. Varma, S.D., Mizuno, I., and Kinoshita, J.H., Flavonoids as inhibitors of lens aldose reductase. *Science*, **188**: 1215–1216, 1975.
77. Varma, S.D., Mizuno, A., and Kinoshita, J.H., Diabetic cataracts and flavonoids. *Science*, **195**: 205–206, 1977.
78. Chaudhry, P.S., Cabrera, J., Juliani, R.H., and Varma, S.D., Inhibition of human lens aldose reductase by flavonoids, sulindac and indomethacin. *Biochem. Pharmacol.*, **32**: 1995–1998, 1983.
79. Okuda, J., Miwa, I., Inagaki, K., Horie, T., and Nakayama, M., Inhibition of aldose reductase from rat and bovine lenses by flavonoids. *Biochem. Pharmacol.*, **31**: 3807–3822, 1982.
80. Whittle, S.R., and Turner, A.J., Anti-convulsants and brain aldehyde metabolism. Inhibitory characteristics of ox brain aldehyde reductase. *Biochem. Pharmacol.*, **30**: 1191–1196, 1981.
81. Suolinna, E-M., Lang, D.R., Racker, E., Quercetin, an artificial regulator of the high aerobic glycolysis of tumor cells. *J. Natl. Cancer Inst.*, **53**: 1515–1519, 1974.
82. Carpenedo, E., Bortignon, C., Bruni, A., and Santi, R., Effect of quercetin on membrane-linked activities. *Biochem. Pharmacol.*, **18**: 1495–1500, 1969.
83. Kuriki, Y., and Racker, E., Inhibition of (N$^+$, K$^+$) adenosine triphosphatase and its partial reactions by quercetin. *Biochemistry*, **15**: 4951–4955, 1976.
84. Suolinna, E-M., Buchsbaum, R.N., and Racker, E., The effect of flavonoids on aerobic glycolysis and growth of tumor cells. *Cancer Res.*, **35**: 1865–1872, 1975.
85. Belt, J.A., Thomas, J.A., Buchsbaum, R.N., and Racker, E., Inhibition of lactate transport and glycolysis in Ehrlich ascites tumor cells by bioflavonoids. *Biochemistry*, **18**: 3506–3511, 1979.
86. Lang D.R., and Racker, E., Effects of quercetin and F₁ inhibitor on mitochondrial ATPase and energy-linked reactions in submitochondrial particles. *Biochim. Biophys. Acta*, **333**: 180–186, 1974.
87. Futai, M., Sternweis, P., and Heppl, L., Purification and properties of reconstitutively active and inactive adenosinetriphosphatase from *Escherichia coli*. *Proc. Natl. Acad. Sci. USA*, **71**: 2725–2729, 1974.
88. Deters, D.W., Racker, E., Nelson, N., and Nelson, H., Partial resolution of the enzymes catalysing photophosphorylation. *J. Biol. Chem.*, **250**: 1041–1047, 1975.
89. Fewtrell C.M.S., and Gomperts, B.D., Effect of flavone inhibitors of transport ATPase on histamine secretion from rat mast cells. *Nature*, **265**: 635–636, 1977.
90. Graziani, Y., and Chayoth, R., Elevation of cyclic AMP level in Ehrlich ascites tumor cells by quercetin. *Biochem. Pharmacol.*, **26**: 1259–1261, 1977.
91. Graziani, Y., Winikoff, J., and Chayoth, R., Regulation of cyclic AMP level and lactic acid production in Ehrlich ascites tumors cells. *Biochim. Biophys. Acta*, **497**: 499–506, 1977.
92. Beretz, A., Anton, R., and Stoclet, J.C., Flavonoid compounds are potent inhibitors of cyclic AMP phosphodiesterase. *Experientia*, **34**: 1054–1055, 1978.
93. Beretz, A., Joly, M., Stoclet J.C., and Anton, R., Inhibition of 3′, 5′-AMP-phosphodiesterase by biflavonoids and xanthones. *Planta Medica*, **36**: 193–195, 1979.
94. Nikaido, T., Ohmoto, T., Sankawa, U., Hamanaka, T., and Totsuka, K., Inhibition of cyclic AMP phosphodiesterase by flavonoids. *Planta Medica*, **46**: 162–166, 1982.
95. Ferrell, J.E. Jr., and Chang Sing, P.D.G., Loew, G., King, R., Mansour, J.M., and Mansour, T.E., Structure/activity studies of flavonoids as inhibitors of cyclic AMP phosphodiesterase and relationship to quantum chemical indices. *Mol. Pharmacol.*, **16**: 556–568, 1979.
96. Petkov, E., Nikolov, N., and Uzunov, P., Inhibitory effect of some flavonoids and flavonoid mixtures on cyclic AMP phsophodiesterase activity of rat heart. *Planta*

Medica, **43**: 183–186, 1981.
97. Ruckstuhl, M., Beretz, A., Anton, R., and Landry, Y., Flavonoids are selective cyclic GMP phosphodiesterase inhibitors. *Biochem. Pharmacol.*, **28**: 535–538, 1979.
98. Ruckstuhl M., and Landry, Y., Inhibition of lung cyclic AMP- and cyclic GMP-phosphodiesterases by flavonoids and other chromone-like compounds. *Biochem. Pharmacol.*, **30**: 697–702, 1981.
99. Raiman, R.J., Later, E.R. and Necheles, H., Effect of rutin on anaphylactic and histamine shock. *Science*, **106**: 368, 1947.
100. Moss, J.N., Beiler, J.M., and Martin, G.J., Inhibition of anaphylaxis in guinea pigs by D-catechin. *Science*, **112**: 16, 1950.
101. Vane, J.R. The inhibition of prostaglandin synthesis as a mechanism of action for aspirin-like drugs. *Nature* (New Biol.), **231**: 232–235, 1971.
102. Ferreira, S.H., Moncada, S., and Vane, J.R., Indomethacin and aspirin abolish prostaglandin release from the spleen. *Nature* (New Biol.), **231**: 237–239, 1971.
103. Smith, J.B., and Willis, A.L., Aspirin selectively inhibits prostaglandin production in human platelets. *Nature* (New Biol.), **231**: 235–237, 1971.
104. O' Flaherty, J.T., Biology of disease. Lipid mediators of imflammation and allergy. *Lab. Invest.*, **47**: 314–329, 1982.
105. Benveniste, J., Tencé, M., Varenne, P., Bidault, J., Boullet, C., and Polonsky, J., Semi-synthèse et structure porposée du facteur activant les plaquettes (P.A.F.): PAF-acether, un alkyl ether analogue de la lysophosphatidylcholine. *C.R. Acad. Sci.*, Paris (D), **289**: 1037–1040, (in French).
106. Demopoulos, C.A., Pinckard, R.N., and Hanahan, D.J., Platelet-activating factor: Evidence for 1-*O*-alkyl-2-acetyl-sn-glycero-3-phosphorylcholine as the active components. *J. Biol. Chem.*, **254**: 9355–9379, 1979.
107. Moncada, S., Gryglewski, R., Bunting, S., Vane, J.R., An enzyme isolated from arteries transforms prostaglandin endoperoxides to an unstable substance that inhibit platelet aggregation. *Nature*, **263**: 663–667, 1976.
108. Ikeda, K., Tanaka, K., and Katori, M., Potentiation of bradykinin-induced vascular permeability increase by prostaglandin E_2 and arachidonic acid in rabbit skin. *Prostaglandins*, **10**: 747–758, 1975.
109. Murota, S-I., and Murota, I., Effect of prostaglandin I_2 and related compounds on vascular permeability response in granuloma tissues. *Prostaglandins*, **15**: 297–301, 1978.
110. Williams, T.J., Prostaglandin I_2 and the vascular changes of inflammation. *Brit. J. Pharmacol.*, **65**: 517–524, 1979.
111. Meck, M.J., Piper, P.J., and Williams, T.J., The effect of leukotrienes C_4 and D_4 on the microvasculature of guinea-pig skin. *Prostaglandins*, **21**: 315–321, 1981.
112. Dahlen, S.E., Bjork, J., Hedquist, P., Arfors, K-E., Hammarstörm, S., Lindgren, J-A., and Samuelsson, B., Leukotrienes promote plasma leakage and leukocyte adhesion in postcapillary venules: *In vivo* effects with relevance to the acute inflammatory response. *Proc. Natl. Acad. Sci. USA*, 3887–3891, **1981**.
113. Turner, S.R., Tainer, J.A., and Lynn, W.S., Biogenesis of chemotactic molecules by the arachidonate lipoxygenase system of platelets. *Nature*, **257**: 680–681, 1975.
114. Goetzl, E.J., and Sun, F.F., Generation of unique mono-hydroxy-eicosatetraenoic acids from arachidonic acid by human neutrophils. *J. Exp. Med.*, **150**: 406–411, 1979.
115. Ford-Hutchinson, A.W., Bray, M.S., Doig, M.V., Shipley, M.E., and Smith, M.J.H., Leukotriene B: a potent chemokinetic and aggregating substance released from polymorphonuclear leukocytes. *Nature*, **268**: 264–265, 1980.
116. Smith, M.J., Ford-Hutchinson, A.W., and Bray, M.A., Leukotriene B: a potential mediator of inflammation. *J. Pharmac. Pharmacol.*, **32**: 517–518, 1980.
117. Palmer, R.M.J., Stepney, R.J., Higgs, G.A., and Eakins, K.E., Chemokinetic activity of arachidonic acid lipoxygenase products on leucocytes of different species. *Prostaglandins*, **20**: 411–418, 1980.
118. Kitchin, E.A., Boot, J.R., and Dawson, W., Chemotactic activity of thromboxane

B_2, prostaglandins and their metabolites for polymorphonuclear leucocytes. *Prostaglandins*, **16**: 239–244, 1978.

119. Flower R.J., and Blackwell, G.J., Anti-inflammatory steroids induce biosynthesis of a phospholipase A_2 inhibitor which prevents prostaglandin generation. *Nature*, **278**: 456–459, 1979.

120. Blackwell, G.J., Carnuccio, R., DiRosa, M., Flower, R.J., Parente, L., and Persico, P., Macrocortin: A polypeptide causing the antiphospholipase effect of glucocorticoids. *Nature*, **287**: 147–149, 1980.

121. Hirata, F., Schiffmann, E., Venkatasubramanian, K., Salomon, D., and Axelrod, J., A phospholipase A_2 inhibitory protein in rabbit neutrophils induced by glucocorticoids. *Proc. Natl. Acad. Sci. USA*, **77**: 2533–2536, 1980.

122. Hirata, F., Carmine, R. der, Nelson, C.A., Axelrod, F., Shiffmann, F., Warabi, A., De Blas, A.L., Nirenberg, M., Managaniello, V., Vaughan, M., Kumagai, S., Green, I., Decker, J.L., and Steinberg, A.D., Presence of autoantibody for phospholipase inhibitory protein, lipomodulin, in patients with rheumatic diseases. *Proc. Natl. Acad. Sci. USA*, **78**: 3190–3194, 1981.

123. Bennett, J.P., Gomperts, B.D., and Wollenweber, E., Inhibitory effects of natural flavonoids on secretion from mast cells and neutrophils. *Arzneim-Forsch./Drug Res.*, **31**: 433–437, 1981.

124. Middleton, E., Jr., Drzewieck, G., and Krishnarao, D., Quercetin: An inhibitor of antigen-induced human basophil histamine release. *J. Immunol.*, **127**: 546–550, 1981.

125. Schneider, C., Berton, G., Spisani, S., Traniello, S., and Romeo, D., Quercetin, a regulator of polymorphonuclear leukocytes (PMNL) functions. *Adv. Exp. Biol. Med.*, **121**: 371–379, 1979.

126. Lee, T.-P., Matteliano, M.L., and Middleton, E. Jr., Effect of quercetin on human polymorphonuclear leukocyte lysosomal enzyme release and phospholipid metabolism. *Life Sci.*, **31**: 2765–2774, 1982.

127. Berton, G., Schneider, C., and Romeo, D., Inhibition by quercetin of activation of polymorphonuclear leucocyte functions. Stimulus-specific effects. *Biochim. Biophys. Acta*, **195**: 47–55, 1980.

128. Long, C.D., DeChatelet, L.R., O'Flaherty, J.T., MacCall, C.E., Bass, D.A., Shirley, P.S., and Parce, J.W., Effect of quercetin on magnesium-dependent adenosine triphosphatase and the metabolism of human polymorphonuclear leukocytes. *Blood*, **57**: 561–567, 1981.

129. Landolfi, R., Mower, R.L., and Steiner, M., Modification of platelet function and arachidonic acid metabolism by bioflavonoids. Structure-activity relations. *Biochem. Pharmacol.*, **33**: 1525–1530, 1984.

130. Mower, R.L., Landolfi, R., and Steiner, M., Inhibition *in vitro* of platelet aggregation and arachidonic acid metabolism by flavone. *Biochem. Pharmacol.*, **33**: 357–363, 1984.

131. Beretz, A., Strierle, A., Anton, R., and Cazenave, J-P., Role of cyclic AMP in the inhibition of human platelet aggregation by quercetin, a flavonoid that potentiates the effect of prostacyclin. *Biochem. Pharmacol.*, **31**: 3597–3600, 1981.

132. Sekiya, K., Okuda, H., Selective inhibition of platelet lipoxygenase by baicalein. *Biochem. Biophys. Res. Commun.*, **105**: 1090–1095, 1982.

133. Yoshimoto, T., Furukawa, M., Yamamoto, S., Horie, T., and Watanabe-Kohno, S., Flavonoid: Potent inhibitors of arachidonate 5-lipoxygenase. *Biochem. Biophys. Res. Commun.*, **116**: 612–618, 1983.

134. Koshihara, Y., Neichi, T., Murota, S-I., Lao, A-N., Fujimoto, Y., and Tatsuno, T., Selective inhibition of 5-lipoxygenase by natural compounds isolated from Chinese plants, *Artemisia rubripes* Nakai. *FEBS Lett.*, **158**: 41–44, 1983.

135. Fiebrich, F., and Koch, H., Silymarin, an inhibitor of lipoxygenase. *Experientia*, **35**: 1548–1550, 1979.

136. Fiebrich, F., and Koch, H., Silymarin, an inhibitor of prostaglandin synthetase. *Experientia*, **35**: 1550–1552, 1979.

137. Kimura, Y., Okuda, J., Tani, T., and Arichi, S., Studies on *Scutellariae Radix*. VI. Effects of flavanone compounds on lipid peroxidation in rat liver. *Chem. Pharm. Bull.*, **30**: 1792–1795, 1982.
138. Agarwal, O.P., The anti-inflammatory action of nepitrin, a flavonoid. *Agents and Actions*, **12**: 298–302, 1982.
139. Cutting, W.C., Dreisbach, R.H., and Neff, B.J., Antiviral chemotherapy III. Flavones and related compounds. *Stanford Med. Bull.*, **7**: 137–138, 1949.
140. Cutting, W.C., Dreisbach, R.H., and Matsushima, F., Antiviral chemotherapy VI. Parenteral and other effects of flavonoids. *Stanford Med. Bull.*, **11**: 227–229, 1953.
141. Apple, M.A., Fischer, P., Wong, W., Paganelli, J., Harasymiv, I., and Osofsky, L., Inhibition of oncorna virus reverse transcriptase by plant flavonols. *Proc. Amer. Assoc. Cancer Res. and Amer. Soc. Clin. Oncol.*, **16**: 198, 1975.
142. Béládi, I., Pusztai, R., Mucsi, I., Bakay, M., and Gábor M., Activity of some flavonoids against viruses. *Ann. N.Y. Acad. Sci.*, **284**: 358–364, 1977.
143. Huang, M-T., Wood, A.W., Newmark, H.L., Sayer, J.M., Yagi, H., Jerina, D.M., and Conney, A.H., Inhibition of the mutagenicity of bayregion diol-epoxides of polycyclic aromatic hydrocarbons by phenolic plant flavonoids. *Carcinogenesis*, **4**: 1631–1637, 1983.
144. Edwards, J.M., Raffauf, R.F., and Le Quesne, P.W., Antineoplastic activity and cytotoxicity of flavones, isoflavones, and flavones. *J. Natural Products*, **42**: 85–91, 1979.
145. Buening, M.K., Chang, R.L., Huang, M-T., Fortner, J.G., Wood, A.W., and Conney, A.H., Activation and inhibition of benzo (α)-pyrene and aflatoxin B_1 metabolism in human liver microsomes by naturally occurring flavonoids. *Cancer Res.*, **41**: 67–72, 1981.
146. Lasker, J.M., Huang, M-T., and Conney, A.H., *In vivo* activation of zoxazolamine metabolism by flavone. *Science*, **216**: 1419–1421, 1982.
147. Kinoshita, T., Sankawa, U., Takuma, T., and Asahi, K-I., Induction of differentiation of cultured tumor cells by flavonoids. *Pro. Fifth Symp. on Development and Application of Naturally Occurring Medicines*. Hiroshima, **1984**.

4
Bracken Fern

Bracken fern, *Pteridium aquilinum*, is widely distributed in many parts of the world and used as a human food in Japan and some other countries. The toxic effect of bracken fern on livestock has attracted the attention of veterinary scientists since the end of the last century. The predominant feature of cattle bracken poisoning is depressed bone marrow activity, which gives rise to severe leucopenia, thrombocytopenia and hemorrhagic syndrome. The carcinogenicity of bracken fern was demonstrated most clearly by the experiment of Evans and Mason showing that rats fed diets containing bracken fern developed multiple intestinal adenocarcinomas. Subsequently, the simultaneous induction of urinary bladder tumors and the occurrence of mammary carcinoma in Sprague-Dawley rats fed bracken diet have been reported. However, neither the causative principle of cattle bracken poisoning nor bracken carcinogen had been isolated until very recently when our group succeeded in isolating a carcinogenic principle, ptaquiloside, a novel norsesquiterpene glucoside of the illudane type. It was also demonstrated that ptaquiloside is a causative principle of cattle bracken poisoning.

4.1 Toxicity of Bracken

Bracken fern, *Pteridium aquilinum* (Figs. 4–1 and –2), is widely distributed in many parts of the world. The toxic effect of bracken fern on livestock has been a concern of veterinary scientists since the end of the nineteenth century. The toxic syndromes induced by ingestion of sufficient quantities of bracken fern differ in horses, cattle and sheep.[1,2] Ingestion of the bracken fern by horses leads to a thiamine deficiency that can be remedied by administering thiamine. The deficiency develops because the fern contains an enzyme, thiaminase, which can cleave the thiamine mole-

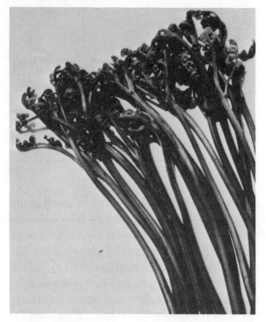

Fig. 4–1. Young bracken frond used as human food in the fiddlehead or crosier stage of growth.

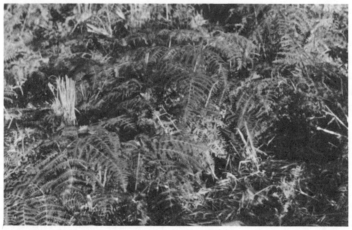

Fig. 4–2. Mature bracken.

cule thereby inactivating it. Affected horses show anorexia, gait disturbance, stagger, and incoordination. They stand with the legs widely spread in a crouching position. It was found that when bracken containing the enzyme thiaminase in the active state was fed to experimental rats they also developed a disease condition which simulated the typical nervous lesions of avitaminosis B_1 and could be cured by vitamin B_1 therapy.[3-5] Evans and coworkers demonstrated the presence of a thiaminase in bracken which was the first of its kind to be found in the plant kingdom.[6,7]

Bracken fern poisoning in cattle develops slowly with signs appearing several weeks after the ingestion begins, and the affected animals do not respond to thiamine therapy. The predominant feature in affected cattle is depressed bone marrow activity, named "bracken poisoning", which gives rise to severe leucopenia, especially of granulocytes, thrombocytopenia, hemorrhagic syndrome, and hematuria.[8] The bracken poisoning is quite dramatic and nearly always fatal. Death occurs within a few weeks or months from the onset of symptoms. The cattle bracken poisoning factor can be extracted from bracken with hot ethanol[9] or hot water.[10] Oral administration of this fraction to a calf produced clinical bracken poisoning. However, in spite of sustained effort and a great deal of work, this factor has not yet been successfully isolated. Sheep are generally resistant. Bright blindness in sheep was first reported as a progressive degeneration of the neuroepithelium of the retina of hill sheep in Yorkshire, and it was suggested that there was a connection between this blindness and grazing on bracken.[11] Subsequently, it was confirmed that all the affected sheep had access to bracken. Experimental feeding of bracken to sheep was also successful in producing bright blindness.[12]

Chronic enzootic hematuria in cattle is well documented by Rosenberger.[13] It is characterized by hemorrhages from the urinary bladder mucosa and, in advanced cases, by tumorous processes of various forms and sizes in the wall of the bladder. Cattle are affected regardless of age and sex. Changes in the blood picture accompanying the hematuria consist of declines in white cell count and hemoglobin content. Thrombocytopenia and leucopenia are present in advanced cases. Necropsy usually shows characteristic bladder lesions consisting of hemorrhagic foci. Histologic examination shows capillary ectasia, angiomatous cavity formation and vascularized epithelial proliferation, which leads to malignant carcinogenic infiltration of the entire bladder wall. Götze[14] reported that bracken fern was regularly found in farms where cattle were affected by this disease, whereas in the same district, pastures where no cases of the disease occurred were also free of bracken fern. Thus he assumed that bracken fern was the cause of the disease. A feeding experiment was carried out by Rosenberger and Heeschen.[15] They succeeded in producing chronic hematuria in cattle by continued feeding of green and dry bracken fern and demonstrated that chronic enzootic bovine hematuria and bracken poisoning with panmyeloid bone marrow damage are two clinical expressions of the one and the same causative factor, bracken fern toxin, depending on the duration and amount of bracken feeding. Evans *et al.*[16] studied the toxicity of bracken rhizomes on cattle. They reported that bracken rhizomes caused bovine bracken poisoning and that the toxic factor was present in the rhizomes in concentrations at least five times those found normally occurring in the fronds.

4.2 Carcinogenic Properties of Bracken

The earliest evidence for the carcinogenicity of bracken fern was reporeted by Rosenberger and Heeschen,[15] who described changes of a polypous-tumorous nature in the urinary bladder mucosa accompanied by hematuria in cattle that had ingested bracken fern for long periods. Georgiev et al.,[17] obtained an ether and chloroform extract from the urine of cattle in a hematuria district, which produced hemangiomatous changes when introduced into the urinary bladder of calves, dogs and rats. Application of the same extract dissolved in acetone produced in the skin of white mice papillomas which later transformed into cancroids and carcinosarcomas. Pamukcu[18] conducted an epidemiologic survey of Turkish cattle with a condition known as chronic enzootic bovine hematuria-associated bladder tumors and found that the geographic distribution of cattle with this condition and that of bracken overlapped.

The carcinogenicity of bracken fern was demonstrated most clearly by the experiment of Evans and Mason,[19] showing that rats fed diets containing bracken fern developed multiple ileal adenocarcinomas. In this experiment rats received a diet which contained dry bracken fern powder at 34% by weight for 64 days and vitamin B_1 was given by sc injection because bracken fern has thiaminase. Pamukcu et al.[20,21] and Price and Pamukcu[22] confirmed that bracken fern was carcinogenic to cows and rats. Tumors induced by bracken fern feeding in cows were hemangiomas, papillomas and transitional-cell carcinomas of the urinary bladder. Histologic features of naturally occurring and bracken fern-induced bladder tumors in cattle were reported in detail by Pamukcu et al.[23] Simultaneous intestinal and urinary bladder tumors were induced in rats fed a diet containing bracken fern (1:3 by weight) until the animals died or were sacrificed.[21] Adenomatous polyps and adenocarcinomas developed predominantly in the ileum. Urinary bladder tumors occurred in 81% of the autopsied rats and were either papillomas or sessile or papillary carcinomas. Histologically, the carcinomas were transitional cell carcinomas and squamous cell carcinomas. The variation in production of bladder tumors in rats seems to depend on the dosing regimen, which is ineffectual if of less than 3 months duration. It is suggested that the highest incidence

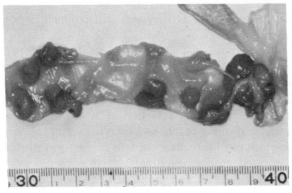

Fig. 4–3. Ileal tumors induced in rats fed bracken diet.

is obtained in cases where relatively small amounts of the carcinogen are given over long periods.[24] In Japan, young bracken fern fronds in the fiddlehead or crosier stage of growth are used as human food.[25,26] However, when rats were given a diet containing powdered young bracken fern, in a proportion of one part by weight of bracken fern to two parts of basal diet for 4 months, all rats that survived for more than 7 months after the start of the experiment had ileal tumors (Fig. 4–3) and some had tumors of the cecum as well. The most common site of intestinal tumors induced by bracken fern was the terminal 20 cm of the ileum. Histologically, the intestinal tumors were not only epithelial tumors, such as adenomas and adenocarcinomas, but also sarcomas.[26] Yunoki *et al.*[27] and Saito *et al.*[28] also reported the occurrence of intestinal tumors in rats fed Japanese bracken fern. The latent period of tumor development was longer and the incidence of intestinal tumors was lower in rats which received a diet containing processed bracken fern (whch had been immersed in boiling water) than in rats which received a diet containing unprocessed bracken fern. However, the incidece of urinary bladder tumors was higher in the former.[26]

In Japan, young bracken fern is usually used as a human food after its astringent taste has been removed by one of the following treatments. 1. Fresh bracken fern is immersed in boiling water containing wood ash or sodium bicarbonate, then seasoned. Sometimes, it is merely boiled before being eaten. 2. Fresh bracken is pickled in salt and immersed in boiling water before use. The carcinogenic activity of processed bracken fern used as a human food was studied in ACI rats.[29] Tumor incidence in rats fed an unprocessed bracken-containing diet was 78.5%. However, it was 25%, 10%, and 4.7% in rats fed a diet containing processed bracken fern treated with wood ash, sodium bicarbonate and NaCl, respectively. Although the carcinogenic activity of bracken fern was markedly reduced by such treatment, weak carcinogenic activity was still retained in the brackern fern thus prepared.

It was mentioned above that rats fed a bracken fern diet developed multiple tumors in the terminal 20 cm of the ileum. Specifically the most preferred site was the terminal 3 cm of the ileum.[29] In order to elucidate the factors which determine such preferential localization, the following experiments were carried out.[30] Surgical resection of 20 cm of the terminal ileum, of the cecum, and of the cecum and terminal ileum together were performed on three groups of rats. Bracken fern feeding was started 10 days later. In all operated groups, intestinal tumors occurred most frequently in a 20-cm section adjacent and proximal to the anastomosis. These results suggest that the preferential site of intestinal tumors induced by a bracken fern diet is the section in which the content of the small intestine is prone to stagnation.

It has been reported that the carcinogenic activity of bracken fern is influenced by the geographic location where the fern is grown.[29,31] Schacham et al.[31] reported that rats given a diet containing 34% bracken fern for 32 weeks developed tumors of the small intestine, which were classed as benign adenomatous polyps. They inferred that geographic, seasonal, or climatic conditions might influence the antihematopoietic and carcinogenic effects of bracken fern. Comparative studies also showed that the carcinogenicity of the curled tops of young bracken fronds was greater than that of the stalks and that the carcinogenic activity of the bracken rhizomes was stronger than that of the young fronds.[32] Furthermore, to study the relationship between the stage of maturation of bracken fern and carcinogenic activity, the carcinogenicity of mature bracken fern was compared with that of immature young fern with curled tops.[24] The mature bracken fern used was collected in September in the same area where the immature fern had been collected in June. Rats received diets containing the mature or immature ferns in proportion by weight of one part bracken fern to two parts basal diet for 4 months. It was evident that the latent period of the tumor in rats fed the diet containing mature bracken fern was longer than in those fed the diet containing young fern; i.e., although the majority of animals fed young bracken fern died of tumors within 11 months and all animals of this group died within 14 months after the start of feeding, the majority of rats fed mature fern were still alive 16 months after the start of the experiment. The incidence of intestinal tumors was significantly different in the two groups. Urinary bladder tumors were induced slightly more frequently in rats fed mature bracken fern. The majority of intestinal tumors in rats fed mature bracken were adenomas, whereas in rats fed young bracken intestinal tumors were predominantly adenocarcinomas. Thus it was evident that the mature bracken still retained fairly strong carcinogenic activity, although it was weak compared with the young bracken. Recently, induction of mammary cancer in female Charles River Sprague-Dawley rats (CD rats) fed a bracken diet was reported.[33] Female 6-week-old CD rats were given a diet containing 30% bracken fronds throughout the experimental period of 260 days. They developed multiple mammary tumors with an incidence of 87% in addition to ileal and urinary bladder tumors. The earliest mammary tumor was detected on day 78, and the last on day 256. The average number of tumors per rat was 5.6. Most mammary tumors were papillary carcinomas and adenocarcinomas.

4.3 Carcinogenicity of Bracken Fern in Laboratory Animals Other Than Rats and Livestock (Table 4–1).

Mice

Bracken fern was found to induce pulmonary adenomas in Swiss mice[34] and dd strain of mice.[24] When non-inbred Swiss white mice (6 weeks old) were fed 33% bracken pellets for 5 weeks there was 100% incidence of pulmonary adenomas, and an average of 16 per animal in 26 experimental mice, compared with 0.57 in 46 control mice.[34,35] Intestinal tumors did not develop in Swiss and dd mice, but developed in mice of the C57BL/6 strain when given bracken fern, and the tumors were consistently found in the terminal region of the jejunum–not, as in rats, in the ileum.[24] Bracken fern did not induce urinary bladder tumors in mice. However, Miyakawa and Yoshida[36] reported that ICR strain of mice developed urinary bladder tumors when fed a bracken fern-containing diet after prior surgical implantation of a glass bead into the bladder, but

Table 4-1. Carcinogenicity of Bracken Fern

Animal[†]	Target organs and histological findings
Rat[19,21,26)]	Ileum, cecum (adenoma, adenocarcinoma, sarcoma) Urinary bladder (papilloma, carcinoma) Sprague-Dawley: mammary cancer[33)]
Mouse[24,34,37)]	Swiss & dd: lung adenoma, lymphatic leukemia C57BL/6: jejunal adenoma
Quail[34)]	Cecum, colon, ileum (adenocarcinoma)
Hamster[34,38)]	Cecum, ileum (adenocarcinoma)
Guinea pig[34,41)]	Small intestine (adenoma, adenocarcinoma) Urinary bladder (carcinoma)
Cattle[20,22)]	Urinary bladder (papilloma, carcinoma, hemangioendothelioma)

† All animals were fed a diet containing dry bracken powder, except quail, which were given ethanol extract of bracken fern.

not in mice on the same bracken fern diet without an implanted glass bead or in animals on a normal diet with an implanted glass bead. Pamukcu et al.[37] reported that when female Swiss mice were given bracken fern every other week over a total period of 60 weeks, they developed lymphatic leukemia and pulmonary tumors. No urinary bladder or intestinal tumors were found.

Japanese quail

Japanese quail (Coturnix coturnix japonica) were fed an active hot ethanol extract of dried June bracken fern mixed with their normal diet for the first 5 months after hatching. Adenocarcinomas were induced predominantly in cecum, colon, and in smaller numbers in the distal ileum.[34]

Hamster

Hamsters fed bracken fern diet developed intestinal adenocarcinomas.[34] However, the incidence of tumors in Syrian golden hamsters fed a bracken fern diet (1:2 by weight) was much less than that in rats in another experiment; i.e., only 4 out of 24 hamsters had cecal or ileal adenocarcinoma; however, young hamsters, 1.5 months old, were used in this study.[38]

Guinea pig

Guinea pigs developed not only intestinal adenocarcinomas, but also urinary bladder carcinomas.[34,39] Among the other small experimental animals fed bracken, guinea pigs were especially noteworthy, since they closely reproduced the conditions described for chronic enzootic bovine hematuria.[39-41] Guinea pigs given concentrated aqueous extracts of bracken frond by stomach intubation develop hemorrhage from the urinary bladder after 2–5 days.[42,43] Ushijima et al.[41] also found that hematuria and edema in the urinary bladder in guinea pigs were prominent on day 5 after the start of feeding of a 30% bracken diet.

Guppy

Matsushima et al.,[44] using the guppy (Lebistes reticulatas), recorded that intestinal hyperplasias developed on a diet containing 33% powdered freeze-dried young bracken shoots for 1 month, or diet containing 10% methanol extracts of freeze-dried young bracken shoots for 5 months.

Egyptian toad

Egyptian toad, Bufo regularis, has been tested as a new model for detecting the carcinogenicity of bracken fern. Tumors were induced in 18 of 98 toads subjected to forced feeding with bracken fern.[45] They comprise 7 cases of adenocarcinomas in the ileum, 16 cases of hepatomas and 6 cases of kidney metastases of the hepatomas. The author emphasized that *B. regularis* can be considered to be an advantageous model for detecting the carcinogenicity of bracken fern since lesions occur faster (2–5 months) than in other experimental animals (1–2 years). Moreover, it is sensitive to small doses (10 mg/50 g body weight, once a week) of the carcinogenic materials.

Farm livestock

The relatively long-term feeding trials by Rosenberger and Heeschen[15] and Pamukcu[18] supported the assumption that bracken may be related the etiology of bovine bladder tumors. Subsequent studies by Pamukcu *et al.*[20,22,23] demonstrated that prolonged low-level ingestion of bracken is a significant factor in the genesis of bovine bladder cancer. The bladder cancers induced in 20 of 30 cows by bracken feeding over long periods of time (mean: 550 days) were indistinguishable from the naturally occurring vesical tumors.[23,46,47] Invasive carcinomas of the bladder developed within 2.5 years after initiation of bracken feeding.[23] In light of these findings it became clear that bracken, as a forage contaminant, was responsible for a high rate of bladder cancer in Turkish cattle. A similar close association between bracken and urinary bladder and intestinal cancer in sheep in Australia and New Zealand[48-50] has been observed. There has been simultaneous occurrence of bladder, intestinal and esophageal cancer in cattle in Brazil and Scotland.[51] Later, Pamukcu *et al.*[20,22] produced experimental bovine enzootic hematuria in 10 of 18 cattle fed varying amounts of bracken over a mean period of 550 days. The majority of bladder neoplasms were papillomas and hemangiomas, and in some animals invasive carcinomas were found as a late development.

Survey studies in Brazil by Döbereiner and Tokarnia[52,53] associated bracken with enzootic hematuria and also with a slower developing epidermoid carcinoma of the upper digestive tract of cattle. The latter condition was found in different breeds of cattle aged 5–15 years, and squamous-cell carcinomas, usually multiple, occurred at different sites including the base of the tongue, palate, pharynx, esophagus, cardia and anterior dorsal sac of the rumen. Jarrett *et al.*[51] reported that cattle in highland areas of Scotland and northern England are substantially more prone to squamous-cell carcinomas of the upper alimentary tract than cattle in neighboring lowlands, and they obtained epidemiological evidence that this was associated with the ingestion of bracken, which transformed pre-existing virus-induced papillomas into squamous-cell carcinomas. The surveys by Döbereiner *et al.*[52] and Neto *et al.*[54] on cattle in Brazil also indicated an association of bracken with the occurrence of squamous-cell carcinoma of the upper alimentary tract as mentioned above. Hirono et al.[55] reported that rats fed a 30% bracken diet developed papillomas of the tongue, pharynx, esophagus and forestomach, and 1 rat also had squamous-cell carcinoma of the pharynx. Thus it is possible that papilloma and squamous-cell carcinoma of the upper alimentary tract in cattle are induced even by consecutive ingestion of bracken alone.

Although tumors in sheep are not common, adenocarcinoma of the intestine has been reported several times in New Zealand[50] and Australia[49] in areas where bracken is incriminated. Harburtt and Leaver[48] reported hematuria and carcinomatous invasive lesions of the urinary bladder in a flock of aged Merino wethers which had access to bracken fern for at least 18 months in northeastern Victoria.

McCrea and Head[56] reported the experimental production of tumors in North Country Cheviot sheep by feeding dried, pelleted bracken frond for periods ranging from 26 to 60 months. One died of acute bracken poisoning after 45 months and all the others developed tumors of the bladder, together with intermittent hematuria in most cases. Bright blindness of Yorkshire hill flocks has been recognized by farmers, and is characterized by stenosis of the blood vessels and progressive retinal atrophy. This condition has been studied by Watson et al.,[57] who have produced it experimentally by feeding whole bracken. The condition has not been recorded in any other species and the agent in bracken responsible for its production is not known.

4.4 Embryotoxic Effects of Bracken Fern

Embryotoxic effects of feeding bracken fern to pregnant mice of ICR-JCL strain were studied by Yasuda et al.[58] Pregnant mice fed a diet containing 33% dried bracken fern showed maternal weight loss, intrauterine growth suppression, and an increase in rib variations, as well as retarded ossification of the sternebrae of the fetuses. The influence of bracken fern diet on pregnant mice was also studied by Fushimi et al.[59] A diet containing 33% bracken material was given to C57BL/6 mice during pregnancy, starting immediately after vaginal plug was confirmed. In a group fed unprocessed bracken fern, abortion was more frequently observed compared with groups fed processed fern treated with sodium bicarbonate. However, the frequency of abortion was not always related to the potency of carcinogenicity of bracken fern.

4.5 Various Effects on Carcinogenic Activity of Bracken

Pamukcu *et al.*[60] reported that the incidence of urinary bladder carcinomas was significantly higher in rats fed a diet supplemented with bracken fern plus thiamine (2 mg of thiamine hydrochloride sc once a week) than in rats given a diet supplemented with only bracken fern. They inferred that this was due to alteration in the absorption, distribution, metabolism, or excretion of the bracken carcinogen induced by thiamine. However, they also showed that phenothiazine significantly inhibited the incidence of intestinal and urinary bladder tumors in rats on a diet containing bracken.[61] The inhibitory effect of butylated hydroxyanisole (BHA), disulfiram, calcium chloride and polyvinylpyrrolidone (PVP) on the intestinal and urinary bladder carcinogenicity of bracken fern was also determined in rats.[62] Dietary BHA, disulfiram and calcium chloride decreased the incidence of intestinal tumors by about 25 to 30%. Similarly, PVP and calcium chloride inhibited bracken-induced urinary bladder carcinogenesis by about 80%. Effect of storage on carcinogenic activity of bracken was studied with ACI rats.[63] Group I received a diet containing fresh dry bracken powder; group II received a diet which contained the same dry bracken powder used in group I but preserved for 1 years at 4°C or room temperature; group III received a diet containing bracken powder preserved for 2 years at 4°C or room temperature. Significant differences in incidence of ileal tumor were observed between group I and both groups of group III, and the latent period of intestinal tumors in groups II and III was longer than that of group I. The results indicate that longer storage times reduced the carcinogenic activity of bracken.

4.6 Epidemiology of the Carcinogenicity of Bracken Fern

Pamukcu and Price[21] suggested that the high incidence of human stomach cancer in Japan may be partially due to bracken fern, since considerable quantities of this plant are eaten in Japan. However, bracken fern is usually eaten after its astringent taste has been removed by boiling water containing wood ash or sodium bicarbonate (processed bracken). Processed bracken fern contains much less carcinogen than unprocessed fern although it still contains a slight amount.[29] Therefore it is difficult to evaluate the significance of bracken fern consumption in relation to the high incidence of human stomach cancer in Japan.

Kamon and Hirayama[64] made an epidemiologic survey of cancer in a mountainous area of central Japan where the people eat much bracken fern. They reported a significantly higher risk of esophageal cancer in people who ate hot tea gruel every day and in those who ate bracken fern every day; the risk was particularly high when both types of food were consumed.

The possible human hazard of bracken fern carcinogen has been indicated by several workers,[65-67] especially the transfer of bracken fern carcinogen to milk. A calf given milk from a cow receiving a sublethal dietary bracken supplement showed evidence of a hematological response which would be typical of a calf directly consuming bracken at a low rate.[65,66] Pamukcu et al.[67] studied the carcinogenicity of the milk of bracken fern-fed cows. The milk obtained was fed to rats as either fresh or freeze-dried powdered milk mixed with a grain diet. Nine of 34 rats fed the whole milk diet and 11 of 56 fed the powdered diet developed small intestinal, renal, or urinary bladder carcinomas within 117 weeks, while none of 70 rats fed either whole or powdered milk from cows receiving a normal diet and none of 20 rats fed a basic grain diet displayed neoplasia of those organs. Milk from cows that have eaten bracken fern may thus be hazardous to humans. Pamukcu and Bryan[68] reported that indirect human exposure to bracken fern through milk and dairy products is most likely to occur in areas of the world such as Turkey, Bulgaria, Yugoslavia, Colombia, and other regions where grazing cattle ingest bracken fern, especially under free range conditions, and where dried bracken fern is used for bedding in winter. It has also been speculated that rain may leach carcinogens from the plant and eventually transport it into human water supplies. Recently, Evans[40] has been studying the carcinogenicity of bracken spores. Bracken is a sporophyte and although not all mature plants shed large quantities of spores annually, many do so, and a single frond alone can produce as much as 1 gm in the summer months. Spores are shot out by a catapult mechanism of the sporangium. It is obvious that they can become airborne and inhaled in the same way as pollen grains and mold spores. Evans has therefore been testing bracken spores by giving them orally, without anaesthesia, to 100 mice (2 different strains) the majority of which have received no more than a total of 0.2 gm in ten doses. At this writing, the experiment has not completed one year, but 50 control mice, dosed only with water are all alive and healthy while 10% of the spore mice have already succumbed to various cancers including lymphocytic leukemia.

4.7 Difficulty of Isolating Bracken Fern Carcinogen

4.7.1 Progress of studies on the nature of the bracken carcinogen (Table 4–2).

The nature of the carcinogen in bracken fern has not yet been elucidated. Flavonoids,[69,70] indanones[71,72] and pterolactam[73] have been isolated from bracken fern. However, there are no data to indicate that these chemicals are carcinogenic.[24,28] Pamukcu et al.[74] separated urine from cattle fed on bracken fern into nonacidic and acidic fractions, and implanted pellets containing each fraction into the urinary bladder of mice; they found that the incidence of tumors was significantly higher in the group

Table 4–2. Historical Background of the Study of Bracken Carcinogen

Extract	Carcinogenicity test	Result	Reference
Acidic fraction of urine from cattle fed on bracken fern	Implantation of pellets containing the fraction into the urinary bladder of mice	+	Pamukcu et al.[74] (1966)
Methanol extract of bracken fern	//	+	Pamukcu et al.[75] (1970)
Shikimic acid	Intraperitoneal injection or intragastric administration in mice	+	Evans & Osman[77] (1974)
Pterosin and pteroside	Feeding experiment in rats	−	Hikino et al.[71] (1970) Fukuoka et al[72] (1972) Saito et al.[28] (1975)
Pterolactam	Urinary bladder implantation in mice, feeding or intragastric administration in rats	−	Takatori et al.[73] (1972) Hirono et al.[24] (1975)
Tannin	Urinary bladder implantation in mice	+	Wang et al.[79] (1976)
Shikimic acid	Feeding experiment in rats	−	Hirono et al.[78] (1977)
Boiling water extract of bracken fern	//	+	Hirono et al.[85] (1978)
Tannin and tannin free fraction of bracken fern	Sc injection of tannin fraction Diet containing tannin fraction, chloroform fraction, and tannin-free fraction given to rats.	+ − + +	Pamukucu et al.[80] (1980) // // //
Quercetin	Feeding experiment (Rats) (Mice) (Rats) (Hamsters) (Rats)	+ − − − −	Pamukcu et al.[96] (198). Saito et al.[97] (1980) Hirono et al.[100] (1981) Morino et al.[102] (1982) Takanashi et al.[101] (1983)

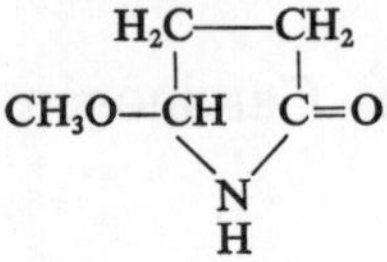

$$
\begin{array}{c}
\text{H}_2\text{C}\!-\!\!-\!\!-\!\text{CH}_2 \\
|\qquad\quad| \\
\text{CH}_3\text{O}\!-\!\text{CH}\quad\text{C}\!=\!\text{O} \\
\diagdown\;\;\diagup \\
\text{N} \\
\text{H}
\end{array}
$$

Fig. 4–4. Chemical structure of pterolactam.

treated with the acidic fraction. They also implanted pellets containing a methanol extract of bracken fern into the urinary bladder of mice, and their findings suggested that the carcinogenic substance is soluble in methanol.[75] Leach et al.[76] briefly reported on the isolation from bracken fern of an active principle that is mutagenic, carcinogenic, and lethal to mice on ip injection and tentatively assigned the molecular formula $C_7H_8O_4$ to this material. Subsequently, Evans and Osman[77] corrected the formula to $C_7H_{10}O_5$ and showed that the isolated compound was shikimic acid, which is carcinogenic and mutagenic in mice. They also suggested that another fraction of bracken contains a strong carcinogen in addition to shikimic acid, and this fraction can also induce the syndrome of acute bovine bracken fern poisoning. However, rats fed a diet containing shikimic acid did not develop tumors.[78] Thus, at least in rats, the carcinogenicity of bracken fern may be attributable to substance(s) other than shikimic acid. Hikino et al.[71] and Fukuoka et al.[72] isolated the indanones pteroside and pterosin from the fronds and rhizomes of bracken, but these compounds were not carcinogenic. Takatori et al.[73] isolated 5-methoxy-2-pyrrolidone from bracken and named it pterolactam (Fig. 4–4). However, the carcinogenic activity of pterolactam could not be experimentally confirmed, neither by implantation into the urinary bladder of Swiss mice, nor by feeding or intragastric administration in rats.[24] Wang et al.[79] isolated a carcinogenic tannin from bracken. The tannin induced bladder tumors in mice when intravesically implanted. However, neither intestinal nor bladder tumors were induced when a diet containing tannin was fed to rats.[80] The cyanogenic glycoside prunasin (O-β-D-glucopyranosyl-D-mandelonitrile) has been isolated from bracken by Kofod and Eyjolfsson.[81] However, the carcinogenicity test of prunasin in rats was negative.[82] Evans and Widdop[35,83,84] reported that the hot ethanol extraction was carcinogenic in rats and mice in addition to cattle toxicity.

Hirono et al. studied the carcinogenicity to rats of a boiling water extract of bracken fern. All the rats fed the concentrated boiling water extract developed urinary bladder carcinomas, and most of them also had ileal tumors. These results show that the carcinogen in bracken fern can be extracted with boiling water, and is thus probably water soluble.[85]

The following observations relevant to the nature of the carcinogenic or toxic substance contained in bracken have also been reported. Mori *et al.*[86] compared the carcinogenic activities of young bracken fern dried at high temperatures of 70 to 90° C with a hot, forced draft, and fern minced to a pastelike consistency using a mechanical chopper with that of unprocessed bracken dried at room temperatures below 30° C. There was no significant difference in the latent period, incidence, histologic types, or multiplicity of the intestinal tumors between groups fed a diet containing bracken fern dried at high temperature or minced fern and the group fed bracken dried at room temperature. These results suggest that the carcinogenic substance contained in bracken is relatively stable to heat. It was evident that mincing of bracken did not inhibit its carcinogenic activity. The authors inferred that there may not be any enzyme present in bracken which inhibits the activity of the bracken carcinogen.

Quercetin has been reported to be mutagenic in the *Salmonella* test system.[87-93] It was also mutagenic to V79 Chinese hamster cells,[94] and induced transformed colonies in Pienta's system with cryopreserved golden hamster embryo cells.[95] Pamukcu *et al.*[96] reported that Norwegian rats fed a 0.1% quercetin diet developed tumors of the ileum and urinary bladder in high incidence, i.e., 80% and 20%, respectively. From these results, they inferred that quercetin contained in bracken is a principal effector of bracken carcinogenesis. Quercetin has been tested for carcinogenicity in mice,[97,98] rats[96,99-101] and hamsters[102] in several experiments by administration in the diet and in mice by skin application[103] and urinary bladder implantation.[79] Induction of ileal and urinary bladder carcinomas has not been observed except in the experiment on rats fed quercetin by Pamukcu *et al.*,[96] even though the other experiments used the same or higher doses of quercetin. ACI rats used in the study by Hirono *et al.*[100] were an inbred strain, which are highly susceptible to the carcinogencity of bracken, i.e., they had tumors in the ileum and urinary bladder in high incidence. Thus, from the available evidence taken as a whole, the carcinogenicity of bracken fern does not appear to be attributable to the quercetin contained in bracken. Morino *et al.*[102] reported that quercetin was not carcinogenic to golden hamsters of either sex when given at concentrations of 4% and 1% of the diet in experiments lasting 735 days. Evans[40] just terminated a similar experiment with Japanese quail, lasting 623 days, which failed to produce any tumors. In this experiment quercetin was added to the diet for 425 days at concentrations of 0.5% and 0.1%. Jarrett[104] produced tumors in all cattle fed bracken in his large cattle feeding trial, but after five years no tumors at all have developed in the quercetin-treated group.

Very recently, Evans and her coworkers[105] published a summary of their study concerning the isolation and chemical characterization of compounds not previously reported from bracken fern. They emphasized that these occur in fractions which have been shown to be carcinogenic in mice.

4.7.2 Obstacles to the isolation of bracken carcinogen

As mentioned above, the nature of the carcinogen contained in bracken fern has long been uncertain. There seem to be several reasons for the difficulty encountered in isolating the bracken fern carcinogen. One important reason was the absence of specific acute toxicity of bracken in small laboratory animals such as rats and mice, whereas bracken fern poisoning is demonstrable upon feeding to cattle. A reliable hematological change cannot be induced by feeding bracken fern to rats and mice.

Needless to say, there is no evidence that the same factor which causes cattle bracken fern poisoning is the bracken fern carcinogen. In addition, the acute toxicity of a substance does not necessarily denote carcinogenic activity. Nevertheless, there are numerous carcinogens which produce signs of acute toxicity, e.g., cycasin and carcinogenic pyrrolizidine alkaloids. It is easier to isolate the acutely toxic substance and test it for carcinogenic activity in plants which are acutely toxic to experimental animals when given in large amounts. Rats fed a diet containing a large amount of dry powder from flower stalks of petasites, a kind of coltsfoot, produced severe liver damage, including centrilobular necrosis, proliferation of intrahepatic bile ducts and megalocytosis of liver cells. These histologic findings strongly suggested that the flower stalks of petasites contain a hepatotoxic pyrrolizidine alkaloid and were considered, therefore, a good candidate for testing for carcinogenic activity. This resulted in the successful isolation of petasitenine, a carcinogenic pyrrolizidine alkaloid contained in flower stalks of petasites.[106, 107] Cycasin was isolated as a toxic glucoside from cycads long before its carcinogenicity was detected.[108] Therefore, using bovine bracken fern poisoning as the criterion may be one approach in the search for the bracken fern carcinogen. However, this approach requires large amounts of extract. The isolation of a carcinogen from a plant such as bracken fern, which produces no acute toxicity in laboratory animals, is difficult. Moreover boiling water extract of bracken, which was proved to be carcinogenic to rats, was not mutagenic in the Ames test using *Salmonella typhimurium*; nor did the extract induce transformation in cryopreserved hamster embryonic cells by the Pienta test. Because results obtained in other short-term tests were also erratic, they could not be used as the endpoint in the extraction of the carcinogen from bracken fern. Consequently, the most reliable available method is to look for carcinogenicity in each fraction using experimental animals as efficiently as possible. Some workers[74,75] applied urinary bladder implantation technique to test the carcinogenic activity of bracken fern extract. Although this technique has the advantage that the amount of extract necessary for testing is relatively small, the results were not always comparable with those obtained by oral administration in the case of the carcinogen tannin.[80]

Accordingly, the most reliable test was considered to be experimental feeding using rats. It takes more than half a year to test carcinogenicity in rats using diets containing bracken fern material. Thus, a large amount of test sample was required, even though the experiment was started using rats as young as possible. An efficient method for carcinogenicity testing using laboratory animals is desirable not only for the isolation of the carcinogens but also for testing many chemicals which have already been proven to be mutagenic by the Ames or other short-term test. Differences in carcinogenic activity of bracken fern obtained from different geographic areas and differences in the susceptibility of various animal strains to the carcinogenic activity must also be considered. Comparison of carcinogenicity in various fractions should be made with the same strain and sex of animals and with the same supply of bracken fern. If not, it is nearly impossible to compare the carcinogenicity of the various fractions and may lead to wrong conclusions. All these factors had to be considered in order to avoid the complications encountered in previous attempts to isolate the bracken fern carcinogen.

4.8 Isolation of Bracken Carcinogen

Based on the carcinogenicity in rats, fractionation of the aqueous extracts of bracken was performed, resulting in the isolation of a bracken carcinogen, ptaquiloside (**1**). The isolation procedure of ptaquiloside (**1**) is outlined in Fig. 4–5.[109,110]

The dried powdered bracken was extracted with boiling water with vigorous agitation for ten minutes and this extraction process was repeated three times. A resin, Amberlite XAD-2, was added to the combined aqueous extract [I-A] and the mixture stirred and filtered. The resin adsorbate was eluted with methanol and the resulting methanol solution concentrated to give the eluate residue [II-B]. The results of the carcinogenicity assay on the aqueous filtrate residue [II-A] and the eluate residue [II-B] clearly revealed that the latter fraction [II-B] was carcinogenic, as shown in Table 4–3. The eluate residue [II-B] was dissolved in *n*-butanol saturated with water and extracted with water saturated with *n*-butanol three times.

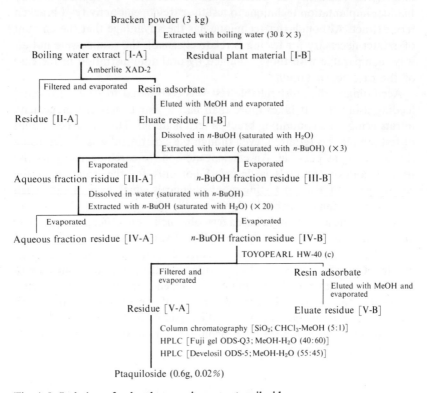

Fig. 4–5. Isolation of a bracken carcinogen, ptaquiloside.

The carcinogenicity of the two fractions thus obtained, the aqueous fraction [III-A] and the n-butanol fraction [III-B], was examined: the former fraction [III-A] was found to show carcinogenic activity which was slightly stronger than the latter fraction [III-B] (Table 4–3). For further fractionation the aqueous fraction [III-A] was dissolved in water saturated with n-butanol and extracted with n-butanol saturated with water twenty times. Again in this stage, studies on the carcinogenicity of the resulting two fractions, the aqueous fraction [IV-A] and the n-butanol fraction [IV-B], were carried out, the results indicating that the latter fraction [IV-B] was markedly carcinogenic (Table 4–3). Subsequently, the n-butanol fraction [IV-B] dissolved in water was treated with a resin, TOYOPEARL HW-40 (c), in order to adsorb flavonoids on the resin, and the mixture was stirred and filtered. The residue [V-A] obtained on concentration of the filtrate showed strong carcinogenicity, whereas the eluate residue [V-B] obtainable

Table 4–3. Carcinogenicity of Bracken Fractions Administered to Rats

Fraction	Rats[1]			Bracken diet		Amount of fraction	Experimental	Incidence of tumor		
	No.	Strain	Age (weeks)	Concentration over usual bracken content	Administration period (days)	ingested per rat (g)	period (days)	Mammary gland	Intestine	Urinary bladder
I-A[2]										
I-B										
II-A	5	ACI	6	×5	174	416.9	174	0/5	0/5	0/5
II-B	5	ACI	6	×5	174	42.9	174	1/5	4/5	4/5
III-A	7	CD	4	×5	133	27.0	192	7/7(83)[3]	7/7	4/7
III-B	7	CD	4	×5	133	16.0	176	7/7	5/7	4/7
IV-A	7	CD	4	×7.5 (7 days)	120	14.1	171	0/7	3/7	0/7
IV-B	7	CD	4	subsequently ×6	127	19.1	164	7/7(105)	7/7	6/7
V-A	7	CD	4	×5 (35 days)	133	9.4	218	7/7 (93)	7/7	5/7
V-B	7	CD	4	subsequently ×3	119	5.1	213	0/7	0/7	0/7

[1] All rats used were female.

[2] Carcinogenicity of boiling water extract was reported previously.

[3] Appearance of the first mammary tumor (in days).

from the resin adsorbate was not carcinogenic (Table 4–3). Thus separation using the resin adsorption and the solvents partition described above provided the fraction [V-A] exhibiting strong carcinogenicity, which was obtained in about 0.3% yield based on the dried powdered bracken.

The fraction [V-A] was analyzed by means of high-performance liquid chromatography (HPLC) and shown to consist of more than ten compounds. As preliminary experiments in the search for bracken carcinogen(s), the compounds in the fraction [V-A] were separated, isolated in minute amounts by HPLC, and subjected to structural analysis. Among them, a new compound, ptaquiloside (1), was isolated as one of the major components of the fraction [V-A] and was found to be unstable. To isolate ptaquiloside (1) on a large scale, the fraction [V-A] was chromatographed on silica gel with chloroform-methanol (5:1); during the column chromatography decomposition of ptaquiloside (1) took place to some extent. Fractions containing ptaquiloside (1) obtained after silica gel chromatography were further separated and purified by repeating reversed phase HPLC [i, Fuji gel ODS-Q3 and methanol-water (40:60); ii, Develosil ODS-5 and methanol-water (55:45)] to afford ptaquiloside (1) which was at least 99% pure and obtained in 0.02% yield based on the dried powdered bracken.

4.9 Structure and Properties of Ptaquiloside (1)

Ptaquiloside (1) is a colorless amorphous compound with the following physical and spectral properties:[110]

molecular formula $C_{20}H_{30}O_8$,
$[\alpha]_D^{22} -188°$ (c 1.00, CH_3OH),
IR (KBr) 3400 (broad), 1724, 1640 (weak) cm^{-1},
SIMS m/z 421 (M + Na)$^+$.

4.9.1 Chemical properties of ptaquiloside (1)[110]

Ptaquiloside (1) is an unstable compound, which gave pterosin B (4)[71,111-113] and D-glucose in both acidic and basic aqueous solutions at room temperature (Fig. 4–6). For example, the half-life of ptaquiloside (1) in 0.01 M sulfuric acid-methanol at 22°C was about two hours. Acetylation of ptaquiloside (1) with acetic anhydride and pyridine yielded crystal-

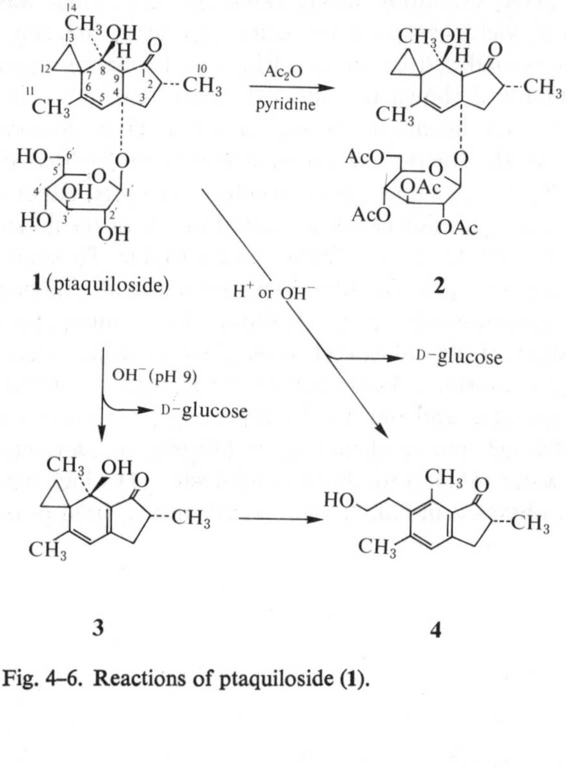

Fig. 4–6. Reactions of ptaquiloside (1).

line ptaquiloside tetraacetate (**2**) (Fig. 4–6). In weakly alkaline aqueous solution (pH 8–10) at room temperature ptaquiloside (**1**) was converted with liberation of D-glucose to an unstable conjugated dienone (**3**), which was found to be particularly unstable in a weakly acidic aqueous solution and immediately transformed into pterosin B (**4**) (Fig. 4–6).

4.9.2 Planar structure of ptaquiloside (**1**)[110]

Tables 4–4 and 4–5 show the NMR spectral data of ptaquiloside (**1**) and the derivatives (**2**) and (**3**). The planar structure of ptaquiloside (**1**) was established by NMR spectral analysis and chemical properties.

The ¹H-NMR and ¹H-NMDR spectra of ptaquiloside (**1**) together with the proton noise-decoupled, off-resonance, and selective proton decoupled ¹³C-NMR spectra disclosed the presence of the partial structures I–VII (cf. Tables 4–4 and 4–5). The partial structures I–VII contain all carbon atoms in ptaquiloside (**1**), and the problem to be solved in the next stage was the correlation of these partial structures, which was made possible by long range selective proton decoupling experiments (LSPD).[114]

Table 4–4. ¹H-NMR Spectral Data[†1]

	1[†2]	2[†3]	3[†3]
2	2.23 (ddq, 12.5, 8.0, 6.9)	2.23 (ddq, 12.2, 8.2, 7.0)	2.47 (ddq, 7.6, 6.7, 2.4)
3a	1.93 (t, 12.5)	1.93 (t, 12.2)	2.18 (dd, 18.6, 2.4)
3b	2.49 (dd, 12.5, 8.0)	2.42 (dd, 12.2, 8.2)	2.85 (dd, 18.6, 6.7)
5	5.76 (dq, 1.3, 1.0)	5.73 (quint, 1.5)	6.11 (q, 1.2)
9	2.64 (d, 1.3)	2.53 (d, 1.5)	—
10	1.07 (d, 6.9)	1.07 (d, 7.0)	1.15 (d, 7.6)
11	1.53 (d, 1.0)	1.55 (d, 1.5)	1.74 (d, 1.2)
12a	0.48 (m)[†4]	0.51 (m)[†5]	0.62 (ddd, 9.8, 7.0, 4.3)[†6]
12b	0.86 (m)[†4]	0.87 (m)[†5]	1.06 (ddd, 9.8, 6.7, 4.9)[†6]
13a	0.69 (m)[†4]	0.71 (m)[†5]	0.92 (ddd, 9.8, 7.0, 4.9)[†6]
13b	0.86 (m)[†4]	0.87 (m)[†5]	1.40 (ddd, 9.8, 6.7, 4.3)[†6]
14	1.29 (s)	1.15 (s)	1.24 (s)
1′	4.60 (d, 7.6)	5.07 (d, 7.9)	—
2′	*	4.90 (dd, 9.7, 7.9)	—
3′	*	5.28 (t, 9.7)	—
4′	3.20 (dd, 8.9, 9.1)	4.98 (t, 9.7)	—
5′	*	3.94 (ddd, 9.7, 5.5, 2.5)	—
6′a	3.66 (dd, 11.9, 5.6)	4.17 (dd, 12.2, 5.5)	—
6′b	3.90 (dd, 11.9, 1.3)	4.25 (dd, 12.5, 2.5)	—
Ac	—	1.95, 1.96, 2.02, 2.07	—

[†1] Chemical shifts are in ppm relative to TMS. The values shown in parentheses are coupling constants in Hz. Spectra were taken in CD₃OD.
[†2] Observed at 270 MHz.
[†3] Observed at 400 MHz.
[†4,5,6] Assignments may be interchanged.
* These signals could not be observed by overlapping with a solvent signal.

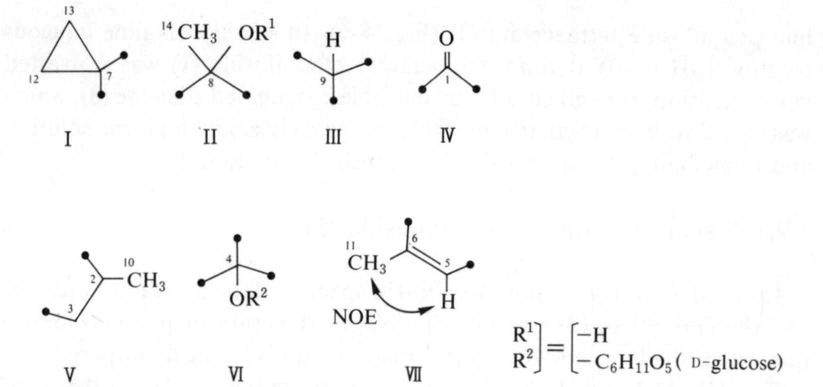

Chart 4.1

A circle [•] denotes a quaternary carbon.

In the proton coupled ^{13}C-NMR spectrum of **1** under the gated decoupling experiment, all quaternary carbon signals at δ_C 31.0 (C-7 in I), 72.9 (C-8 in II), 224.9 (C-1 in IV), 83.0 (C-4 in VI), and 145.3 (C-6 in VII) were observed as broad singlets with fine splittings arising from two and/or three bond C-H couplings ($^2J_{C-H}$ and/or $^3J_{C-H}$).   (a) LSPD irradiating H-14 (δ_H 1.29) in II collapsed the C-7 (δ_C 31.0) and C-8 (δ_C 72.9) carbon signals to the better defined broad singlets, indicating that the protons (H-14) of the methyl group in II are three bonds away from the C-7 quaternary carbon in I: the cyclopropane ring in I is therefore connected to the C-8 carbon in II.   (b) The splitting pattern of the C-7 carbon signal in I also became simple on irradiation of H-11 (δ_H 1.53) in VII, revealing that the C-6 carbon is bonded to the C-7 carbon. These findings, (a) and (b), made it possible to correlate three partial structures, I, II, and VII, leading to a new partial structure VIII, which was further supported by NOE experiments between H-14 in II and H-13a in I, and between H-11 in VII and two proton signals of the cyclopropane ring [H-12a and H-13b (or H-12b)] in I.   (c) LSPD irradiating H-10 (δ_H 1.07) in V simplified the C-1

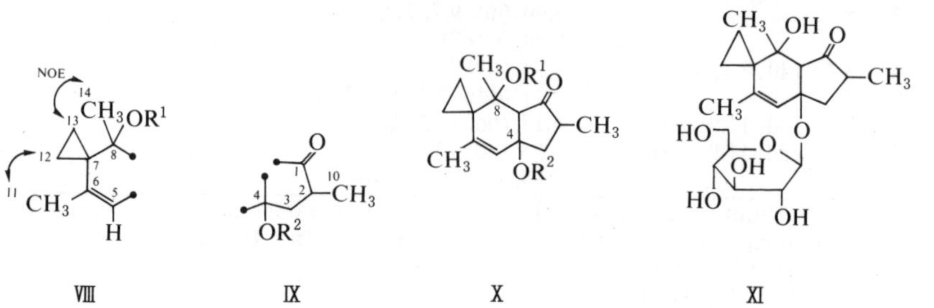

VIII   IX   X   XI

Chart 4.2

Table 4–5. ^{13}C-NMR Spectral Data[†1]

	1[†2]		2[†3]	
1	224.9	(s)	221.7	(s)
2	46.1	(d, 120.4)	43.9	(d, 125.0)
3	46.1	(t, 130.8)	44.5	(t, 130.0)
4	83.0	(s)	81.4	(s)
5	124.2	(d, 161.1)	120.0	(d, 159.5)
6	145.3	(s)	145.6	(s)
7	31.0	(s)	29.4	(s)
8	72.9	(s)	70.0	(s)
9	63.5	(d, 129.2)	61.4	(d, 130.0)
10	14.5	(q, 125.5)	13.4	(q, 125.2)
11	20.3	(q, 125.0)	19.6	(q, 126.3)
12	6.8	(t, 159.5)	5.6	(t, 160.0)
13	11.5	(t, 159.5)	10.6	(t, 160.0)
14	27.9	(q, 126.0)	26.4	(q, 126.5)
1′	100.2	(d, 159.9)	95.9	(d, 159.0)
2′	76.2	(d, 143.1)	71.6[†5]	(d, 149.4)
3′	78.7[†4]	(d, 141.2)	71.8[†5]	(d, 149.0)
4′	72.9	(d, 143.5)	69.1	(d, 149.9)
5′	79.2[†4]	(d, 141.5)	73.2	(d, 148.5)
6′	63.9	(t, 143.6)	62.5	(t, 148.9)
			170.4, 170.2	
Ac	—		169.4, 169.0	
			20.8, 20.6	

[†1] Chemical shifts are in ppm relative to TMS.
    The values shown in parentheses are $^1J_{C-H}$.
[†2] Spectra were taken in CD_3OD at 67.8 MHz.
[†3] Spectra were taken in $CDCl_3$ at 22.5 MHz.
[†4,5] Assignments may be interchanged.

carbonyl carbon signal in IV, indicating that the C-2 carbon in V is connected to the C-1 carbon in IV. (d) Since the C-2 and C-3 carbons in V must be connected to quaternary carbons as described above, the remaining quaternary carbon C-4 (δ_C 83.0) in VI is necessarily bonded to the C-3 carbon in V. Based on these observations, (c) and (d), correlation of three partial structures, IV, V, and VI could be made to give a new partial structure IX. (e) LSPD of H-9 (δ_H 2.64) in III greatly simplified three quaternary carbon signals (C-1, C-4, and C-8), showing that the C-9 carbon in III is bonded to C-8 in VIII and to C-1 and C-4 in IX as well to afford the planar structure X for ptaquiloside (1). The planar structure X was chemically confirmed by the formation of pterosin B (4) from ptaquiloside (1) as described above.

The location of D-glucose and stereochemistry of the glycosidic linkage in ptaquiloside (1) were determined as follows. The β-configuration of the glycosidic linkage in ptaquiloside (1) was established by the coupling constant of the anomeric proton signal H-1′ [δ_H 4.60 (1H, d, $J = 7.6$ Hz)] and the C-H coupling constant of the anomeric carbon signal C-1′ (δ_C

100.2, $J_{C-H} = 159.9$ Hz). The location of the glycosidic linkage was determined by LSPD of the anomeric proton signal H-1' in ptaquiloside (1): irradiation of H-1' in 1 eliminated a long range coupling from the C-4 carbon signal, indicating unambiguously that D-glucose is bonded to the hydroxyl group at C-4. Further evidence showing the location of the glycosidation linkage in ptaquiloside (1) is the formation of the conjugated dienone (3) with concomitant liberation of D-glucose on treatment of 1 with aqueous base. Therefore, the planar structure of ptaquiloside (1) was determined to be XI.

4.9.3 Stereochemistry of ptaquiloside (1)[115]

From the NOE experiment in the ^{1}H-NMR spectrum of ptaquiloside (1) the tertiary methyl group (H-14) and the methine (H-9) at the ring juncture were shown to be *cis*.

The whole stereostructure including absolute stereochemistry of ptaquiloside was determined to be represented by 1 in terms of X-ray crystallographic analysis of ptaquiloside tetraacetate (2).

4.9.4 Structure and chemical reactivity of ptaquiloside (1)

Ptaquiloside (1) is a glucoside of the norsequiterpene belonging to the illudane type. Although sesquiterpenes of this type occur rather rarely in nature, illudin-S (5)[116−118] isolated as a toxic compound from the bioluminescent mushroom is worthy of mention as an example of the illudane type sesquiterpenes so far known. Whereas ptaquiloside (1) shows prominent carcinogenicity, illudin-S (5) is known to have antitumor activity.

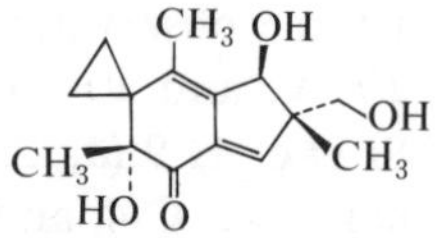

5

Chart 4.3

As described above, ptaquiloside (1) readily undergoes aromatization by the action of acids or bases to give stable aromatic compounds having the indanone skeleton, e.g., pterosin B (4): a number of aromatic sesquiterpenes named pterosins and pterosides have been isolated as characteristic constituents of bracken.[112, 113] Biogenetically, ptaquiloside (1) can be regarded as a precursor of these aromatic sesquiterpenes, pterosins and pterosides.

The instability of ptaquiloside (1) is evidently due to the ready conversion to various aromatic compounds as described. There seem to be two possible pathways for the conversion of ptaquiloside (1) into stable aromatic compounds. One plausible pathway is the facile conversion of ptaquiloside (1) with concomitant elimination of D-glucose to the unstable dienone (3), which is further transformed rapidly into stable aromatic compounds. The extreme instability of the dienone (3) can be ascribed to the presence of the highly reactive cyclopropane ring, which is conjugated with the keto group and constitutes a cyclopropylcarbinol system as well: the cyclopropane ring in the dienone (3) can react with various nucleophiles (e.g., water, methanol, amines, thiols, etc.) quite readily. The other possible pathway is the direct conversion of ptaquiloside (1) accompanied by elimination of D-glucose into stable aromatic compounds without intervention of the dienone (3): ptaquiloside (1) possesses the cyclopropylcarbinol group, which is well known to generate a non-classical cation capable of reacting with a variety of nucleophiles under solvolytic conditions.

4.10 Carcinogenicity Test of Ptaquiloside (PT)[119]

Female CD rats were used for carcinogenicity testing of PT. Group 1 consisted of 12 female CD rats, each of which was given an intragastric administration of 780 mg of PT/kg body weight on day 25 after birth. They were then administered 100 mg PT/kg body wt 17 days after the first administration. Subsequently, they were given consecutive intragastric administration once a week for 7 weeks as shown in Table 4–6. Group

Table 4–6. Administration Schedule of PT

Week	Dose of PT by intragastric administration (mg/kg body wt)†	
	Group 1	Group 2
1	780	100 ($\times$2)
2	—	100 ($\times$2)
3	100	150 ($\times$2)
4	200	150 ($\times$2)
5	200	100 ($\times$2)
6	200	100 ($\times$2)
7	150	100 ($\times$2)
8	100	100 ($\times$2)
9	100	100
10	100	

† Group 1 was administered once weekly and group 2 twice weekly, escept for a single administration made in week 9.

2, consisting of 12 female CD rats, 28 days old, received intragastric administration of PT twice a week for 8 weeks and only a single administration in week 9. The administration schedule of PT in experiment group 2 is also shown in Table 4–6. The average total doses of PT per rat in groups 1 and 2 were 300 mg and 339 mg, respectively. PT was freshly dissolved in 1 ml of physiological saline each time and administered by means of a metal gastric tube. Food and water were withheld from 10:00 to 15:00 h prior to administration of PT. Then, PT was given to rats between 15:00 h and 16:00 h when their stomachs were nearly empty. After administration of PT, food and water were given ad libitum. Since PT is unstable at room temperature under both acidic and basic conditions, it was kept at -20°C in a freezer. Another group of 15 female CD rats, 25 days old, without treatment, served as controls. The experiment was terminated 300 days after the start of administration of PT.

All rats of group 1 had severe hematuria and urinary incontinence after the first intragastric administration of 780 mg PT/kg body wt and 2 of 12 rats died 3 days after the administration. Five rats in group 1 died within 83 days after the start of the experiment. The remaining 7 rats survived more than 190 days and all had mammary cancer (Table 4–7). The earliest

Table 4–7. Incidence of Tumor Induced by PT in Female CD Rats

Group	Initial No. of rats	Effective No. of rats[1]	No. of rats with tumors of		
			Mammary gland	Ileum	Urinary bladder
Group 1	12	7	7 (4.8)[2]	4	0
Group 2	12	11	10 (3.9)	10	1
Control	15	15	0	0	0

[1] No. surviving for more than 165 days after the start of the experiment.
[2] Figure in parentheses is the average number of tumors per rat.

mammary tumor was detected by palpation on day 82. The average number of mammary tumors per rat was 4 8. Histologically, the tumors were adenocarcinoma, papillary carcinoma and anaplastic carcinoma, i.e., the same as those induced in CD rats fed a bracken diet. Mammary cancer induced in a rat which was sacrificed 265 days after the start of experiment showed metastasis in the lung. Furthermore, 4 of these 7 rats (57%) also had multiple ileal adenocarcinomas. No urinary bladder tumors were induced. However, squamous metaplasia or preneoplastic hyperplasia of the urinary bladder mucosa was present in 8 of 10 rats which survived more than 40 days. In group 2, all rats, except one which died 60 days after the start of experiment, survived more than 165 days and 8 rats survived beyond 270 days. Mammary cancers were induced in 10 of 11 (effective number) rats (91%). The earliest mammary tumor was detected on day 94 after the start of PT administration. The average number of mammary tumors per rat was 3.9. The histological types and incidence were similar to those in group 1. One animal which died 276 days after the start of the experiment showed lung metastasis of the mammary cancer. Multiple ileal adenocarcinomas were also observed in 10 of 11 rats (91%). Although urinary bladder papilloma was induced only in one rat, hyperplasia of the bladder mucosa was encountered in 7 of 11 rats. No tumors were found in rats of the control group.

Since PT is unstable under both acidic and basic conditions, it was administered into the empty stomach in order to have the compound transit the stomach as rapidly as possible and minimize decomposition. The low incidence of urinary bladder tumor in this experiment was considered to be due to the short period of PT administration and relatively early death of the animals from mammary cancer. The incidences of mammary cancer were 100% and 91% in groups 1 and 2, respectively. Ileal tumor was also induced in high incidence, 57% and 91%, and the terminal 20 cm of the ileum was the most common site, as in the case of rats fed bracken diet. From these results, it is evident that PT is one of the carcinogenic principles of bracken fern. Van der Hoeven *et al.*[120] isolated from bracken fern a new mutagenic compound which has the same planar structure as PT and named it aquilide A.

A previous experiment by our group indicated no significant difference in the incidence of intestinal tumors between germ-free and conventional rats fed a diet containing bracken, suggesting that gut microflora does not play a definite role in bracken tumorigenesis.[121] Since it is assumed that PT is converted with concomitant elimination of glucose into an unstable dienone under particular alkaline conditions,[110] it is logical that no significant difference was observed in the incidence of intestinal tumors between germ-free and conventional rats fed a bracken diet.

4.11 Reproduction of Acute Bracken Poisoning with PT[122]

Very recently, it was demonstrated that the causative principle of cattle bracken poisoning is also ptaquiloside.

A female Holstein-Friesian, six-month-old calf was given PT. The PT was dissolved in 500 ml of 0.9% saline and administered by drench, once in the morning before feeding. Since PT is unstable at room temperature, it was kept at $-20°C$ and dissolved just before administration.

The PT was administered six of every seven days as follows: 400mg/day for the first 24 days, 800 mg/day for 14 days and 1600 mg/day for 4 days.

The total amount of PT administered was 27.2 g. Blood samples were taken twice a week from the jugular vein, using a Vacutainer tube containing EDTA. Red and white blood cells were counted in a Coulter counter. Thrombocytes were counted by the direct counting method.

Leucocyte counts increased greatly upon PT administration and reached maximum ($25.3 \times 10^3/mm^3$) on day 17 after start of administration, following large fluctuations. Subsequently, they decreased and reached a level of $4.7 \times 10^3/mm^3$ on day 64 after the start of the experiment. Neutrophilic granulocyte numbers followed a pattern similar to that of leucocytes. They began to decrease rapidly about 50 days after the start of administration, reaching a minimum of $0.1 \times 10^3/mm^3$. The granulocytopenia continued for about 35 days until the autopsy, despite cessation of PT administration. The erythrocyte level remained between 6 and $8 \times 10^6/mm^3$ during the course of the study. Thrombocyte levels showed a relatively slow depression accompanied by mild fluctuations, and reached a minimum level of $1 \times 10^5/mm^3$ 50 days after the beginning of the administration of PT (Fig. 4–7). After the PT administration was stopped, the thrombocyte count gradually began to recover, but still remained

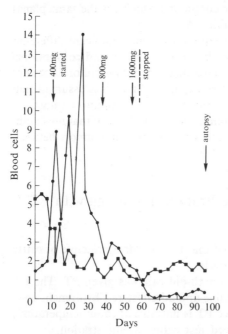

Fig. 4–7. Neutrophilic granulocyte and thrombocyte counts of a calf receiving drench of ptaquiloside. ● Neutrophilic granulocytes ($\times 10^3/mm^3$), ■ thrombocytes ($\times 10^5/mm^3$)

less than $2 \times 10^5/\text{mm}^3$ one month later. The calf was autopsied 86 days after the start of administration of PT. Sternal bone marrow was found to be mostly replaced with fat marrow and only small foci of erythropoietic cells and a small number of megakaryocytes remained.

REFERENCES

1. Radeleff, R.D., *Veterinary Toxicology*, Lea and Febiger, Philadelphia, pp. 74–77, 1970.
2. Evans, W.C., Patel, M.C. and Koohy, Y., Acute bracken poisoning in homogastric and ruminant animals., *Proc. Royal Soc. Edinburgh*, **81B**: 29–64, 1982.
3. Weswig, P.H., Freed, A.M. and Haag, J.R., Antithiamine activity of plant materials, *J. Biol. Chem.*, **165**: 737–738, 1946.
4. Evans, W.C., and Evans, E.T.R., The effects of the inclusion of bracken (*Pteris aquilina*) in the diet of rats, and the problem of bracken poisoning in farm animals. *Br. Vet. J.*, **105**: 175–186, 1949.
5. Thomas, B., and Walker, H.F., The inactivation of thiamine by bracken (*Pteris aquilina*), *J. Soc. Chem. Ind. Lond.*, **68**: 6–9, 1949.
6. Evans, W.C., Jones, N.R., and Evans, R.A., The mechanism of the anti-aneurin activity of bracken (*Pteris aquilina*), *Biochem. J.* (Proc. Biochem. Soc.), **46**: 38–39, 1950.
7. Evans, W.C., and Jones, N.R., Plant thiaminases, *Biochem. J.* (Proc. Biochem. Soc.), **50**: 28, 1952.
8. Evans, W.C., Evans, E.T.R., and Hughes, L.E., Studies on bracken poisoning in cattle, Part 1. *Brit. Vet. J.*, **110**: 295–306, 1954.
9. Evans, W.C., Evans, I.A., Thomas, A.J., Watkins, J.E., and Chamberlain, A.G., Studies on bracken poisoning in cattle. (Part IV) *Brit. Vet. J.*, **114**: 180–198, 1958.
10. Evans, W.C., Evans, I.A., Chamberlain, A.G., and Thomas, A.J., Studies on bracken poisoning in cattle. (Part VI) *Brit. Vet. J.*, **115**: 83–85, 1959.
11. Watson, W.A., Barlow, R.M., and Barnett, K.C., Bright blindness—A condition prevalent in Yorkshire hill sheep, *Vet. Rec.*, **77**: 1060–1069, 1965.
12. Barnett, K.C., and Watson, W.A. Bright blindness in sheep, A primary retinopathy due to feeding bracken (*Pteris aquilina*), *Res. Vet. Sci.*, **11**: 289–290, 1970.
13. Rosenberger, G., Nature, manifestations, cause and control of chronic enzootic haematuria in cattle, *Veterinary med. rev.*, No. 2/3, 189–206, **1971**.
14. Götze, R. Über das chronische Blutharnen des Rindes, *Dtsch. tierarztl. Wschr.*, **50**: 57–61, 1942(in German).
15. Rosenberger, G., and Heeschen, W., Adlerfarn (*Pteris aquilina*) — die Ursache des sog. Stallrotes der Rinder (Haematuria vesicalis bovis chronica), *Dtsch. tierarztl. Wschr.*, **67**: 201–208, 1960 (in German).
16. Evans, W.C., Evans, I.A., Axford, R.F.E., Threlfall, G., Humphreys, D.A., and Thomas, A.J., Studies on bracken poisoning in cattle Part VII. — The toxicity of bracken rhizomes, *Vet. Rec.*, **73**: 852–853, 1961.
17. Georgiev, R., Antonov, S., Vrigasov, A., Dimitrov, A., and Goranov, C., Über die Ätiologie der chronischen vesikalen Hämaturie der Rinder 1. Mitteilung, Zur Frage des Karzinomatösen Charakters der chronischen vesikalen Hämaturie der Rinder, *Wien. tierarztl. Msch.* **51**: 641–657, 1964 (in German).
18. Pamukcu, A.M., Epidemiologic studies on urinary bladder tumors in Turkish cattle, *Ann. NY Acad. Sci.*, **108**: 938–947, 1963.
19. Evans, I.A., and Mason, J., Carcinogenic activity of bracken, *Nature* (London) **208**: 913–914, 1965.

20. Pamukcu, A.M., Göksoy, S.K., and Price, J.M., Urinary bladder neoplasms induced by feeding bracken fern (*Pteris aquilina*) to cows, *Cancer Res.*, **27**: 917–924, 1967.
21. Pamukcu, A.M., and Price, J.M. Induction of intestinal and urinary bladder cancer in rats by feeding bracken fern (*Pteris aquilina*), *J. Natl. Cancer Inst.*, **43**: 275–281, 1969.
22. Price, J.M., and Pamukcu, A.M., The induction of neoplasms of the urinary bladder of the cow and the small intestine of the rat by feeding bracken fern (*Pteris aquilina*), *Cancer Res.*, **28**: 2247–2251, 1968.
23. Pamukcu, A.M., Price, J.M., and Bryan, G.T., Naturally occurring and bracken-fern-induced bovine urinary bladder tumors. *Vet. Pathol.*, **13**: 110–122, 1976.
24. Hirono, I., Sasaoka, I., Shibuya, C., Shimizu, M., Fushimi, K., Mori, H., Kato, K., and Haga, M., Natural carcinogenic products of plant origin, *GANN Monograph on Cancer Research*, **17**: 205–217, 1975.
25. Hodge, W.H., Fern foods of Japan and the problem of toxicity. *Am. Fern. J.*, **63**: 77–80, 1973.
26. Hirono, I., Shibuya, C., Fushimi, K., and Haga, M., Studies on caricinogenic properties of bracken, *Pteridium aquilinum*. *J. Natl. Cancer Inst.*, **45**: 179–188, 1970.
27. Yunoki, K., Hayashi, T., and Morita, N., Induction of intestinal tumors in rats with feeding of bracken fern, *Acta. Med. Univ. Kagoshima*, **14**: 249–254, 1972.
28. Saito, M., Umeda, M., Enomoto, M., Hatanaka, Y., Natori, S., Yoshihira, K., Fukuoka, M., and Kuroyanagi, M., Cytotoxicity and carcinogenicity of pterosins and pterosides, 1-indanone derivatives from bracken (*Pteridium aquilinum*), *Experientia*, **31**: 829–831, 1975.
29. Hirono, I., Shibuya, C., Shimizu, M., and Fushimi, K., Carcinogenic activity of processed bracken used as human food, *J. Natl. Cancer Inst.*, **48**: 1245–1250, 1972.
30. Hirono, I., Shibuya, C., and Fushimi, K., Experimental studies on sites of tumor development in the intestine by chemical carcinogens, In "Pathophysiology of carcinogenesis in digestive organs," eds. Farber E. *et al.* Univ. Tokyo Press, Tokyo, pp. 285–295, **1977**.
31. Schacham, P., Philp. R.B., and Gowdey, C.W., Antihematopoietic and carcinogenic effects of bracken fern (*Pteridium aquilinum*) in rats. *Am. J. Vet. Res.*, **31**: 191–197, 1970.
32. Hirono, I., Fushimi, K., Mori, H., Miwa, T., and Haga, M,, Comparative study of carcinogenic activity in each part of bracken, *J. Natl. Cancer Inst.*, **50**: 1367–1371, 1973.
33. Hirono, I., Aiso, S., Hosaka, S., Yamaji, T., and Haga, M., Induction of mammary cancer in CD rats fed bracken diet, *Carcinogenesis*, **4**: 885–887, 1983.
34. Evans, I.A., The radiomimetic nature of bracken toxin, *Cancer Res.*, **28**: 2252–2261, 1968.
35. Evans, I.A., and Widdop, B., Carcinogenic activity of bracken, British empire cancer campaign for research, Annual Report, p. 377, **1966**.
36. Miayakwa, M., and Yoshida, O., Induction of tumors of the urinary bladder in female mice following surgical implantation of glass beads and feeding of bracken fern, *Gann*, **66**: 437–439, 1975.
37. Pamukcu, A.M., Ertüuk, E., Price, J.M., and Bryan, G.T., Lymphatic leukemia and pulmonary tumors in female Swiss mice fed bracken fern (*Pteris aquilina*), *Cancer Res.*, **32**: 1442–1445, 1972.
38. Kawai, T., Nakayama, M., Takanashi, H., Uchida, E., Ueno, I., Hosaka, S., Mori, H., and Hirono, I., Carcinogenicity of bracken fern to Syrian golden hamsters, unpublished.
39. Ushijima, J., Matsukawa, K. and Yuasa, R., Oncogenic activity of bracken fern, *Jap. J. Vet. Sci.*, **33**: 129–130, 1971, (in Japanese).
40. Evans, I.A. Bracken carcinogenicity, In "Chemical carcinogens, ACS Monograph 182" (ed. C.E. Searle), pp. 1171–1204, American Chemical Society, Washington, D.C., 1984.
41. Ushijima, J., Matsukawa, K., Yuasa, A., and Okada, M., Toxicities of bracken fern

in Guinea pigs, *Jpn. J. Vet. Sci.*, **45**: 593–602, 1983.

42. Evans, I.A., Bracken fern toxin. In Oncology 1970: Proc. 10th Int. Cancer Cong. Vol. 5, Part A Environmental Cancer, pp. 178–195, Year Book Med. Pub., Chicago, Ill., 1972.
43. Evans, I.A., Prorok, J.H., Cole, R.C., Al-Salmani, M.H., AL-Samarrai, A.M.H., Patel, M.C., and Smith R.M.M., The carcinogenic, mutagenic and teratogenic toxicity of bracken, *Proc. Royal. Soc. Edinburgh*, **81B**: 65–77, 1982.
44. Matsushima, T., Sato, S., Hara, K., Sugimura, T., and Takashima, F., Bioassay of environmental carcinogens with the guppy, *Lebistes reticulatas, Mutat. Res.*, **31**: 265, 1975.
45. El-mofty, M.M., Sadek, I.A., and Bayoumi, S., Improvement in detecting the carcinogenicity of bracken fern using an Egyptian toad. *Oncology*, **37**: 424–425, 1980.
46. Pamukcu, A.M., Investigations on the pathology of enzootic bovine hematuria in Turkey, *Zentralbl. Vet. Med.*, **2**: 409–429, 1955.
47. Pamukcu, A.M., Tumors of the urinary bladder in cattle, with special reference to etiology and histogenesis, *Acta Unio. Int. Contra Cancrum*, **18**: 625–638, 1962.
48. Harburtt, R.P., and Leaver, D.D., Carcinoma of the bladder of sheep, *Aust. Vet. J.*, **45**: 473–475, 1969.
49. McDonald, J.W., and Leaver, D.D., Adenocarcinoma of the small intestine of Merino sheep, *Aust. Vet. J.*, **41**: 269–271, 1965.
50. Dodd, D.C., Adenocarcinoma of the small intestine of sheep, *New Zealand Vet. J.*, **8**: 100–112, 1960.
51. Jarrett, W.F.H., McNeil, P.E., Grimshaw, W.T.R., Selman, I.E., and McIntyre, W.I.M., High incidence area of cattle cancer with a possible interaction between an environmental carcinogen and a papilloma virus, *Nature* (London), **274**: 215–217, 1978.
52. Döbereiner, J., Tokarnia, C.H., and Canella, C.F.C., Occurrence of enzootic haematuria and epidermoid carcinoma of the upper digestive tract of cattle in Brazil, *Pesqi. Agropec. Brasil*, **2**: 489–504, 1967.
53. Tokarnia, C.H., Döbereiner, J., and Canella, C.F.C. Occurrence of enzootic hematuria and epidermoid carcinoma of the upper digestive tract of cattle in Brazil. II. Complementary studies, *Pesq. Agropec. Brasil*, **4**: 209–234, 1969.
54. Neto, O.C., Barros, H.M., and Bicudo, P.L., Study of the carcinoma of upper digestive tract and of the enzootic haematuria in cattle in the region of Botucatu, State of Sao Paulo. *Arq. Esc. Vet. Univ. Fed. Minas Gerais*, **27**: 125–139, 1975.
55. Hirono, I., Hosaka, S., and Kuhara, K. Enhancement by bracken of induction of tumors of the upper alimentary tract by *N*-propyl-*N*-nitrosourethan, *Br. J. Cancer*, **46**: 423–427, 1982.
56. McCrea, C.T., and Head, K.W., II. Experimental production of tumors, *Brit. Vet. J.*, **137**: 21–30, 1981.
57. Watson, W.A., Barnett, K.C., and Terlecki, S., Progressive retinal degeneration (bright blindness) in sheep: a review, *Vet. Rec.*, **91**: 665–670, 1972.
58. Yasuda, Y., Kihara, T., and Nishimura, H. Embryotoxic effects of feeding bracken fern (*Pteridium aquilinum*) to pregnant mice, *Toxicol. Appl. Pharmacol.*, **28**: 264–268, 1974.
59. Fushimi, K., Kato, T., and Hirono, I., Influence of bracken meal on pregnant mice, *Acta Schol. Med. Univ. Gifu*, **21**: 448–452, 1973.
60. Pamukcu, A.M., Yalciner, S., Price, J.M., and Bryan, G.T., Effects of coadministration of thiamine on the incidence of urinary bladder carcinomas in rats fed bracken fern, *Cancer Res.*, **30**: 2671–2674, 1970.
61. Pamukcu, A.M., Wattenberg, L.W., Price, J.M., and Bryan, G.T., Phenothiazine inhibition of intestinal and urinary bladder tumors induced in rats by bracken fern, *J. Natl. Cancer Inst.*, **47**: 155–159, 1971.
62. Pamukcu, A.M., Yalciner, S., and Bryan, G.T., Inhibition of carcinogenic effect of bracken fern (*Pteridium aquilinum*) by various chemicals, *Cancer*, **40**: 2450–2454, 1977.

63. Kawai, T., Takanashi, H., Nakayama, M., Mori, H., and Hirono, I., Effect of storage on carcinogenic activity of bracken fern, *Cancer Lett.*, **12**: 29–35, 1981.

64. Kamon, S., and Hirayama, T. Epidemiology of cancer of the oesophagus in Miye, Nara and Wakayama prefectures with special reference to the role of bracken fern, *Proc. Jpn. Cancer Assoc.*, **34**: 211, 1975.

65. Evans, I.A., Widdop, B., Jones, R.S., Barber, G.D., Leach, H., Jones, D.L., and Mainwaring-Burton, R., The possible human hazard of the naturally occurring bracken carcinogen, *Biochem. J.*, **124**: 28–29, 1971.

66. Evans, I.A., Jones, R.S., and Mainwaring-Burton, R., Passage of bracken fern toxicity into milk, *Nature* (London), **237**: 107–108, 1972.

67. Pamukcu, A.M., Ertürk, E., Yalciner, S., Milli, U., and Bryan, G.T., Carcinogenic and mutagenic activities of milk from cows fed bracken fern (*Pteridium aquilinum*), *Cancer Res.*, **38**: 1556–1560, 1978.

68. Pamukcu, A.M., and Bryan, G.T., Bracken fern, a natural urinary bladder and intestinal carcinogen, In "Naturally occurring carcinogens–Mutagens and modulators of carcinogenesis," eds. Miller, E.C. *et al.* Jpn. Sci. Soc. Press, Tokyo/Univ. Park Press, Baltimore, pp. 89–99, **1979**.

69. Nakabayashi, T., Isolation of astragalin and isoquercitrin from bracken, *Pteridium aquilinum, Bull. Aqric. Chem. Soc. Jpn.*, **19**: 104–109, 1955.

70. Wang, C.Y., Pamukcu, A.M., and Bryan, G.T., Isolation of fumaric acid, succinic acid, astragalin, isoquercitrin and tiliroside from *Pteridium aquilinum, Phytochemistry*, **12**: 2298–2299, 1973.

71. Hikino, H., Takahashi, T., Arihara, S., and Takemoto, T., Structure of pteroside B, glycoside of *Pteridium aquilinum* var. *latiusculum, Chem. Pharm. Bull.*, **18**: 1488–1489, 1970.

72. Fukuoka, M., Kuroyanagi, M., Toyama, M., Yoshihira, K., and Natori, S., Pterosins J, K and L and six acylated pterosins from bracken, *Pteridium aquilinum* var. *latiusclum, Chem. Pharm. Bull.*, **20**: 2282–2285, 1972.

73. Takatori, K., Nakano, S., Nagata, S., Okumura, K., Hirono, I., and Shimizu, M., Pterolactam, a new compound isolated from bracken, *Chem. Pharm. Bull.*, **20**: 1087, 1972.

74. Pamukcu, A.M., Olson, C., and Price, J.M., Assay of fractions of bovine urine for carcinogenic activity after feeding bracken fern (*Pteris aquilina*), *Cancer Res.*, **26**: 1745–1753, 1966.

75. Pamukcu, A.M., Price, J.M., and Bryan, G.T., Assay of fractions of bracken fern (*Pteris aquilina*) for carcinogenic activity, *Cancer Res.*, **30**: 902–905, 1970.

76. Leach, H., Barber, G.D., Evans, I.A., and Evans, W.C., Isolation of an active principle from the bracken fern that is mutagenic, carcinogenic and lethal to mice on intraperitoneal injection, *Biochem. J.*, **124**: 13–14, 1971.

77. Evans, I.A., and Osman, M.A., Carcinogenicity of bracken and shikimic acid, *Nature* (London), **250**: 348–349, 1974.

78. Hirono, I., Fushimi, K., and Matsubara, N., Carcinogenicity test of shikimic acid in rats, *Toxicology Letters*, **1**: 9–10, 1977.

79. Wang, C.Y., Chiu, C.W., Pamukcu, A.M., and Bryan, G.T., Identification of carcinogenic tannin isolated from bracken fern (*Pteridium aquilinum*), *J. Natl. Cancer Inst.*, **56**: 33–36, 1976.

80. Pamukcu, A.M., Wang, C.Y., Hatcher, J., and Bryan, G.T., Carcinogenicity of tannin and tannin-free extracts of bracken fern (*Pteridium aquilinum*) in rats, *J. Natl. Cancer Inst.*, **65**: 131–136, 1980.

81. Kofod, H., and Eyjolfsson, R., The isolation of the cyanogenic glycoside prunasin, *Tetrahedr. Lett.*, 1289–1291, **1966**.

82. Hirono, I., Hosaka, S., Uchida, E., Takanashi, H., Haga, M., Sakata, M., Mori, H., Tanaka, T., and Hikino, H., Safety examination of some edible or medicinal plants and plant constituents, Part 3, *J. Food Safety*, **4**: 205–211, 1980.

83. Evans, I.A., Widdop, B., and Barber, G.D., Carcinogenic activity of bracken, British empire cancer campaign for research, Annual Report, p. 411, 1967.

84. Evans, I.A., Bracken carcinogenicity, *Res. Vet. Science*, **26**: 339–348, 1979.
85. Hirono, I., Ushimaru, Y., Kato, K., Mori, H., and Sasaoka, I., Carcinogenicity of boiling water extract of bracken, *Pteridium aquilinum Gann*, **69**: 383–388, 1978.
86. Mori, H., Kato, K., Ushimaru, Y., Kato, T., and Hirono, I., Effect of drying with hot forced draft and of mincing bracken fern on its carcinogenic activity, *Gann*, **68**: 517–520, 1977.
87. Wang, C.Y., Pamukcu, A.M., and Bryan, G.T., Bracken fern, a naturally occurring carcinogen, In: C.C. Stock, L. Santamaria, P. Mariani and S. Gorini (eds.), *Ecological Perspectives on Carcinogens and Cancer Control*, Medicine Biologie Environment, **4**: 565–572, Basal, Karger, 1976.
88. Bjeldanes, L.F., and Chang, G.W., Mutagenic activity of quercetin and related compounds, *Science*, **197**: 577–578, 1977.
89. Brown, J.P., Dietrich, P.S., and Brown, R.J., Frameshift mutagenicity of certain naturally occurring phenolic compounds in "the *Salmonella*/microsome" test: Activation of anthraquinone and flavonol glycosides by gut bacterial enzymes, *Biochem. Soc. Trans.*, **5**: 1489–1492, 1977.
90. Sugimura, T., Nagao, M., Matsushima, T., Yahagi, T., Seino, Y., Shirai, A., Sawamura, M., Natori, S., Yoshihira, K., Fukuoka, M., and Kuroyanagi, M., Mutagenicity of flavone derivatives, *Proc. Jpn. Acad.*, **53**: Ser. B 194–197, 1977.
91. Hardigree, A.A., and Epler, J.L., Comparative mutagenesis of plant flavonoids in microbial systems, *Mutat. Res.*, **58**: 231–239, 1978.
92. McGregor, J.T., and Jurd, L., Mutagenicity of plant flavonoids: Structural requirements for mutagenic activity in *Salmonella typhimurium*, *Mutat. Res.*, **54**: 297–309, 1978.
93. Brown, J.P., and Dietrich, P.S., Mutagenicity of plant flavonols in the *Salmonella*/mammalian microsome test. Activation of flavonol glycosides by mixed glycosidases from rat cecal bacteria and other sources, *Mutat. Res.*, **66**: 223–240, 1979.
94. Maruta, A., Enaka, K., and Umeda, M., Mutagenicity of quercetin and kaempferol on cultured mammalian cells, *Gann*, **70**: 273–276, 1979.
95. Umezawa, K., Matsushima, T., Sugimura, T., Hirakawa, T., Tanaka, M., Katoh, Y., and Takayama, S., In vitro transformation of hamster embryo cells by quercetin, *Toxicol. Lett.*, **1**: 175–178, 1977.
96. Pamukcu, A.M., Yalciner, S., Hatcher, J.F., and Bryan, G.T. Quercetin, a rat intestinal and bladder carcinogen present in bracken fern (*Pteridium aquilinum*), *Cancer Res.*, **40**: 3468–3472, 1980.
97. Saito, D., Shirai, A., Matsushima, T., Sugimura, T., and Hirono, I., Test of carcinogenicity of quercetin, a widely distributed mutagen in food, *Teratogenesis, Carcinogenesis, and Mutagenesis*, **1**: 213–221, 1980.
98. Hosaka, S., and Hirono, I. Carcinogenicity test of quercetin by pulmonary-adenoma bioassay in strain A mice, *Gann*, **72**: 327–328, 1981.
99. Ambrose, A.M., Robbins, D.J., and DeEds, F., Comparative toxicities of quercetin and quercitrin, *J. Am. Pharm. Assoc.*, **41**: 119–122, 1952.
100. Hirono, I., Ueno, I., Hosaka, S., Takanashi, H., Matsushima, T., Sugimura, T., and Natori, S., Carcinogenicity examination of quercetin and rutin in ACI rats, *Cancer Lett.* **13**: 15–21, 1981.
101. Takanashi, H., Aiso, S., Hirono, I., Matsushima, T., and Sugimura, T., Carcinogenicity test of quercetin and kaempferol in rats by oral administration, *J. Food Safety*, **5**: 55–60, 1983.
102. Morino, K., Matsukura, N., Kawachi, T., Ohgaki, H., Sugimura, T., and Hirono, I., Carcinogenicity test of quercetin and rutin in golden hamsters by oral administration, *Carcinogenesis*, **3**: 93–97, 1982.
103. Van Duuren, B.L., and Goldschmidt, B.M., Carcinogenic and tumor-promoting agents in tobacco carcinogenesis, *J. Natl. Cancer Inst.*, **56**: 1237–1242, 1976.
104. Jarrett, W.F.H., personal communication.
105. Evans, I.A., Al-Samarrai, A.M.H., and Smith, R.M.M., Bracken toxicology: Identification of some water-soluble compounds from crozier and rhizome, *Res.*

Vet. Sci., **37**: 261–265, 1984.
106. Yamada, K., Tatematsu, H., Suzuki, M., Hirata, Y., Haga, M., and Hirono, I., Isolation and the structures of two new alkaloids, petasitenine and neopetasitenine from *Petasites japonicus* Maxim., *Chem. Lett.*, 461–464, **1976**.
107. Hirono, I., Mori, H., Yamada, K., Hirata, Y., Haga, M., Tatematsu, H., and Kanie, S., Carcinogenic activity of petasitenine, a new pyrrolizidine alkaloid isolated from *Petasites japonicus* Maxim., *J. Natl. Cancer Inst.*, **58**: 1155–1157, 1977.
108. Nishida, K., Kobayashi, A., and Nagahama, T., Cycasin, a new toxic glycoside of *Cycas revoluta* Thunb. I., Isolation and structure of cycasin, *Bull. Agric. Chem. Soc. Jpn.*, **19**: 77–84, 1955.
109. Hirono, I., Yamada, K., Niwa, H., Shizuri, Y., Ojika, M., Hosaka, S., Yamaji, T., Wakamatsu, K., Kigoshi, H., Niiyama, K., and Uosaki, Y., Separation of carcinogenic fraction of bracken fern, *Cancer Lett.*, **21**: 239–246, 1984.
110. Niwa, H., Ojika, M., Wakamatsu, K., Yamada, K., Hirono, I., and Matsushita, K., Ptaquiloside, a novel norsesquiterpene glucoside from bracken, *Pteridium aquilinum* var. *latiusculum*, *Tetrahedron Lett.*, **24**: 4117–4120, 1983.
111. Yoshihira, K., Fukuoka, M., Kuroyanagi, M., and Natori, S., 1-Indanone derivatives from bracken, *Pteridium aquilinum* var. *latiusculum*, *Chem. Pharm. Bull.*, **19**: 1491–1495, 1971.
112. Yoshihira, K., Fukuoka, M., Kuroyanagi, M., Natori, S., Umeda, M., Morohoshi, T., Enomoto, M., and Saito, M., Chemical and toxicological studies on bracken fern, *Pteridium aquilinum* var. *latiusculum*. I., Introduction, extraction and fractionation of constituents, and toxicological studies including carcinogenicity tests, *Chem. Pharm. Bull.*, **26**: 2346–2364, 1978.
113. Fukuoka, M., Kuroyanagi, M., Yoshihira, K., and Natori, S., Chemical and toxicological studies on bracken fern, *Pteridium aquilinum* var. *latiusculum*. II., Structures of pterosins, sesquiterpenes having 1-indanone skeleton, *Chem. Pharm. Bull.*, **26**: 2365–2385, 1978.
114. Seto, H., Sasaki, T., Yonehara, H., and Uzawa, J. Studies on the biosynthesis of pentalenolactone. Part I., Application of long range selective proton decoupling (LSPD) and selective ^{13}C-{^{1}H} NOE in the structural elucidation of pentalenolactone G., *Tetrahedron Lett.*, 923–926, **1978**.
115. Niwa, H., Ojika, M., Wakamatsu, K., Yamada, K., Ohba, S., Saito, Y., Hirono, I., and Matsushita, K., Stereochemistry of ptaquiloside, a novel norsesquiterpene glucoside from bracken, *Pteridium aquilinum* var. *latiusculum*, *Tetrahedron Lett.*, **24**: 5371–5372, 1983.
116. McMorris, T.C., and Anchel, M., Fungal metabolites, The structures of the novel sesquiterpenoids illudin-S and -M, *J. Am. Chem. Soc.*, **87**: 1594–1600, 1965.
117. Nakanishi, K., Ohashi, M., Tada, M., and Yamada, Y., Illudin S (lampterol), *Tetrahedron*, **21**: 1231–1246, 1965.
118. Matsumoto, T., Shirahama, H., Ichihara, A., Fukuoka, Y., Takahashi, Y., Mori, Y., and Watanabe, M., Structure of lampterol (illudin-S), *Tetrahedron*, **21**: 2671–2676, 1965.
119. Hirono, I., Aiso, S., Yamaji, T., Mori, H., Yamada, K., Niwa, H., Ojika, M., Wakamatsu, K., Kigoshi, H., Niiyama, K., and Uosaki, Y., Carcinogenicity in rats of ptaquiloside isolated from bracken, *Gann*, **75**: 833–836, 1984.
120. Van der Hoeven, J.C.M., Lagerweij, W.J., Posthumus, M.A., van Veldhuizen, A., and Holterman, H.A.J. Aquilide A, a new mutagenic compound isolated from bracken fern (*Pteridium aquilinum* (L.) Kuhn), *Carcinogenesis*, **4**: 1587–1590, 1983.
121. Sumi, Y., Hirono, I., Hosaka, S., Ueno, I., and Miyakawa, M., Tumor induction in germ-free rats fed bracken (*Pteridium aquilinum*), *Cancer Res.*, **41**: 250–252, 1981.
122. Hirono, I., Kono, Y., Takahashi, K., Yamada, K., Niwa, H., Ojika, M., Kigoshi, H., Niiyama, K., and Uosaki, Y., Reproduction of acute bracken poisoning in a calf with ptaquiloside, a bracken constituent, *Vet. Rec.*, **115**: 375–378, 1984.

5

Carrageenan

5.1 Chemical and Physical Properties of Carrageenan

Carrageenan is a sulfated polysaccharide extracted from various red seaweeds and consisting mainly of varying amounts of the ammonium, calcium, magnesium, potassium or sodium salts of sulfate esters of galactose and 3,6-anhydrogalactose copolymers. The principal copolymers are designated κ-, λ-, and ι- (Fig. 5–1) and differ both in structure and in their ability to form gels upon the addition of potassium ions to dilute solutions of carrageenan.[1] Native carrageenan is used in foods, cosmetics,

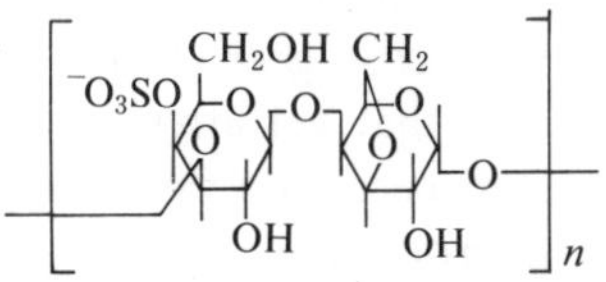

κ-Carrageenan

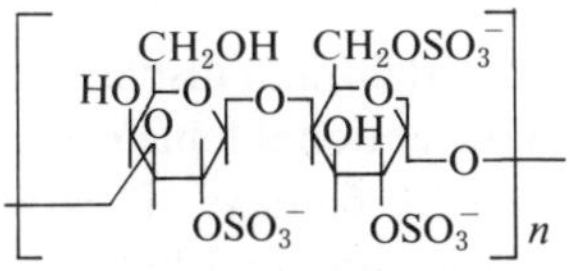

λ-Carrageenan

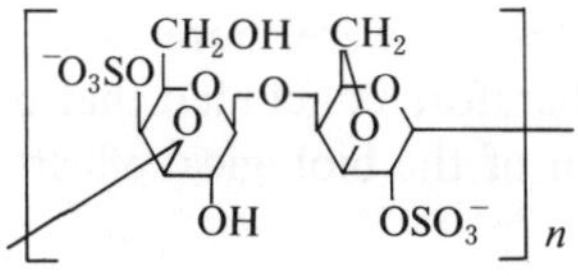

ι-Carrageenan

Fig. 5–1. Chemical structure of carrageenan.

pharmaceuticals and other products in which their ability to stabilize mixtures, emulsify ingredients and thicken or gel solutions are utilized. Degraded carrageenan has been produced from extracts of *Eucheuma spinosum*, the principal component of which is iota-carrageenan, by treatment with dilute hydrochloric acid. It has an average molecular weight of 20,000–40,000. Degraded carrageenan has long been used as an antipeptic agent in Europe.

5.2 Toxic Effect of Carrageenan

It has been reported that oral administration of degraded carrageenan induced hyperplastic mucosal changes in the rabbit colon,[2] as well as ulcerative lesions of the large intestine in guinea pigs,[3] rabbits,[4] rats,[5] and rhesus monkeys.[6] Furthermore, Fabian *et al.*[7] induced colorectal squamous metaplasia and colon adenomatous polyps in rats by prolonged oral administration of degraded carrageenan. Van Der Waaij *et al.*[8] reported that ulcerative lesions of the large intestine induced by degraded carrageenan in guinea pigs were significantly mitigated by selective elimination of aerobic gram-negative intestinal microflora. Onderdonk *et al.*[9] found that pretreatment with metronidazole, an antimicrobial active primarily against anaerobic bacteria, prevented carrageenan-induced colitis in guinea pigs. Furthermore, they reported that germfree guinea pigs given degraded carrageenan did not develop cecal ulceration, but that animals associated with a conventional microflora acquired cecal ulcerations during carrageenan challenge.[10] They inferred from these findings that carrageenan alone is not responsible for cecal ulceration and that bacteria are important in the development of cecal ulcerations. Hirono *et al.*[11] studied the role of intestinal bacterial flora in display of the effect of degraded carrageenan. Germfree and conventional female Wistar rats were fed a diet containing 10 % carrageenan for 63 days. They were sacrificed 7, 20, 35 and 63 days after the start of feeding and histological changes induced by carrageenan were studied. The germfree rats showed mucosal lesions, such as macrophage aggregates, erosion and squamous metaplasia of the large intestine, and these lesions were more extensive than those in the conventional rats. It was therefore concluded that bacterial flora are not essential for manifestation of the biological effects of degraded carrageenan.

5.3 Carcinogenicity of Carrageenan.

Carcinogenicity has been studied in both the native and degraded forms of carrageenan. Rustia *et al.*[12] reported that no significant increase in tumor incidence was seen in MRC rats and Syrian golden hamsters fed a diet containing 0.5, 2.5 or 5% native (undegraded) carrageenan with a high molecular weight of approximate 800,000 for the animal's life span. It has been reported by Cater[13] that subcutaneous injections of native carrageenan induced sarcomas only at the injection site in rats. The effect of dietary native carrageenan upon colon carcinogenesis was studied in female Fischer 344 rats. Carrageenan enhanced the incidence of colonic tumors in azoxymethane- and *N*-nitrosomethylurea-treated rats.[14] As mentioned above, it has been reported that oral administration of degraded carrageenan induces ulcerative lesions of the large intestine in various laboratory animals. The effects of prolonged oral administration of degraded carrageenan was studied in rats.[15] Degraded carrageenan was given to Sprague-Dawley rats through the diet (10, 5, or 1%), in drinking water (5%) or by stomach intubation (5 or 1 g/kg body weight) for up to 24 months. Carrageenan-induced ulcerative lesions, squamous metaplasia and tumors such as squamous cell carcinoma, adenoma and adenocarcinoma were found in the colon and rectum. Some rats had metastases of squamous cell carcinomas to the regional lymph nodes. Final incidences of tumors in rats given 10% diet and 5% diet were 31.7% and 20%, respectively. In rats given a 5% aqueous solution as drinking water or those given 5g/kg body weight by stomach tube, the incidences of tumors were 27.5% and 27.6%, respectively. These results show that degraded carrageenan is carcinogenic to the colorectum of the rat. Oohashi *et al.*[16] have undertaken studies on carcinogenesis arising from precancerous lesions, e.g. squamous metaplasia and ulcerative lesions of the rat colorectum, after termination of degraded carrageenan administration. Rates of tumor incidence in groups that were given a 10% diet of degraded carrageenan for 2, 6, and 9 months were 12.8%, 19.0% and 40.5%, respectively. The colorectal squamous metaplasia persisted in all rats and progressed irreversibly. Kawaura *et al.*[17] studied the effect of dietary degraded carrageenan on intestinal carcinogenesis initiated by 1,2-dimethylhydrazine (DMH) in Sprague-Dawley rats. The rats fed degraded carrageenan diet and treated with DMH had a higher incidence of colorectal tumors. Thus, degraded carrageenan enhanced intestinal carcinogenesis induced by DMH, in rats.

5.4 Carcinogenicity of Dextran Sulfate Sodium

Degraded carrageenan involves a polydisperse material of variable composition that is difficult to obtain and standardize. Some of these problems can be avoided by the use of a readily available, well-studied and well-characterized poly-anionic substitute, dextran sulfate sodium. Dextran sulfate sodium is a synthetic sulfated polysaccharide composed of dextran with sulfated glucose, whereas the carrageenans contain sulfated galactose and anhydrous galactose moieties. The biologic effects of dextran sulfate sodium were compared with those of degraded carrageenan by oral administration in inbred ACI rats.[18] All rats given a 10% dextran sulfate sodium diet died of severe diarrhea within 2 weeks after the start of the feeding. However, rats fed a 5% dextran sulfate sodium diet developed intestinal tumors between 134 and 215 days. These tumors were induced in the colon and cecum and consisted of adenomas, adenocarcinomas and papillomas. In another experiment, ACI rats fed a diet containing 1% dextran sulfate sodium developed colorectal papillomas and squamous cell carcinomas, in addition to adenoma and adenocarcinomas.[19] Antecedent pathological changes in the colorectal mucosa, such as ulceration and squamous metaplasia, and tumors in the large intestine induced by dextran sulfate sodium were virtually the same as those induced by degraded carrageenan. Thus, the difficulty of standardizing carrageenan, a natural product, can be avoided by the use of dextran sulfate. The mechanism of carcinogenesis and the pathogenesis of other effects brought about by sulfated poly-saccharides is still unknown. In a further study, the carcinogenicity was compared in rats fed diets containing 2.5% of dextran or one of 3 kinds of dextran sulfate sodium, with different molecular weights and almost the same sulfur content.[20] The average daily intake per rat of 3 kinds of dextran sulfates sodium during the 150 days after the start of feeding was almost the same. Dextran sulfate sodium of molecular weight 54,000 showed potent carcinogenic activity, whereas dextran sulfate sodium of molecular weight 520,000 and 9500 and dextran showed no significant carcinogenicity, i.e., the peak of carcinogenic activity of dextran sulfate sodium appeared at molecular weight 54,000, and dextran sulfate with larger or smaller molecular weight had no carcinogenic activity. Squamous metaplasia of the colorectal mucosa was present in all or almost all rats of each experimental group, except the group given dextran diet. Severe metaplasia was most frequently observed at molecular weight 54,000 and moderate metaplasia was most frequent at 520,000.

Since degraded carrageenan and dextran sulfate sodium yielded negative results in the Ames test for mutagenicity,[21-23] these compounds were assumed to be nongenotoxic carcinogens, probably tumor promoters, rather than genotoxic carcinogens. In this context, the effect of dextran sulfate sodium on colorectal carcinogenesis by 1,2-dimethylhydrazine (DMH) in rats was studied.[24] Male ACI rats received a single subcutaneous injection of 20 mg/kg body weight and then, starting one week later, were fed a diet containing 1% dextran sulfate sodium (DS-M-1), sulfur content 18.9% and weight-average molecular weight 54,000, until the termination of the experiment. The experiment was terminated after 40 weeks. The incidence of colorectal carcinoma in rats given DMH and DS-M-1 was significantly higher than that of the group which received DMH alone. Thus, the results of this study suggest that DS-M-1 acts as a promoter for colorectal carcinogenesis by DMH and that the carcinogenic activity of dextran sulfate sodium may be an expression of nongenotoxic carcinogenicity as a promoter.

REFERENCES

1. National Research Council (1981), Food Chemicals Codex, 3rd ed., Washington DC, National Academy Press, pp. 74–75.
2. Watt, J. and Marcus, R., Hyperplastic mucosal changes in the rabbit colon produced by degraded carrageenan, *Gastroenterology*, **59**: 760–768, 1970.
3. Watt, J., and Marcus, R., Carrageenan-induced ulceration of the large intestine in the guinea pig, *Gut*, **12**: 164–171, 1971.
4. Watt, J., and Marcus, R., Ulcerative colitis in rabbits fed degraded carrageenan, *J. Pharm. Pharmacol.*, **22**: 130–131, 1970.
5. Marcus, R., and Watt, J., Colonic ulceration in young rats fed degraded carrageenan, *Lancet*, **2**: 765–766, 1971.
6. Benitz, K.F., Golberg, L., and Coulston, F., Intestinal effects of carrageenans in the rhesus monkey (*Macaca mulatta*), *Food Cosmet. Toxicol.*, **11**: 565–575, 1973.
7. Fabian, R.J., Abraham, R., Coulston, F., and Golberg, L., Carrageenan-induced squamous metaplasia of the rectal mucosa in the rat, *Gastroenterology*, **65**: 265–276, 1973.
8. Van Der Waaij, D., Cohen, B., and Anver, M., Mitigation of experimental inflammatory bowel disease in guinea pigs by selective elimination of the aerobic gram-negative intestinal microflora, *Gastroenterology*, **67**: 460–472, 1974.
9. Onderdonk, A.B., Hermos, J.A., Dzink, J.L., and Bartlett, J.G., Protective effect of metronidazole in experimental ulcerative colitis, *Gastroenterology*, **74**: 521–526, 1978.
10. Onderdonk, A.B., and Bartlett, J.G., Bacteriological studies of experimental ulcerative colitis, *Am. J. Clin. Nutr.*, **32**: 258–265, 1979.
11. Hirono, I., Sumi, Y., Kuhara, K., and Miyakawa, M., Effect of degraded carrageenan on the intestine in germfree rats, *Toxicol. Lett.*, **8**: 207–212, 1981.
12. Rustia, M., Shubik, P., and Patil, K., Lifespan carcinogenicity tests with native carrageenan in rats and hamsters, *Cancer Lett.*, **11**: 1–10, 1980.
13. Cater, D.B., The carcinogenic action of carrageenan in rats, *Br. J. Cancer*, **15**: 607–614, 1961.

14. Watanabe, K., Reddy, B.S., Wong, C.Q., and Weisburger, J.H., Effect of dietary undegraded carrageenan on colon carcinogenesis in F344 rats treated with azoxymethane or methylnitrosourea, *Cancer Res.*, **38**: 4427–4430, 1978.
15. Wakabayashi, K., Inagaki, T., Fujimoto, Y., and Fukuda, Y., Induction by degraded carrageenan of colorectal tumors in rats, *Cancer Lett.*, **4**: 171–176, 1978.
16. Oohashi, Y., Ishiko, T., Wakabayashi, K., and Kuwabara, N., A study on carcinogenesis induced by degraded carrageenan arising from squamous metaplasia of the rat colorectum, *Cancer Lett.*, **14**: 267–272, 1981.
17. Kawaura, A., Shibata, M., Togei, K., and Otsuka, H., Effect of dietary degraded carrageenan on intestinal carcinogenesis in rats treated with 1,2,-dimethylhydrazine dihydrochloride, *Tokushima J. Exp. Med.*, **29**: 125–129, 1982.
18. Hirono, I., Kuhara, K., Hosaka, S., Tomizawa, S., and Golgerg, L., Induction of intestinal tumors in rats by dextran sulfate sodium, *J. Natl. Cancer Inst.*, **66**: 579–583, 1981.
19. Hirono, I., Kuhara, K., Yamaji, T., Hosaka, S., and Golberg, L., Induction of colorectal squamous cell cacinomas in rats by dextran sulfate sodium, *Carcinogenesis*, **3**: 353–355, 1982.
20. Hirono, I., Kuhara, K., Yamaji, T., Hosaka, S. and Golberg, L., Carcinogenicity of dextran sulfate sodium in relation to its molecular weight, *Cancer Lett.*, **18**: 29–34, 1983.
21. Nagoya, T., Hattori, Y. and Kobayashi, F., Mutagenicity and cytogenicity studies of dextran sulfate, *Pharmacometrics*, **22**: 621–627, 1981.
22. Wakabayashi, K., A study on carcinogenesis of degraded carrageenan, a polysaccharide-sulphate, derived from seaweeds, *Juntendo Med. J.*, **27**: 159–171, 1981.
23. Mori, H., Ohbayashi, F., Hirono, I., Shimada, T., and Williams, G.M., Absence of genotoxicity of the carcinogenic sulfated polysaccharides carrageenan and dextran sulfate in mammalian DNA repair and bacterial mutagenicity assays, *Nutr. Cancer*, **6**: 92–97, 1984.
24. Hirono, I., Ueno, I., Aiso, S., Yamaji, T, and Golberg, L., Enhancing effect of dextran sulfate sodium on colorectal carcinogenesis by 1,2-dimethylhydrazine in rats, *Gann*, **74**: 493–496, 1983.

Mushroom Hydrazines

6.1 Occurrence and Biochemistry of Mushroom Hydrazines

Hydrazines and their derivatives, hydrazides and hydrazones, are well known in organic chemistry since the 19th century. The high chemical reactivity of this class of compounds imparts a vast range of biological activities and hydrazines have numerous industrial uses. Many of these compounds are employed as rocket propellants, antioxidants, herbicides, and chemotherapeutic agents. However, the compound containing a nitrogen-nitrogen bond in nature had not been reported until 1951, when a toxic azoxy compound, macrozamin, was characterized. Since then more than forty compounds containing a nitrogen-nitrogen bond have been discovered from bacteria, actinomycetes, fungi, mushroom, and higher plants.[1,2]

Hydrazine is detected in tobacco smoke and is assumed to arise due to pyrolysis of nitrogen-containing compounds in tobacco.

In the early 1960s agaritine (1) was characterized as the first example of naturally occurring hydrazines in the course of studies on non-protein amino acid metabolism.[3] From the press juice of a basidimycetes, *Agaricus bisporus* (Agaricaceae, Basidiomycetes), the commonly eaten cultivated mushroom in North America and Europe, a new glutamic acid derivative was isolated, designated agaritine, and characterized as β-*N*-(γ-L(+)-glutamyl)-4-hydroxymethylphenylhydrazine (L-glutamic acid 5-[2-(4-hydroxymethyl)-phenylhydrazide] (1),[3,4] Buttons from two- to three-day old mushrooms were homogenized and extracted in methanol or water and the extract was applied to ion-exchange chromatography. Further purification by preparative paper chromatography and recrystallization affaorded in 0.04% yield a colorless compound of mp 203–208° C, $[\alpha]_D^{25} +7°$ (water), showing characteristics of amino acid.[3–6] Cleavage of agaritine with acid or enzyme obtained from the same mushroom resulted

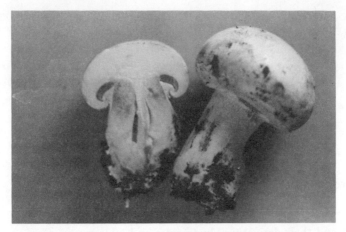

Fig. 6–1. *Agaricus bisporus* (LANGE) SING. (Agaricaceae)

in L-glutamic acid and 4-hydroxybenzyl alcohol.[3,6] The presence of the di-substituted hydrazine function, suspected from the analytical data and the reducing property, was substantiated by the hydrolysis of agaritine using a highly active enzyme to 4-(hydroxymethyl) phenylhydrazine (**2**) and L-glutamic acid.[3,6] Degradation of agaritine with ferric chloride yielded glutamic acid and benzyl alcohol.[4,5] The proposed structure was confirmed by synthesis from γ-azide of *N*-carbobenzoxy-L-glutamic acid and α-hydroxy-*p*-tolylhydrazine.[4,5] An improved method of synthesis, used to produce materials in amounts sufficient for biological testing, was also reported.[7]

The content of agaritine in the fresh mushroom is about 0.4 g/kg and the concentration diminishes with age of the mushroom.[6] Agaritine has also been found in boiled press juice preparation in quantities comparable to those found in *Agaricus bisporus* in ten other species of the genus: *A. argentatus, A. campestris, A. comptulis, A. crocodilinus, A. edulis, A. hortensis, A. micromegathus, A. pattersonii, A. perrarus,* and *A. xanthodermus.*[6]

CH_2OH

NH
|
NH NH_3^+
| |
$COCH_2CH_2CH-COO^-$

Agaritine(β-*N*-(γ-L(+)-glutamyl)-
4-hydroxymethylphenylhydrazine) (**1**)

CH_2OH

$NHNH_2$

(**2**)

CH_2OH

$N{\equiv}N^+$

(**3**)

An enzyme, γ-glutamyl transferase, purified from the mushroom, catalyzes the breakdown of agaritine (1) to 4-(hydroxymethyl)phenylhydrazine (2) and L-glutamic acid. A variety of β-N-acylphenylhydrazine analogues were prepared and the substrate specificity of the enzyme examined.[3,8] Substantial evidence was provided that 4-hydroxymethylbenzene diazomium ion (3) exists in the fungus, although it was not certain whether it resulted from the metabolism of agaritine (1) or formed directly.[9,10] Stability and decomposition of agaritine were also examined.[11]

p-Aminobenzoic acid (4) and glutamic acid were proved to be the efficient precursors of agaritine in the mushroom,[12] suggesting the biosynthetic sequence shown below. Recently *p*-hydrazinobenzoic acid (5) was identified in the mushroom.[13]

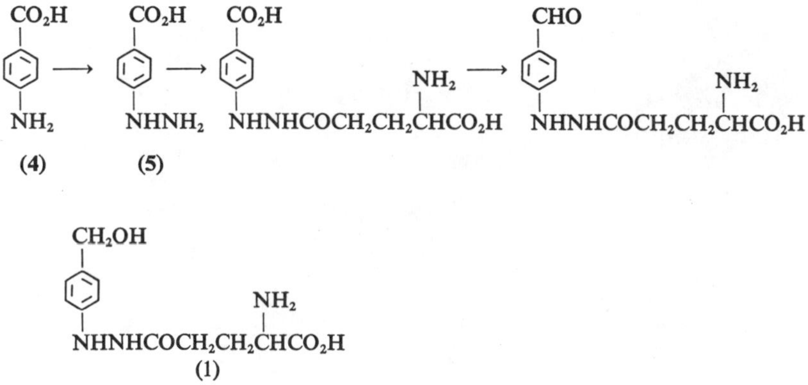

Possible biosynthesis of agaritine

The presence of agaritine in *Cortinellus shiitake*, one of the most popularly eaten mushrooms in Japan, has been reported,[14] but has not been confirmed by reexamination.

Another example of mushroom hydrazine derivatives is *N*-methyl-*N*-formylhydrazones from false morel, *Gyromitra esculenta* (Pers.) Fr. (Helvellaceae, Ascomycetes). The mushroom is widely distributed throughout the world, usually in sandy soil under pine trees, and eaten, after drying and boiling, as a choice foodstuff in northern Europe. Fresh false morel is poisonous, and raw or incompletely processed mushrooms have caused many deaths. From the fungus, gyromitrin (ethylidene gyromitrin) was isolated as the major poisonous principle and characterized as acetaldehyde formylmethylhydrazone (2-ethylidene-1-methylhydrazinecarboxaldehyde) (6).[16]

$$R-CH=N-N\begin{array}{c}CHO\\CH_3\end{array}$$

R : CH_3 — gyromitrin (9)
CH_3CH_2 (7)
$CH_3CH_2CH_2$ (8)
$CH_3\underset{\underset{CH_3}{|}}{CH}CH_2$ (9)

$CH_3CH_2CH_2CH_2$ (10)
$CH_3CH_2CH_2CH_2CH_2$ (11)
$CH_3CH_2CH_2CH_2CH_2CH_2$ (12)

$CH_3CH_2CH_2CH_2CH_2\underset{H}{\overset{H}{-C=C-}}$ (13)

$CH_3CH_2CH_2CH_2CH_2\underset{H\ H}{-C=C-}$ (14)

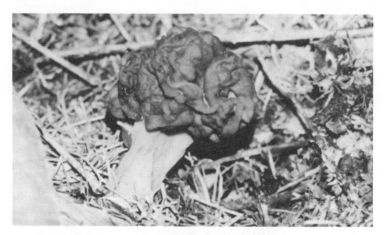

Fig. 6–2. *Gyromitra esculenta* (PERS.) FR. (Helvellaceae)

The ethanol extract of the fresh fungus was partitioned, chromatographed, and distilled under reduced pressure to afford gyromitrin, colorless liquid, bp 143° C. The structure was established by physical data, especially ¹H-NMR and mass spectroscopy, and hydrolysis to methylformylhydrazine (15) and acetaldehyde.[16] By gas chromatography-mass spectrometry comparison with synthetic homologues, the minor constituents of the fungus were identified as N-methyl-N-formylhydrazones of propanal (7), butanal (8), 3-methylbutanal (9), pentanal (10), hexanal (11), octanal (12), *trans*-2-octenal (13), and *cis*-2-octenal (14).[17–19] The content of gyromitrin was 49.9 mg/kg, while the total of the higher homologues was 7.1 mg/kg.[19] These N-methyl-N-formylhydrazones were also found in mycelia obtained from the culture of isolated ascospores.[20] The hydrazones were synthesized by the reaction of methylhydrazine and ethyl formate to afford *N*-methyl-*N*-formylhydrazine (**15**) and subsequent condensation with the respective aldehydes.[16] It is estimated that 99.0% of gyromitrin is lost by boiling and 99% by drying.[18]

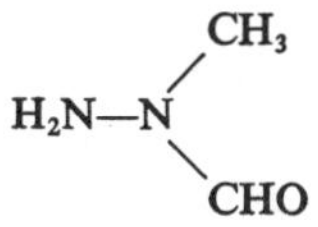

$$H_2N-N\begin{matrix} \diagup CH_3 \\ \diagdown CHO \end{matrix} \qquad\qquad H_2N-NH-CH_3$$

$$\text{(15)} \qquad\qquad\qquad\qquad \text{(16)}$$

N-Methyl-*N*-formylhydrazine (**15**) has been postulated to be hydrolysis product of gyromitrin.[16] Gyromitrin (**6**) at 37°C under acidic conditions reproducing those found in the human stomach is converted to methylhydrazine (**16**). In addition, methylhydrazine is formed in the mouse stomach after p. o. administration of gyromitrin.[21] The two metabolites were also detected in the extract of the fungus and are assumed to form during maceration or cooking. If the mushrooms are heated in an open vessel, methylhydrazine is lost by steam distillation, but if they are cooked in a closed container, methylhydrazine remains to cause the poisoning.[22]

6.2 Carcinogenicity of Mushroom Hydrazines

Carcinogenic potentialities of synthetic hydrazines was first reported in 1962, when the basic compound hydrazine sulfate was found to induce lung neoplasms in mice.[23] The following studies clearly demonstrated that nearly forty alkyl, aryl, and acyl substituted hydrazines are indeed potential tumorigenic substances in mice, hamsters and rats due to their tumor-inducing abilities in the intestines, brain, lungs, blood vessels, liver, breasts, kidneys, etc.[24]

These studies received particular attention because synthetic hydrazines are widely used and present in the environment, and some hydrazine derivatives are found in the commonly eaten mushrooms. Thus the systematic studies on the carcinogenicity of synthetic hydrazines by Toth were applied to the naturally occurring hydrazines.

Carcinogenicity of methylhydrazine (**16**) in mice was first reported in 1972,[25] although the formation of the compound from gyromitrin was not known at that time.[21] Groups of random-bred Swiss mice of each sex, six weeks old, were given 0.01% *N*-methylhydrazine in drinking water for life. Female and male treated animals died by 70 and 80 weeks of age, respectively, and control survivors were sacrificed at 120 weeks of age. The compound showed a marked effect on the survival rates when compared with respective controls. Lung adenomas were found in 12/50 (24%) (17 tumors) and in 11/50 (22%) (12 tumors) female and male treated animals, respectively.[25]

Next, the same solution was administered daily in drinking water to male and female 6-week-old randomly bred Syrian golden hamsters for the remainder of their life span. All control survivors were sacrificed at 120 weeks of age; all treated animals had died by 110 weeks. The treatment substantially reduced the survival compared with the controls. The treatment gave rise to malignant histiocytomas (Kupffer-cell sarcomas) of liver and tumors of the cecum. Thirty-two percent of the females and 54% of the males developed malignant histiocytomas, whereas among the controls no such lesions were observed. The incidence of tumors of the cecum was 18% and 14% in females and males respectively, compared to 1% in the controls. Macroscopic, microscopic and histochemical investigations of the liver lesions showed the characteristic appearance of malignant histiocytomas.[26]

Using the synthetic sample of N-methyl-N-formylhydrazine (15), the hydrolysis product of gyromitrin and a constituent of the mushroom, carcinogenicity was again confirmed in mice[27] and hamsters[28] as follows. Continuous administration of 0.0078% solution in drinking water to 6-week-old outbred Swiss mice for life produced tumors of the liver, lung, gall bladder and bile duct. The incidences of tumors in these four tissues were 33, 50, 9 and 7%, whereas in the untreated controls they were 1, 18, 0, and 0%, respectively. A higher does (0.0156%) given under the same conditions had no tumorigenic effect, since it was too toxic for the animals. Histopathologically, the lesions were classified as benign hepatomas, liver cell carcinomas, adenoms and adenocarcinomas of the lung, adenomas of gall bladder, cholangiomas and cholagiocarcinomas.[27]

The same compound in the same concentration was administered in drinking water to randomly bred Syrian golden hamsters for life beginning at 6 weeks of age. The treatment gave rise to benign and malignant liver cell tumors, malignant histiocytoas and tumors of the gall bladder and bile ducts. The tumor incidence in these four tissues was 43, 34, 11, and 8%, while in controls it was 0, 0, 0, and 0%, respectively. Histological examination showed that tumors were classified as benign hepatomas, liver cell carcinomas, malignant histiocytomas, adenomas and adenocarcinomas of the gall bladder, cholagiomas and cholangiocarcinomas.[28] It is worth noting that lung tumors were induced in mice but not in hamsters, while malignant histiocytomas were evoked in hamsters but not in mice.

Carcinogenicity testing of the major constituent of false morel mushroom, gyromitrin (6), was performed using different route of administration, because of the instability and insolubility in water of the compound. It was administered to noninbred Swiss mice in propylene glycol in 52 weekly intragastric instillations as 100 μg/g body weight. The treatment induced tumors of the lung, preputial gland, forestomach and clitoral glands. Tumor incidences in the four tissues in treated females were 70, 0, 16, and 12%, respectively, while in the treated males they were 40, 90, 0, and 0%. The corresponding incidences in the solvent controls were 26, 0,0, and 0% in females and 22, 0, 0, and 0% in males, respectively. Histopathologically, the neoplasms were classified as adenomas and adenocarcinomas of the lung; squamous cell papillomas and carcinomas, adenocarcinomas, undifferentiated carcinomas, angiosarcomas and fibrosarcomas of the preputial glands; squamous cell papillomas and carcinomas of the forestomach; and squamous cell papillomas and carcinomas and keratoacanthomas of the clitoral glands.[29]

There are several reports in the literature of poisoning cases resulting from the ingestion of inadequately cooked false morel.[30] The poisoning is characterized by nausea, vomiting and sometimes diarrhea. About 38–48 hours after consuming the fresh mushroom, varying degrees of jaundice may develop, with enlargement of the liver and often also of spleen.[31] Acute toxicity tests of gyromitrin and related compounds on experimental animals have been performed.[32-35] The LD_{50} values by oral administration in rabbits, rats, mice and chickens were reported to be 70, 320, 344, and 400 mg/kg, respectively.[32]

In the case of agaritine (1), tumorigenic effect was first examined by 4-methylphenylhydrazine (17), which was postulated to be a metabolite of 4-(hydroxymethyl)-phenylhydrazine (2),[8] since a sufficient amount of sample of agaritine for testing was not available. 4-Methylphenylhydrazine hydrochloride was administered as 10 weekly subcutaneous injections of 140 μg/g body weight and as 7 weekly intragastric instillations of 250 μg/g body weight in physiological saline to randomly bred Swiss mice. Treatments given subcutaneously resulted in induction of lung tumors in incidence of 36% in females and 44% in males, while intragastric treatment caused a 40% incidence in females. In addition, it gave rise to blood vessel tumors by the latter route in incidences of 32% in females and 18% in males. In the control groups lung tumor incidence was 20% in females and 21% in males, while blood vessel tumor incidence was 7% in females and 6% in males. Histopathologically, the lesions were classified as adenomas and adenocarcinomas of the lungs, and angiomas and angiosarcomas of the blood vessels.[36]

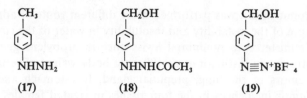

$$CH_3 \quad\quad CH_2OH \quad\quad CH_2OH$$

NHNH₂ ... (structures)

$$NHNH_2 \quad\quad NHNHCOCH_3 \quad\quad N{\equiv}N^+BF^-_4$$

(17)   **(18)**   **(19)**

4-(Hydroxymethyl)phenylhydrazine (2) is a hydrolysis product of agaritine.[3,8] Since the compound is relatively unstable, N'-actate (18) was prepared and tumor induction in mice examined. The compound was administered as a 0.0625% solution in drinking water for the life span of albino Swiss mice, from 6 weeks of age. The survival of experimental and control animals did not differ significantly. Compared to that in untreated controls, in treated animals the lung tumor incidence rose from 15 to 34% in females and from 22 to 48% in males, while the incidence of blood vessel tumors increased from 8 to 32% in females and from 5 to 30% in males. Histopathologically, the tumors were classified as adenomas and adenocarcinomas of the lungs and angiomas and angiosarcomas of the blood vessels.[37]

Then carcinogenicity test of agaritine (1) itself was performed but a negative result was obtained as follows: Groups of 50 outbred albino Swiss mice of each sex, six weeks old, were administered agaritine at a concentration of 625 mg/1 in the drinking water daily for life; a group of 50 male mice was administered 312 mg/1. Groups of 100 mice of each sex, five weeks old, served as controls. All survivors were sacrificed at 120 weeks of age. A significant difference in the survival rate was observed between the groups: at 50 weeks of age 24/50 high-dose males, 39/50 low-dose males, 80/100 male controls, 48/50 high-dose females and 88/100 femal controls were still alive. No compound-related increase in the incidence of tumors was observed.[38]

4-(Hydroxymethyl)benzenediazonium ion (3) exists in *Agaricus bisporus*.[9,10] Water-soluble 4-methylphenylhydrazine (17) induced soft-tissue tumors at injection sites when given by repeated s.c. injection in mice as described above. Since none of the other known water-soluble hydrazines had induced tumors at application sites, it was postulated that a corresponding diazonium ion may have formed locally and was ultimately responsible for cancer induction.[24] 4-(Hydroxymethyl)benzenediazonium tetrafluoroborate (19) was prepared and administered as 26 weekly s.c. injections of 50 μg/g body weight to randomly bred Swiss mice. In addition, as a solvent control, sodium tetrafluoroborate was given as 26 weekly s.c. injections at 25 μg/g body weight in 0.9% NaCl solution to another group of mice. The 4-(hydroxymethyl)benzenediazonium tetrafluoroborate treatment induced tumors in the subcutis and skin in incidences of 20 and 12%, respectively, while in the solvent sodium tetrafluoro-borate-injected mice, the corresponding tumor incidences were 6 and 0%, respectively. Histopathologically, the tumors were classified as a fibroma, fibrosarcomas, rhabdomyosarcomas and angiosarcoma in the subcutis and also as squamous cell papillomas and carcinomas of the skin.[39]

The same compound was administered as a single intragastric instillation at 400 $\mu g/g$ to Swiss albino mice. The treatment gave rise to glandular stomach tumors in incidences of 30% in females and 32% in males. Histopathologically, the tumors were polypoid adenomas and adenocarcinomas.[40]

As far as the author is aware reports on feeding experiments of the mushrooms containing the hydrazine derivatives themselves have not yet been published.

Recently, short-term tests for carcinogenicity such as Ames' test have been frequently employed for preliminary examinations. Clearly positive results have not been reported for the naturally occurring hydrazine derivatives by these methods.[41]

Although evidence of carcinogenicity of agaritine to experimental animals has not been provided, the two metabolites of agaritine have been shown to be carcinogenic. Agaritine itself is rather unstable and can be removed nearly completely by cooking, but the remaining metabolites cannot. Results of studies on gyromitrin itself, supported by studies on two of its metabolites, provided sufficient evidence for proving carcinogenicity in experimental animals. Gyromitrin, like agaritine, is destroyed by proper preparation before eating, but the possibility of human exposure to gyromitrin and the metabolites remains.[41] Considering the worldwide consumption of the mushrooms in question, it has been proposed that human populations abandon their consumption.[27-29,36,37]

REFERENCES

1. LaRue, T.A., Naturally occurring compounds containing a nitrogen-nitrogen bond. *Lloydia*, **40**: 307–321, 1977.
2. Turner, W.B., Agaritine and related compounds. In: *Fungal Metabolites*, pp. 307–308, Academic Press, London and New York, 1971; Turner, W.B., and Aldridge, D.C., Agaritine and related compounds. In: Fungal Metabolites II, pp. 395–396, Academic Press, London and New York, **1983**.
3. Levenberg, B., Structure and enzymatic cleavage of agaritine, a phenylhyrazide of L-glutamic acid isolated from *Agaricaceae*. *J. Am. Chem. Soc.*, **83**: 503–504 (1961).
4. Daniels, E.G., Kelly, R.B., and Hinman, J.W., Agaritine: an improved isolation procedure and confirmation of structure by synthesis. *J. Am. Chem. Soc.*, **83**: 3333–3334, 1961.

5. Kelly, R.B., Daniels, E.G., and Hinman, J.W., Agaritine: Isolation, degradation, and synthesis. *J. Org. Chem.*, **27**: 3229–3231, 1962.
6. Levenberg, B., Isolation and structure of agaritine, a γ-glutamyl-substituted arylhydrazine derivative from *Agaricaceae. J. Biol. Chem.*, **239**: 2267–2273, 1964.
7. Wallcave, L., Nagal, D.L., Raha, C.R., Jae, H.-S., Bronczyk, S., Kupper, R., and Toth, B., An improved synthesis of agaritine. *J. Org. Chem.*, **44**: 3752–3755, 1979.
8. Gigliotti, H.J., and Levenberg, B., Studies on the γ-glutamyltransferase of *Agaricus bisporus. J. Biol. Chem.*, **239**: 2274–2284, 1964.
9. Levenberg, B., An aromatic diazonium compound in the mushroom *Agaricus bisporus. Biochem. Biophys. Acta*, **63**: 212–214, 1962.
10. Ross, A.E., Nagel, D.L., and Toth, B., Evidence for the occurrence and formation of diazonium ions in the *Agaricus bisporus* mushroom and its extracts. *J. Agric. Food Chem.*, **30**: 521–525, 1982.
11. Ross, A.E., Nagel, D.L., and Toth, B., Occurrence, stability and decomposition of β-N[γ-L(+)-glutamyl]-4-hydroxymethylphenylhydrazine (agaritine) from the mushroom *Agaricus bisporus. Fd. Cosmet. Toxicol.*, **20**: 903–907, 1982.
12. Shütte, H.R., Liebisch, H.W., Mersch, O., and Senf, L., Untersuchungen zur Biosynthese des Agaritins in *Agaricus bisporus. Anales de Quimica*, **68**: 899–903, 1972 (in German).
13. Chauhan, Y., Nagel, D., Issenberg, P., and Toth, B., Identification of *p*-hydrazinobenzoic acid in the commercial mushroom *Agaricus bisporus. J. Agric. Food Chem.*, **32**: 1067–1069, 1984.
14. Issenberg, P., personal communication cited in ref. 15.
15. Toth, B., Mushroom hydrazines: Occurrence, metabolism, carcinogenesis, and environmental implications. In: *Naturally Occurring Carcinogens-Mutagens and Modulators of Carcinogenesis.* (E.C. Miller *et al.*, eds.), Japan Sci. Soc. Press, Tokyo, and University Park Press, Baltimore, pp. 57–65, 1979.
16. List, P.H., and Luft, P., Gyromitrin, das Gift der Frühjahrslorchel. *Arch Pharm.* **301**: 294–305, 1968; *idem*: Detection and determination of gyromitrin in the fresh *Gyromitra esculenta. ibid.*, **302**: 143–146, 1969.
17. Pyysalo, H., Some new toxic compounds in false morels, *Gyromitra esculenta. Naturwiss.*, **62**: 395, 1975.
18. Pyysalo, H., and Honkanen, E., Mass spectra of some *N*-methyl-*N*-formylhydrazones. *Acta Chem. Scand.*, **30**: 792–793, 1976.
19. Pyysalo, H., and Niskanen, A., On the occurrence of *N*-methyl-*N*-formylhydrazones in fresh and processed false morel, *Gyromitra esculenta. J. Agric. Food Chem.*, **25**: 644–647, 1977.
20. Raudaskoski, M., and Pyysalo, H., Occurrence of *N*-methyl-*N*-formylhydrazones in mycelia of *Gyromitra esculenta. Z. Naturforsch.*, **33c**: 472–474, 1978.
21. Nagel, D., Wallcave, L., Toth, B., and Kupper, R., Formation of methylhydrazine from acetaldehyde *N*-methyl-*N*-formylhydrazone, a component of *Gyromitra esculenta. Cancer Res.*, **37**: 3458–3460, 1977.
22. Wright, A. von, Pyysalo, H., and Niskanen, A., Qualitative evaluation of the metabolic formation of methylhydrazine from acetaldehyde *N*-methyl-*N*-formylhydrazone, the main poisonous compound of *Gyromitra esculenta. Toxicol. Lett.*, 2: 261–265, 1978.
23. Biancifiori, C., and Ribacchi, R., Pulmonary tumors in mice induced by isoniazid and its metabolites. *Nature*, **194**: 488–489, 1962.
24. Toth, B., Synthetic and naturally occurring hydrazines as possible cancer causative agents. *Cancer Res.*, **35**: 3693–3694, 1962.
25. Toth, B., Hydrazine, methylhydrazine and methylhydrazine sulfate carcinogenesis in Swiss mice. Failure of ammonium hydroxide to interfere in the development of tumors. *Int. J. Cancer*, **9**: 109–118, 1972.
26. Toth, B., and Shimizu, H., Methylhydrazine tumorigenesis in Syrian hamsters and the morphology of malignant histiocytomas. *Cancer Res.*, **33**: 2774–2753, 1973.
27. Toth, B., and Nagel, D., Tumors induced in mice by *N*-methyl-*N*-formylhydrazine

of the false morel *Gyromitra esculenta*. *J. Natl. Cancer Inst.*, **60**: 201–204, 1978.

28. Toth, B., and Patil, K., Carcinogenic effects in the Syrian golden hamster of *N*-methyl-*N*-formylhydrazine of the false morel mushroom *Gyromitra esculenta*. *J. Cancer Res. Clin. Oncol.*, **93**: 109–121, 1979.

29. Toth, R., Smith, J.W., and Patil, K.D., Cancer induction in mice with acetaldehyde methylformylhydrazone of the false morel mushroom. *J. Natl. Cancer Inst.*, **67**: 881–887, 1981.

30. Franke, S., Freimuth, U., and List, P.H., On the virulence of the mushroom *Gyromitra esculenta Fr. Arch. Toxikol.*, **22**: 293–332, 1967.

31. Garnier, R., Conso, F., Efthymiou, M.L., Riboulet, G., and Gaultier, M. Poisoning by *Gyromitra esculenta*. *Toxicol. Eur. Res.*, **1**: 359–364, 1978.

32. Mäkinen, S.M., Kreula, M., and Kauppi, M., Acute oral toxicity of ethylidene gyromitrin in rabbits, rats, and chickens. *Fd. Cosmet. Toxicol.*, **15**: 575–578, 1977.

33. Niskanen, A., Pyysalo, H., Rimaila-Pärnanen, E., and Hartikka, P., Short-term peroral toxicity of ethylidene gyromitrin in rabbits and chickens. *Fd. Cosmet. Toxicol.*, **14**: 409–415, 1976.

34. Braun, R., Greff, U., and Netter, K.J., Liver injury by the false morel poison gyromitrin. *Toxicology*, **12**: 155–163, 1979.

35. Wright, A. von, Niskanen, A., Pyysalo, H., and Korpela, H., The toxicity of some *N*-methyl-*N*-formylhydrazones from *Gyromitra esculenta* and related compounds in mouse and microbial tests. *Toxicol. Appl. Pharmacol.*, **45**: 429–434, 1978.

36. Toth, B., Tompa, A., and Patil, K., Tumorigenic effect of 4-methylphenylhydrazine hydrochloride in Swiss mice. *Z. Krebsforsch.*, **89**: 245–252, 1977.

37. Toth, B., Nagel, D., Patil, K., Erickson, J., and Antonson, K., Tumor induction with *N'*-acetyl derivative of 4-hydroxymethylphenylhydrazine, a metabolite of agaritine of *Agaricus bisporus*. *Cancer Res.*, **38**: 177–180, 1978.

38. Toth, B., Raha, C.R., Wallcave, L., and Nagel, D., Attempted tumor induction of with agaritine in mice. *Anticancer Res.*, **1**: 255–258, 1981.

39. Toth, B., Patil, K., and Jae H.-S., Carcinogenesis of 4-(hydroxymethyl)benzene-diazonium ion (tetrafluoroborate) of *Agaricus bisporus*. *Cancer Res.*, **41**: 2444–2449, 1981.

40. Toth, B., Nagel, D., and Ross, A., Gastric tumorigenesis by a single dose of 4-(hydroxymethyl)benzenediazinium ion of *Agaricus bisporus*. *Br. J. Cancer*, **46**: 417, 1982.

41. International Agency for Research on Cancer: Agaritine and gyromitrin. In: *IARC Monographs on the Evaluation of the Carcinogenic Risk of Chemicals to Humans*, Vol. 31, p. 63–69, p. 163–170, IARC, Lyons, **1983**.

Safrole is one of many allylic and propenylic benzene-derivatives with ring methoxy and/or ring methylenedioxy substituents which occur naturally in plants and are contained in various foods including spices, herbs and vegetables. These natural alkenylbenzenes as well as synthetic ones are used largely as flavoring agents in food and as perfumes.

The hepatic toxicity following the ingestion of large amounts of sassafras oil by humans, which has been known for over a hundred years, brought safrole to the attention of toxicologists as well as pharmacologists. Its carcinogenic properties for rats and/or mice were reported in 1960, and the use of safrole as an oil and food additive was banned in the United States in that year.

Extensive studies on the metabolism, especially on the activation of safrole and other related substances, have been carried out by the group led by James A. Miller and Elizabeth C. Miller of the University of Wisconsin. Starting with the identification of 1'-hydroxysafrole as a proximate carcinogenic metabolite of safrole,[1] they have established the outlines of the critical metabolic activation steps of alkenylbenzene carcinogens, including safrole and estragole, over the past fifteen years.

7.1 Chemical Properties, Natural Occurrence and Use of Safrole: 1-allyl-3,4-methylenedioxybenzene

Chem. Abst. Name: 5-(2-Propenyl)-1,3-Benzodioxole

Safrole is a major component (80 %) of sassafras oil, obtained by steam distillation from the roots and bark of *Sassafras officinale* or *albidum*. Pure safrole (melting point: around 11°C, boiling point: 232–234°C) is a colorless or slightly yellow liquid with an odor of sassafras. Sassafras oil also contains small amounts of eugenol, elemicin, pinene, phellandrene, sesquiterpene and d-camphor.[2] Safrole is also present in sweet basil and is contained in the distilled oil from *Ocotea pretiosa* in Brazil and the oils from the *Heterotropa* genus.[3] It is a minor component of oils from nutmeg, mace (*Asarum hooyamum* var. *nipponicum*), star anise *(Illicium religiosum* or *amisatum* Linn), ginger, black pepper and cinnamon leaf (*Cinnamonim canyhora*).

Safrole was first isolated in 1890 by Knoll. Sassafras oil was used for medicinal purposes as a topical antiseptic, pediculicide and carminative. It was also used as a flavoring agent for soft drinks such as root beer in the United States. Although its use as a food additive is no longer permitted,[4] safrole is still used as a fragrance in soaps and toiletries and may be ingested by humans in food at levels of no more than low parts per million.[5]

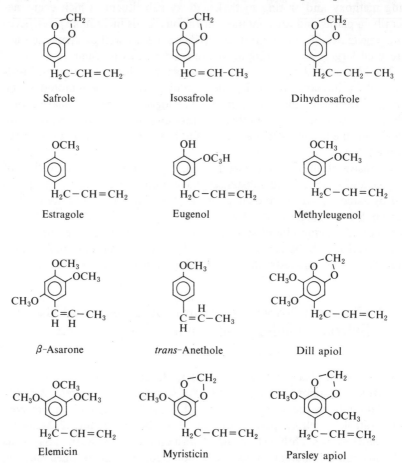

Fig. 7–1. Structures of safrole and related compounds.

Except for dihydrosafrole, the following compounds are naturally occurring alkenylbenzene derivatives and have been found as components of many plants and their essential oils[6,7] (Fig. 7–1).

Anethole: *trans*-4-methoxy-1-propenylbenzene. Contained in oil of anise, fennel and coriander.

β-Asarone: *cis*-1-propenyl-2,4,5-trimethoxybenzene. A major constituent of oil of calamus *(Acorus calamus)*, a bitters flavoring agent.

Clinnamaldehyde: 3-phenylpropenal. Present in cinnamon.

Dihydrosafrole: 1-*n*-propyl-3,4-methylenedioxybenzene. Chem. Abstr. Name: 5-Propyl-1,3-benzodioxole. Dihydrosafrole is a synthetic derivative produced from safrole or isosafrole by catalytic hydrogenation.[8] It is a chemical intermediate in the manufacture of piperonyl butoxide and was formerly used as a flavoring agent.

Dill apiol: 1-allyl-2,3-dimethoxy-4,5-methylenedioxybenzene. Present in dill and indian dill.

Elemicin: 1-allyl-3,4,5-trimethoxybenzene. A constituent of oils from nutmeg, elemigum and sassafras.

Estagole: 1-allyl-4-methoxybenzene. A major component of oils of several spices and herbs, it is contained in tarragon oil and the oils of sweet basil, anise and fennel.

Eugenol: 1-allyl-4-hydroxy-3-methoxybenzene. A constituent of oil of cloves, allspice and artichoke.

Isosafrole: 3,4-methylenedioxy-1-propenyl benzene. Contains a propenyl group instead of the isomeric allyl group of safrole. It is rarely found in essential oils and is a constituent of ylang ylang oil. Like safrole, isosafrole was used in perfumery and as a flavoring agent.

Methyleugenol: 1-allyl-3,4-dimethoxybenzene. Contained in sweet bay, cloves and lemongrass.

Myristicin: 1-allyl-5-methoxy-3,4-methylenedioxybenzene. A constituent of oil of nutmeg or mace, black pepper, dill, celery, carrots, parsley, mint and parsnips.

Parsley apiol: 1-allyl-2,5-dimethoxy-3,4-methylenedioxybenzene. Contained in parsley, fennel and sassafras.

Sinapaldehyde: 4-hydroxy-3,5-dimethoxy-cinnamaldehyde. Extracted from wood lignin.

7.2 Toxicity of Safrole and Related Compounds

Human intoxication by safrole and oil of sassafras, which is 80% safrole, was reported in 1885, although no fatal cases have been recorded.[3]

The first significant study on the pharmacologic effects of safrole and iso-safrole was done by Heffter.[9] In 1961, Abbott *et al.* reported on the chronic oral toxicity of oil of sassafras and safrole.[10] Sassafras oil (Southern) N.F.X. and safrole were each fed at concentrations of 390 and 1170 ppm in the dry diet of rats for 22 months. An appreciable precentage of the animals in all experimental groups showed cellular changes in the liver, compatible with carcinoma. However, routine blood and urine examinations were within normal limits. In the same year, Powers *et al.* studied the toxic effects of cinnamon oil.[11] The intraperitoneal LD_{50} values (Litchfield and Wilcox) in albino Swiss male mice were: cinnamon oil, 0.5 gm/kg; cinnamaldehyde, 0.46 gm/kg; sodium cinnamate, 2.0 gm/kg: and cinnamyl acetate, 1.2 gm/kg. Administration of cinnamon oil, 100 mg/kg, in adult mongrel dogs caused an increase in isometric systolic tension, respiratory stimulation, hypotension and pulmonary edema. Death occurred within two hours. Cinnamaldehyde caused similar effects, but the other compounds investigated were less toxic in these dogs.

The comparative toxicities of aliphatic allyl and propyl esters and many related compounds with the allyl, propenyl, or propyl groups, which are used as flavoring agents in foods and beverages, were studied in rats by Taylor *et al.*[12] to clarify the relationship between structure and toxicity. As already known, some allyl compounds such as allyl alcohol and allyl formate produced peripheral necrosis of the liver. Allyl heptylate, allyl acetate, allyl butyrate and allyl caproate also appeared to be hepatotoxic. Repeated treatment with allyl formate caused cirrhosis. In contrast, aliphatic propyl compounds (propanol and propyl esters) showed no hepatotoxic lesions.

Aromatic propenyl compounds such as anethole and propenylbenzene were usually, but not always, more toxic than aromatic allyl compounds including allylbenzene. Benzaldehyde, anisole, vanillin and isoeugenol were not hepatotoxic. Aromatic allyl compounds were more toxic than aromatic propyl compounds like propylbenzene. Severe liver lesions consisting of discoloration, enlargement and loss of normal texture in the case of the aromatic compounds were found only with safrole, isosafrole, and dihydrosafrole — the allyl, propenyl and propyl derivatives of methylenedioxybenzene, respectively. The hepatotoxicity of these compounds appeared to be independent of the nature of the 3-carbon side chain (propyl, allyl and propenyl groups) and the methylenedioxy group appeared to be necessary for the hepatotoxic action. Mild liver lesions discoloration, mottling and blunting of the lobe edges were seen with a number of the other aromatic compounds tested including compounds with no 3-carbon side chain (guaiacol, methylenedioxybenzene), or with the allyl side chain (estragole, eugenol), the propenyl side chain (anethole), the propyl side chain (dihydroanethole), and the aldehyde group (ani-saldehyde, piperonal), but the occurrence of these lesions was not related to a particular structure.

The acute oral toxicity, LD_{50}, and slope functions of allyl, propenyl, propyl and related compounds examined in the rat by Taylor *et al.*[12] and of allylbenzene and emylendioxybenzene in the rat, mouse and guinea pig by Hagan *et al.*[13] are summarized in Table 7-1. Subacute oral and chronic oral toxicity studies were also performed in rats on some of these compounds by Taylor *et al.*[12] and by Hagan *et al.*[13] respectively. Results of chronic feeding of safrole, dihydrosafrole and isosafrole are described in the following section on the carcinogenicity of safrole and related compounds because these compounds induced tumors.

Benzaldehyde, anisaldehyde, eugenol, isoeugenol or piperonal fed at a level of 1% in the diet of rats for 15–19 weeks caused no liver damage. Anethole induced slight hydropic changes of the liver cells in males when fed at a level of 1% in the diet to rats for 15 weeks, but no liver injury was seen at a level of 0.25% for 1 year. Allyl heptylate caused degeneration of hepatic cells and appearance of new bile ducts at dietary levels of 0.1 to 1% for 17 weeks. Allyl caproate caused no liver injury when fed at a level of 0.19% in the diet of rats for 1 year.[12]

Safrole, isosafrole and dihydrosafrole given to rats at 250, 500 and 750 mg/kg/day subacutely by stomach tube caused liver enlargement and adrenal enlargement with yellow discoloration. Histologically, the livers showed enlargement due to an increase in cytoplasm in all three groups. The increases in cytoplasm of the liver cells may reflect the induction of the hepatic microsomal enzymes or microsamal hemoprotein by safrole. Focal fat degeneration, bile duct proliferation and irregularity in arrangement of liver cell cords were found. Focal necrosis of the liver cells and slight fibrosis were seen in safrole- and isosafrole-treated rats.

The adrenals of rats given safrole and dihydrosafrole showed an increase in lipid in cortical cells. Daily administration of eugenol at 2,000 mg/kg and later at 4,000 mg/kg caused liver changes typical of those observed in rats treated with isosafrole, but to a lesser degree then those in rats treated with safrole and dihydrosafrole. The forestomach showed hyperplasia and hyperkeratosis of the stratified squamous epithelium with focal ulceration. Allyl heptylate given to rats at 10,000, 2,500 and 1,000 ppm in the diet produced enlargement of the liver and kidneys. Hydropic degeneration and bile duct proliferation were seen histologically in the liver.

In contrast to other hepatotoxic alkenylbenzenes, myristicin shows neurological toxicity. As little as 500 mg of raw nutmeg may cause a detectable psychic response such as hallucination. Myristicin acts as both an insecticide and an insecticide synergist.[14]

Table 7-1. Acute Oral Toxicity of Compounds Related to Safrole[12,13]

Compound	Rat LD$_{50}$ (mg/kg)	(M&F) Slope function	Mouse LD$_{50}$ (mg/kg)	Slope function	Main clinical symptoms in rat
Aliphatic allyl compounds					
Allyl alcohol	70	1.6			depression, scrawny appearance, diarrhea
Allyl formate	124	1.3			depression, scrawny appearance
Allyl caproate	218	1.3			depression, scrawny appearance
Allyl heptylate	500	1.7	630	1.5	depression, ataxia
Aliphatic propyl compounds					
n-Propanol	6500	1.2			comatose, scrawny appearance
Propyl formate	3980	1.5			depression
Benzene derivatives					
Allylbenzene	5540	1.5	2900	1.4	depression
Propenylbenzene	3600	2.2			scrawny appearance
Propylbenzene	6040	1.5			depression, scrawny appearance
Benzaldehyde	1300	1.4			depression, comatose
Methoxybenzene derivatives					
Anisole	3700	1.2			depression, blood in urine
Estragole	1820	1.2			depression, comatose
Anethole	2090	1.8			depression, comatose
Anisaldehyde	1510	1.2			depression
Methylenedioxybenzene derivatives					
Methylenedioxybenzene	580	1.4	1220	1.4	depression, comatose
Safrole	1950	1.3	2350	1.4	depression, ataxia diarrhea
Isosafrole	1340	1.4	2470	1.7	depression, comatose, scrawny appearance
Dihydrosafrole	2260	1.7	3700	1.2	depression, scrawny appearance
Piperonal	2700	1.5			exciteness, then depression, ataxia
Hydroxymethoxybenzene derivatives					
Eugenol	2680	1.2	3000	1.8	comatose
Isoeugenol	1560	1.4			comatose, scrawny appearance
Vanillin	1580	1.3			comatose, scrawny appearance

Table 7-2A. Carcinogenicity in Rats of Compounds Related to Safrole (Oral Administration)

(Osborne Mendel rats, male and female)

Experiment	(1)[3]			(2)[13]	
Dose and Tumors Compound	Dose in diet	Liver Tumors	(Exp. period)	Dose in diet	Liver Tumor
Safrole	0.5% 0.1 0.05 0.01	19/47 (24 mo). 8/50 3/50 1/50		(no details)	
Isosafrole				0.5%	5/20 24 mo.
Dihydro-safrole				Esophageal tumor 1% 15/20 0.5 37/50 0.25 4/20 0.1 0/20	
None	0%	3/40 (24 mo.)		0%	0/20

(Charles River CD, random bred, male rats)

Experiment	(3)[1]		(4)[1]		(5)[1]	
Compound	Dose in diet	(fed for 10 mo) Liver carc.	Dose in diet	(fed for 11 mo) Liver carc.	Dose in diet	(fed for 8 mo) Liver carc.
Safrole	0.5% 0/12 (16 mo.)		0.5% 0.3%	1/18 (16 mo.) 0/18 (16 mo.)	0.5%	1/18 (12 mo.)
1'-Hydroxy-safrole	0.55%	11/12 (16 mo.)			0.55%	16/18 (12 mo.)
1'-Acetoxy-safrole					0.41%	1/18 (12 mo.)
None	0%	0/12 (16 mo.)	0%	0/18 (16 mo.)	0%	0/18 (12 mo.)

Experiment	(6)[16]		(7)[16]	
Dose and Tumors Compound	Dose in diet	(fed for 17 mo.) Liver Carc.	Dose in diet	(fed for 22 mo.) Liver Carc.
Safrole	0.22%	0/18 (22 mo.)	0.5%	3/18 (22 mo.)
1'-Hydroxysafrole	0.55% 0.25%	16/18 (22 mol.) 7/18 (22 mo.)		
1'-Acetoxysafrole None	0%	0/18 (22 mo.)	0%	0/18 (22 mo.)

7.3 Carcinogenicity

The earliest evidence suggesting the carcinogenicity of safrole was obtained in male CFN rats by Homburger et al.,[15] who observed development of liver adenomas in 4 out of 5 and 9 out of 9 rats fed 1 % safrole for about 200 days on two types of protein-deficient diet. The following study by Long et al. (1963)[3] using groups of 25 male and 25 female Osborne-Mendel rats fed 0, 100, 500, 1,000 or 5,000 mg safrole per kg of diet for two years revealed the development of liver carcinoma in 14 out of 47 autopsied rats fed the 5,000 ppm level. Liver cell adenoma also occurred in 4 rats. There were 8 cases of liver cell adenoma at 1,000 ppm, one case each of liver cell carcinoma and adenoma at 500 ppm and one case of liver cell adenoma at 100 ppm. Two liver cell caricinomas and one adenoma were seen in the controls. In addition to tumors, the liver showed either diffuse or nodular enlargement of liver cells, variation in cell size, fatty degeneration, bile duct proliferation, and focal cystic necrosis. Other major effects of safrole, at 5,000 ppm only, included retardation of growth, mild anemia and slight atropy of the bone marrow.[3] Similar changes, including tumors, were observed in the livers of rats fed safrole for chronic periods, although the incidence of these changes was not described (Hagan et al.).[13]

A low incidence of liver carcinomas was induced after 12 to 22 months in CD rats (Charles River) by the oral administration of safrole in diets in experiments conducted by the Millers' group at the University of Wisconsin. The carcinogenic activities of compounds related to safrole, especially some known and possible metabolites of safrole, were demonstrated in comparison to the activity level of safrole tested at the same time and under the same conditions[1,16] (Table 7–2A). Local development of sarcomas at the injection site of these known or possible metabolites was also compared in the rats (Table 7–2B).[1,16] As a result, 1'-hydroxysafrole was suggested as a proximate carcinogenic metabolite of safrole, based on the greater hepatocarcinogenic activity upon oral administration to adult rats. The evident carcinogenicity of 1'-acetoxysafrole at the site of subcutaneous injection into the adult rat suggested that any ester formed in vivo may be an ultimate carcinogen of safrole.

A similar comparison of the carcinogenic activities of safrole-related compounds was more extensively investigated, almost exclusively by the Millers' group, in mice, which appeared to be more susceptible than rats to the carcinogenic activity of these compounds (Table 7–3A).[1,16–18] Safrole, isosafrole, dihydrosafrole, estragole, 1'-hydroxysafrole and

Table 7–2B. Carcinogenicity in Rats of Compounds Related to Safrole

(Charles River CD, random bred, male rats)

(Subcutaneous injections)

Compound	Dose	Exp. 1[1] No. of rats with sarcomas at injection site	Exp. 2[1] No. of rats with sarcomas at injection site	Exp. 3[16] No. of rats with sarcomas at injection site	Exp. 3[16] No. of rats with sarcomas at injection site
Solvent only	0.2 ml × 2/week × 20	0/18			
Safrole	18.6μmoles (3mg of safrole) × 2/week × 20	0/18 (18 mo.)	0/18 (17 mo.) 0/18 (17 mo.)	1/18 (21 mo.)	0/18 (21 mo.)
Isosafrole	18.6μmoles × 2/week × 20	0/18 (18 mo.)			
1'-Hydroxysafrole	18.6μmoles × 2/week × 20	2/18 (18 mo.)	1/18 (17 mo.)		
3'-Hydroxyisosafrole	18.6μmoles × 2/week × 20	0/18 (18 mo.)	0/18 (17 mo.)		
3'-Bromoisosafrole	18.6μmoles × 2/week × 20	2/18 (18 mo.)			
1'-Acetoxysafrole	18.6μmoles × 2/week × 20	6/18 (18. mo.)	5/18 (17 mo.)	5/18 (21 mo.)	6/18 (21 mo.)
3'-Acetoxyisosafrole	18.6μmoles × 2/week × 20	0/18 (18 mo.)	0/18 (17 mo.)		
1'-Methoxysafrole	18.6μmoles × 2/week × 20	0/18 (18 mo.)			
3'-Methoxyisosafrole	18.6μmoles × 2/weeks × 20	0/18 (18 mo.)			
1'-Oxosafrole	18.6μmoles × 2/week × 20			1/18 (21 mo.)	2/18 (21 mo.)

1'-hydroxyestragole were carcinogenic in mice by oral administration for more than one year. They were mostly hepatocarcinogenic in mice, including (C57BL/6 × C3H/Anf) F_1, (C57BL/6 × AKR)F_1 and Charles River CD-1 mice, except 1'-hydroxysafrole, which showed development in high incidence of interscapular angioma or angiosarcomas.

The first experiment with infant mice by Epstein et al.[19] demonstrated the induction of liver tumors in 58% of male Swiss mice sacrificed one year after 4 s.c. injections of safrole (total dose 6.6 mg) in infancy as compared to a 0% incidence in female mice treated with the same dose of safrole and a 6% incidence in control male mice. Carcinogenicity studies by the Millers' group using infant mice treated by four subcutaneous injections, by repeated oral administration or by a single intraperitoneal injection of the test substances showed hepatocarcinogenicity for safrole, estragole, methyleugenol, 1'-hydroxysafrole, 1'-acetoxysafrole, 1'-hydroxyestragole, 1'-hydroxymethyleugenol and 1'-hydroxy-2',3'-dehydroestragole (Table 7–3B). Elemicin, myristicin, anethole, eugenol, dill apiol, parsley apiol, 1'-oxosafrole, safrole-2',3'-oxide, 1'-hydroxysafrole-2',3'-oxide, 1'-acetoxysafrole 2',3'-oxide, estragole 2',3'-oxide, eugenol 2',3'-oxide, 1'-hydroxyelemicin and 3'-hydroxyanethole appeared to have little or no hepatocarcinogenic activity when administered to mice at doses at which safrole and estragole showed hepatocarcinogenicity.

As for carcinogenicity of the other methoxybenzene derivatives, high dose levels of the naturally occurring derivative β-asarone in the diets of rats induced leiomyosarcomas of the small intestine.[21] The synthetic compound 3,4,5-trimethoxycinamaldehyde, a derivative of the naturally occurring sinapaldehyde extracted from wood lignin, appeared to induce nasal tumors in rats.[22] As suggested by Miller and Miller,[23] this finding is interesting in light of the fact that possible carcinogenic factors in lignin may be responsible for the excess nasal cancer among furniture workers exposed to wood dust.

Table 7-3A. Carcinogenicity of Compounds Related to Safrole in Mice
(adult mice)

No. of mice with liver cell tumor/No. of mice at start of the experiments

Exp.	1[17]				2[1]	3[1]	4[16]		5[18]		6[18]
Strain	X†1		Y†1		CD-1 (Charles River)	CD-1	CD-1		CD-1		CD-1
Dose and Adm. Route	Gavage for 28 days,†2 then in diet for up to 82 weeks†3				0.5% 0.4% in diet for 13 mo.	0.4% in diet for 13 mo.	0.075% for day 1 to 10; 0.15% for day 11 to 20; 0.5% up to 12 mo.		0.5% 0.25% in diet		0.5% in diet
Sex	m	f	m	f	m	m	m	f	f	f	f
Compound											
Control	8/79	0/87	5/90	1/82	4/50	3/35	0/55	0/55	0/50 (20 mo.)		0/30 (20 mo.)
Safrole	11/17 (19 mo.)	16/16	3/17 (19 mo.)	16/17	8/40; 11/40 (16 mo.)	4/35 (16 mo.)	11/46	25/50 (17 mo.)	39/50 (19 mo.)	34/50 (19 mo.)	21/30 (18 mo.)
Isosafrole	5/18	1/16	2/17	0/16							
Dihydrosafrole	10/17†4	0/17	8/17†4	1/18							
1'-Hydroxysafrole					3/40†5 (0.55%); 3/25†5 (0.44%)		0/45	30/50			
1'-Acetoxysafrole						0/35 (0.5%); 0/35 (0.03%)					
Estragole									35/50 (0.46%)	27/50 (0.23%)	
1'-Hydroxyestragole										24/43 (0.25%)	
Eugenol											0/30 (0.50%)
Anethole											0/50 (0.46%)

†1 X: (C57BL/6 × C3H/Anf)F₁   Y: (C57BL/6 × AKR)F
†2 Safrole & Dihydrosafrole 464 mg/kg, Isosafrole 215 mg/kg
†3 Safrole 1112, Isosafrole 517, Dihydrosafrole 1400 ppm
†4 Incidence of liver cell tumors was significantly different from those in controls ($p = 0.01$).
†5 Interscapular angioma and angiosarcomas were 13/40 (0.55%) and 7/25 (0.44%).

Table 7–3B. Carcinogenicity in Infant Mice of Compounds Related to Safrole

Experiment	(1)[19]		(2)[1]		(3)[16]		(4)[20]	
Strain	Swiss albino mice		Charles River CD⁻¹		Charles River CD⁻¹		Charles River CD⁻¹	
Sex		m f		m f		m		m
Dose and Tumors Compound	Total dose	No. with liver tumors	Total dose	No. with liver carcinomas	Total dose	No. with liver carcinomas	Total dose	No. with liver carcinomas
Safrole	0.66 mg	6/12 0/9 (49–53 w)	10.5 μmoles (15.6 mg of safrole)	14/35 0/27 (16 mo.)	3.18 μmoles	18/35 (16 mo.)		
	6.6 mg	18/31 0/29 (49–53 w)						
1'-Hydroxysafrole			10.5 μmoles	26/31 3/31 (16 mo.)	3.18 μmoles	33/40 (16 mo.)	4.4 μmoles	30/60 (15 mo.)
1'-Acetoxysafrole			10.5 μmoles	27/33 2/22 (16 mo.)	3.18 μmoles	25/34 (16 mo.)		
1'-Oxosafrole					3.18 μmoles	5/31 (16 mo.)		
Estragole							5.2 μmoles	7/19 (15 mo.)
							4.4 μmoles	14/79 (15 mo.)
1'-Hydroxyestragole							4.4 μmoles	35/67 (15 mo.)
Solvent	0	4/78 (78w)	0	3/56 0/31 (16 mo.)	0	6/45 (16 mo.)	0	6/66 (15 mo.)

Table 7-3B. (continued)

Experiment	(5)[18]			(6)[18]			(7)[18]	
Strain	B6C3F₁			Charles River CD⁻¹			Charles River CD⁻¹	
Sex	m			m		f	m	
Dose & Tumors / Compound	Compound	Total dose (μmoles)	No. with liver tumors m (13 mo.)	Compound	p.o. (μmoles)	No. with Liver tumors m	f	i.p. (μmoles)	No. with Liver tumors m
	Elemicin	4.75	15/44	Safrole	2.5/g × 10	30/49	7/48	9.45	32/48
	1'-Hydroxyelemicin	4.75	26/63	1'-Hydroxysafrole				9.45	30/46
	Myristicin	4.75	14/45	Safrole-2',3'-oxide				9.45	6/44
	Anethole	4.75	15/47	1'-Hydroxysafrole 2',3' oxide				9.45	28/51
	3'-Hydroxyanethole	4.75	11/53						
	Dill apiol	4.75	12/52						
	Parsley apiol	4.75	11/55	1'-Acetoxysafrole 2',3'-oxide				9.45	16/41
	Methyleugenol	4.75	55/58	Estragole	2.5/g × 10	35/49	4/44	9.45	30/46
	1'-Hydroxymethyl eugenol	2.85	38/44	Estragole-2',3'-oxide				9.45	19/48
	Estragole	4.75	34/41	Eugenol	2.5/g × 10	13/51	0/52	9.45	11/45
	1'-Hydroxyestragole	4.65	45/46	Eugenol-2',3'-oxide				9.45	15/49
		2.85	40/40						
		1.90	59/60						
	1'-Hydroxy-2',3'-dehydroestragole	1.86	29/30	Anethole	5.0/g × 10	18/59	4/50	9.45	14/42
					2.5/g × 10	9/51	1/56		
	Solvent	0	24/58	Solvent		14/59	9/47		11/42

7.4 Metabolism of Safrole and Some Related Compounds

7.4.1 Metabolic fate

Earlier studies on the *in vivo* oxidation of alkylbenzenes including toluene, ethylbenzene, *n*-propylbenzene and *n*-butylbenzene, which were carried out by R. T. William's group in 1954–1956 demonstrated oxidation of side chains.

Urinary matabolites of safrole were identified by Stillwell *et al.*[24] after i.p. injections of safrole to male Sprague-Dawley rats and guinea pigs. These included 1,2-dihydroxy-4-allylbenzene, conjugated 1'-hydroxysafrole, 1',2'-methylenedioxy-4-'(2',3'-dihydroxypropyl)-benzene and 1,2-dihydroxy-4-'(2',3'-hydroxypropyl)-benzene. Ketosafrole was not detected in urine. 3'-*N*,*N*-1'-Dimethylamino-1'-'(3,4-methylenedioxyphenyl)-1'-propanone was detected also in guinea pigs as a urinary metabolite after oral or intraperitoneal administration of safrole to guinea pigs. Rats excreted it only as a minor urinary metabolite.[25] In contrast to this qualitative understanding of safrole metabolism in several animal species, through quantitative assessments of the urinary metabolites formed from safrole in the rat were first done by Klungsayr and Scheline.[26] They demonstrated that demethylation is the most prominent pathway, and that allylic hydroxylation leading to 1'-hydroxysafrole and derivatives and epoxide-diol formation contribute less to metabolite formation. The value for excretion of 4-allyl-1,2-dihydroxybenzene was about 77% of the measured urinary metabolites, while the value for 1'-hydroxysafrole's excretion was 4%.

Oral administration of C^{14}-labeled safrole or dihydrosafrole to mice revealed 64 and 61% of the ^{14}C in the exhaled CO_2, 18 and 25% in urine, 6 and 5% in intestine and feces, 2 and 2.5% in liver and 6 and 9% in carcasses, respectively.[27]

7.4.2 Metabolic activation of safrole and estragole

Since 1'-hydroxysafrole was demonstrated to be a proximate carcinogen in 1973 by Borchert *et al.*[1] it has come to be recognized as a critical intermediate in the carinogenic activation of safrole. 1'-Hydroxyestragole was also isolated from β-glucuronidase-treated urine from 21-day-old mice as well as adult mice (CD_1) injected i.p. with estragole.[20]

As suggested in the first work on the metabolic activation of safrole,[1]

J.A. Miller and Elizabeth C. Miller pointed to the 1'-carbon atoms in the allyl groups of these carcinogens as the site of formation of metabolic allylic and benzylic esters. Esters of this type, like the pyrrole metabolites of the hepatocarcinogenic pyrrolizidine alkaloids, had been strongly implicated as the reactive alkylating forms of these alkaloids.[28] Similarly, the carcinogenic diaryl acetylenic carbamates[29,5] are benzylic esters containing leaving groups attached to an electron-deficient carbon atom. However, a simple aliphatic allyl ester, allyl formate, showed no evidence of carcinogenicity, even though it is a well-known acinus-peripheral necrotic and cirrhogenic compound. Foci of basophilic liver cells were observed in a part of cirrhogenic liver after repeated s.c. injection of allyl formate.[30]

The greater carcinogenic activity of the allylic alcohol metabolite of safrole, 1'-hydroxysafrole, as compared to safrole in the liver of rat and mouse was shown by the Millers' group as described in section 7.3 on carcinogenesis by safrole and related compounds. The urinary excretion of 1'-hydroxysafrole after administration of safrole to rat, mouse, guinea pig and hamster is shown in Table 7–4.[31] The urinary excretion of 1'-hydroxysafrole by adult male hamsters and guinea pigs was similar to that of rats. However, male mice excreted in urine around 33%, and female mice excreted around 13%, of safrole dose as conjugated 1'-hydroxysafrole. When safrole was fed continuously in the diet to male rats, the urinary excretion of 1'-hydroxysafrole was 5 to 10% of the daily intake of safrole during the first 18 days and thereafter averaged 3 to 4%. Male mice fed 0.5% of safrole in the diet for 2 weeks excreted 17% of the ingested safrole as 1'-hydroxysafrole. There was no evident increase in the urinary excretion of 1'-hydroxysafrole conjugates in rats, guinea pigs and hamsters when their bile ducts were ligated 24 h prior to the injection of safrole[31] (Table 7–4).

Table 7–4. Urinary Excretion of 1'-Hydroxysafrole After Administration of Safrole to Various Animals[31]

Species	Sex	Age	Urinary 1'-hydroxysafrole (% of dose)†
Rat	M	Adult	1.6 ± 0.7 (4)
	F	Adult	1.1, 1.3
	M	4 weeks	2.1 ± 0.8 (4)
Mouse	M	Adult	33 ± 2.7 (4)
	F	Adult	13, 12
Guinea pig	M	Adult	2.1, 2.5
Hamster	M	Adult	3.5 ± 0.3 (4)

† 30 mg/100g body weight of safrole in trioctanoin was injected.

Estragole was metabolized to 1'-hydroxyestragole, similar to the metabolism of safrole to its 1'-hydroxy derivative. The urinary excretion of

1'-hydroxyestragole was around 20% of the dose of estragole in outbred CD-1 mice (Charles River). 1'-Hydroxyestragole was more hepatocarcinogenic than estragole, as noted in section 7.3. Further, the carcinogenicities of many of the known and possible electrophilic metabolites of safrole and estragole were examined in rats and/or mice (Table 7–2A,B and 7–3A,B). Among the possible electrophilic metabolites of safrole, estragole and their 1'-hydroxy metabolites, acetoxy[31] and epoxy[24] derivatives showed carcinogenic activity, especially at site of application, e.g., the forestomach upon feeding and subcutaneous tissue upon injection (Tables 7–2 and 7–3). However, the activities were generally lower than those of 1'-hydroxy metabolites of safrole and estragole.[16,23] 1'-Oxosafrole[25] and 1'-oxoestragole[32] showed no carcinogenic activity.[16]

Wislocki et al.[33] were not able to detect enzymatic acetylation of 1'-hydroxysafrole by mouse or rat liver microsomes, mitochondria or cytosols in the presence of acetyl CoA and with RNA as a nucleophilic acceptor. However, they obtained evidence for the formation of the sulfuric acid ester of 1'-hydroxysafrole by 3'-phosphoadenisine-5'phosphosulfate-dependent sulfotransferase activity in mouse and rat liver cytosols. Their presumption that the sulfuric acid ester of 1'-hydroxysafrole is a major ultimate carcinogenic metabolite of this proximate carcinogen was further evidenced by investigations on the effect of pentachlorophenol, which is known as an inhibitor of sulfotransferase activity, in the formation of a sulfuric acid ester of 1'-hydroxysafrole and in hepatocarcinogenesis by 1'-hydroxysafrole[34] and by the use of brachymorphic[35] mice which are deficient in sulfate ester formation[36] and resistant to hepatocarcinogenesis by 1'-hydroxysafrole[34] (Fig. 7–2).

7.4.3 Adduct formation in vitro and in vivo

Covalent binding of a wide variety of carcinogens to DNA and other macromolecules of target cells has been demonstrated and is generally accepted as a significant event in chemical carcinogenesis. The molecular interactions of carinogens with DNA in vivo involve strong bonds which lead to the formation of adducts that are sufficiently stable to be retained for prolonged periods so that lesions in DNA develop which may eventuate in alterations of gene expression.

The formation of DNA adducts in vivo and in vitro by derivatives of safrole and estragole and the characterization of the major hepatic DNA adducts has been studied extensively by the Miller group in recent years. [37-9] [2',3'-³H]1'-Hydroxysafrole, [2',3'-³H]1'-hydroxyestragole and [1'-³H]-1'-hydroxy-2',3'-dehydroestragole were used in the in vivo formation and characterization of these adducts. Comparisions were made of the nucleo-

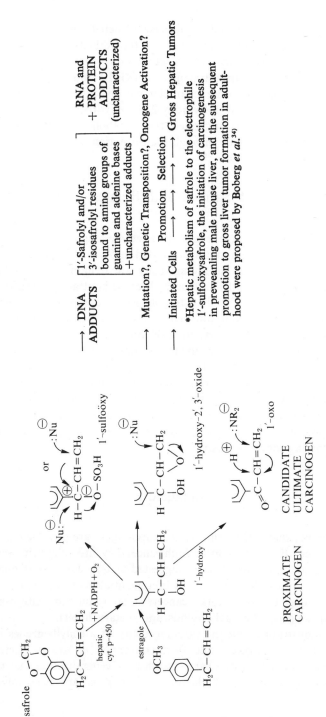

Fig. 7-2. Some possible pathways of metabolic activation *in vivo* of safrole and estragole to form carcinogenic electrophiles.[5,34]

side adducts derived by enzymatic hydrolysis of hepatic DNA from mice injected with these tritiated carcinogens and the adducts formed *in vitro* by reaction of deoxynucleosides with acetoxy and epoxy derivatives. As an example, N^2-(2',3'-dehydroestragole-1'-yl)dGMP and N^7-(2',3'-dehydroestragole-1'-yl)-guanine, were characterized by NMR spectroscopy as hepatic DNA adducts of 1'-hydroxy-2',3'-dehydroestragole in male $B6C3F_1$ mice. These results suggested the metabolic activation of 1'-hydroxy-2',3'-dehydroestragole through the formation of an electrophilic 1'-ester in mouse liver *in vivo*.[40]

7.5 Mutagenicity of Safrole and Related Compounds

Mutagenic activity of safrole, estragole, anethole, eugenol and some of their known or possible metabolites was tested in *Salmonella typhimurium* TA1513, TA100 and TA98. No mutagenicity was demonstrated for safrole, eugenol or 1'-acetoxyallylbenzene with or without added NADPH-fortified liver preparations.[20,41-3] Estragole and *trans*-anethole showed low but significant increases in mutagenic activity in the presence of liver activation systems (S-13 liver fraction). 1'-Hydroxysafrole and 1'-hydroxyestragole were mutagenic, especially in the presence of liver-activating enzymes. The 2',3'-oxides of safrole, estragole, eugenol, 1'-hydroxysafrole, and 1'-hydroxyestragole were strongly mutagenic in TA100. 1'-Acetoxysafrole, 1'-acetoxyestragole, 1'-acetoxysafrole-2'3'-oxide and 1'-oxasafrole-2',3'-oxide were mutagenic in TA1535 with or without an activating system. However, none of these compounds except 1'-oxasafrole-2',3'-oxide demonstrated mutagenicity in TA98.[20,41]

7.6 Conclusion

The probability that safrole and related carcinogens are possible causes of human cancer does not appear high since they are relatively weak carcinogens in animals. However, as suggested by Drs. James and Elizabeth Miller,[5] it is possible that even low lifetime intakes of these naturally occurring carcinogens could induce cancers in some humans with especially predisposing genetic backgrounds and dietary habits.

Studies demonstrating that the carcinogenicity of alkenylbenzenes including safrole and estragole results from conversion *in vivo* to electrophilic allylic and benzylic esters have extended the generalization that the ultimate carcinogenic forms of chemical carcinogens are electrophilic reactants. Further studies elucidating the susceptibility of humans to these naturally occurring carcinogens and clarifying their metabolic pathways in the human should contribute much to a closer understanding of human carcinogenesis and the prevention of cancer.

Acknowledgment

The author wishes to express his great appreciation to Drs. James A. Miller and Elizabeth C. Miller for supplying him with many papers of the work done in their laboratory over the past 15 years and for their critical reading of the manuscript.

REFERENCES

1. Borchert, P., Miller, J.A., Miller, E.C., and Shires, T.K., 1'-Hydroxysafrole, a proximate carcinogenic metabolite of safrole in the rat and mouse, *Cancer Res.*, **33**: 590–600, 1973.
2. Stecher, P. G., *The Merck Index*. 8th ed. Rahway, pp. 592, 761, 928, N.J. Merck & Co., 1968.
3. Long, E.L., Nelson, A.A., Fitzhugh, O.G., and Hansen, W.H., Liver tumors produced in rats by feeding safrole, *Arch. Pathol.*, **75**: 595–604, 1963.
4. Furia, T.E., and Bellanca, N., (eds.) *Fenaroli's Handbook of Flavour Ingredients*, p. 610, Cleveland, Ohio, Chemical Rubber Company, (Cited in Ref. 8) 1971.
5. Miller, J.A., and Miller, E.C., The metabolic activation and nucleic acid adducts of naturally-occurring carcinogenes, Recent results with ethyl carbamate and the spice flavors safrole and estragole (The 1983 Walter Hubert Lecture), *Br. J. Cancer*, **48**: 1–15, 1983.
6. Miller, J.A., Miller, E.C., and Phillips, D.H., The metabolic activation and carcinogenicity of alkenylbenzenes that occur naturally in many spices. In: *Carcinogens and Mutagens in the Environment*, Vol. 1. Food Products (ed. H.F. Stich), pp. 83–96, CRC Press, Boca Raton, Florida, 1982.
7. Leung, A.Y., *Encyclopedia of Common Natural Ingredients Used in Food, Drugs and Cosmetics*, p. 409, New York, Wiley-Interscience, 1980.
8. *IARC Monographs in the Evaluation of Carcinogenic Risk of Chemicals to Man*. Safrole, Isosafrole, and Dihydrosafrole, vol. 10, pp. 231–244, International Agency for Research on Cancer, Lyons, France, 1976.
9. Heffer, A., Zur Pharmakologie der Safrole Gruppe. *Arch. Exp. Path. Pharmakol*, **35**: 342–374, 1894–1895, (in German).
10. Abbott, D.D., Packman, E.W., Wagner, B.M., and Harrisson, J.W.E., Chronic oral toxicity of oil of sassafras and safrole, *Pharmacologist*, **3**: 62, 1961.
11. Powers, M.F., Darby, T.D., and Schueler, F.W., A study of the toxic effects of cinnamon oil, *Pharmacologist*, **3**: 62, 1961.
12. Taylor, J.M., Jenner, P.M., and Jones, W.I., A comparison of the toxicity of some allyl, propenyl and propyl compounds in the rat, *Toxicol. Appl. Pharmacol.*, **6**: 378–387, 1964.
13. Hagen, E.C., Jenner, P.M., Jones, W.I., Fitzhugh, O.G., Long, E.L., Brouwer, J.G., and Webb, W.K., Toxic properties of compounds related to safrole, *Toxicol. Appl. Pharmacol.*, **7**: 18–24, 1965.
14. Crosby, D.G. Natural toxic background in the food of man and his animals, *J. Agr. Food Chem.*, **17**: 532–538, 1969.

15. Homburger, F., Kelly, Jr., T., Friedler, G., and Russfield, A.B., Toxic and possible carcinogenic effects of 4-allyl-1,2-methylene dioxybenzene (safrole) in rats on deficient diets, *Med. Exptl.*, **4**: 1–11, 1961.
16. Wislocki, P.G., Miller, E.C., Miller, J.A., McCoy, E.C., and Rosenkranz, H.S., Carcinogenic and mutagenic activities of safrole, 1'-hydroxysafrole and some known or possible metabolites, *Cancer Res.*, **37**: 1883–1891, 1973.
17. Innes, J.R.M., Ulland, B.M., Valerio, M.G., Petrucelli, L., Fishbein, L., Hart, E.R., Pallotta, A.J., Bates, R.R., Falk, H.L., Gart, L.L., Klein, M., Mitchell, I., and Peter, J., Bioassay of pesticides and industrial chemicals for tumorigenicity in mice: a preliminary note, *J. Natl. Cancer Inst.*, **42**: 1101–1114, 1969.
18. Miller, E.C., Swanson, A.B., Phillips, D.H., Fletcher, T.L., Liem, A., and Miller, J.A., Structure-activity studies of the carcinogenicities in the mouse and rat of some naturally occurring and synthetic alkenylbenzene derivatives related to safrole and estragole, *Cancer Res.*, **43**: 1124–1134, 1983.
19. Epstein, S.S., Fujii, K., Andrea, J., and Mantel, N., Carcinogenicity testing of selected food additives by parenteral administration to infant Swiss mice, *Toxicol. Appl. Pharmacol.*, **16**: 321–334, 1970.
20. Drinkwater, N.R., Miller, E.C., Miller J.A., and Pitot, H.C., The hepatocarcinogenicity of estragole (1-allyl-4-methoxybenzene) and 1'-hydroxyestragole in the mouse and the mutagenicity of 1'-acetoxyestragole in bacteria, *J. Natl. Cancer Inst.*, **57**: 1232–1331, 1976.
21. Gorss, M.A., Jones, W.I., Cook, E.L., and Boone, C.C., Carcinogenicity of oil of calamus, *Proc. Am. Assoc. Cancer Res.*, **8**: 24, 1970.
22. Schoental, R., and Gibbard, S., Nasal and other tumors in rats given 3,4,5-trimethoxycinnamaldehyde, a derivative of sinapaldehyde and other α,β-unsaturated aldehydic wood lignin constituents, *Br. J. Cancer*, **26**: 504–505, 1972.
23. Miller, J.A., Swanson, A.B., and Miller, E.C., The metabolic activation of safrole and related naturally occurring alkenylbenzenes in relation to carcinogenesis by these agents. In: *Naturally Occurring Carcinogens-Mutagens and Modulators of Carcinogenesis* (E.C. Miller et al., eds.) pp. 111–125, Japan Sci. Soc. Press, Tokyo, **1979**.
24. Stillwell, W.G., Carman, J.J., Bell, L., and Horning, M.G., The metabolism of safrole and 2',3'-epoxysafrole in the rat and guinea pig, *Drug. Metab. Disp.*, **2**: 489–489, 1974.
25. Oswald, E.O., Fishbein, L., Corbett, B.J., and Walker, M.P., Identification of tertiary aminomethylenedioxypropiophenones as urinary metabolites of safrole in the rat and guinea pig, *Biochim. Biophy. Acta*, **230**: 237–247, 1971.
26. Klungsayr, J., and Scheline, R.S., Metabolism of safrole in the rat, *Acta Pharmacol. Toxicol.*, **52**: 211–216, 1983.
27. Kamienski, F.X., and Casida, J.E., Importance of demethylation in the metabolism *in vivo* and *in vitro* of methylenedioxyphenyl synergists and related compounds in mammals, *Biochem. Pharmacol.*, **19**: 91–112, 1970.
28. Mattocks, A.R., Toxicity of pyrrolizidine alkaloids, *Nature*, **217**: 723–728, 1968.
29. Harris, P.N., Gibson, W.R., and Dillard, R.D., Oncogenicity of 1-(4-chlorophenyl)-1-phenyl-2-propynyl carbamate for rats, *Toxicol. Appl. Pharmacol.*, **21**: 414–418, 1972.
30. Miller, J.A., Miller, E.C., and Enomoto, M., Unpublished data.
31. Borchert, P., Wislocki, P.G., Miller, J.A., and Miller, E.C., The metabolism of naturally occurring hepatocarcinogen safrole to 1'-hydroxysafrole and electrophilic reactivity of 1'-acetoxysafrole, *Cancer Res.*, **33**: 575–589, 1973.
32. Solheim, E., and Scheline, R.R., Metabolism of alkenebenzene derivatives in the rat, *Xenobiotica*, **3**: 493–498, 1973.
33. Wislocki, P.G., Borchert, P., Miller, J.A., and Miller, E.C., The metabolic activation of the carcinogen 1'-hydroxysafrole *in vivo* and *in vitro* and the electrophilic reactivities of possible ultimate carcinogens, *Cancer Res.*, **36**: 1686–1695, 1976.
34. Boberg, E.W., Miller, E.C., Miller, J.A., Poland A., and Liem, A., Strong evidence

from studies with brachymorphic mice and pentachlorophenol that 1'-sulfooxysafrole is the major ultimate electrophilic and carcinogenic metabolite of 1'-hydroxysafrole in mouse liver, *Cancer Res.*, **43**: 5163–5173, 1983.

35. Sugahara, K., and Schwartz, N.B., Defect in 3'-phosphoadenosine-5'-phosphosulfate formation in brachymorphic mice, *Arch. Biochem. Biophys.*, **214**: 602–609, 1982.
36. Lyman, S.D., and Poland, A., Effect of the brachymorphic trait in mice on xenobiotic sulfate ester formation, *Biochem. Pharmacol.*, **32**: 3345–3350, 1983.
37. Phillips, D.H., Hanawalt, P.C., Miller, J.A., and Miller, E.C., The *in vivo* formation and repair of DNA adducts from 1'-hydroxysafrole, *J. Supramolecular Struct. Cellular Bioch.*, **16**: 83–90, 1981.
38. Phillips, D.H., Miller, J.A., Miller, E.C., and Adams, B., Structures of the DNA adducts formed in mouse liver after administration of the proximate hepatocarcinogen 1'-hydroxyestragole, *Cancer Res.*, **41**: 176–186, 1981.
39. Phillips, D.H., Miller, J.A., Miller, E.C., and Adams, B., The N^2-atom of guanine and the N^6-atom of adenine residues as sites for covalent binding of metabolically activated 1'-hydroxysafrole to mouse liver DNA *in vivo*, *Cancer Res.*, **41**: 2664–2671 1981.
40. Fennell, T.R., Miller, J.A., and Miller, E.C., Characterization of the major hepatic DNA adduct of the strong hepatocarcinogen 1'-hydroxy-2',3'-dehydroestragole in male B6C3F$_1$ mice, *Proc. Amer. Assoc. for Cancer Research*, **25**: 88, 1984.
41. Swanson, A.B., Chambliss, D.D., Blomquist, J.C., Miller, E.C., and Miller, J.A., The mutagenicities of safrole, estragole, eugenol, *trans*-anethole, and some of their known or possible metabolites for *Salmonella typhimurium* mutants, *Mutat. Res.*, **60**: 143–153, 1979.
42. Dorange, J.L., Janiaud, P., Delaforge, M., Levi, P., and Padieu, P., Comparative survey of microsomal activation systems for mutagenic studies of safrole, *Mutat. Res.*, **53**: 179–180, 1978.
43. Green, N.R., and Savage, J.R., Screening of safrole, eugenol, their ninhydrin positive metabolites and selected secondary amines for potential mutagenicity, *Mutat. Res.*, **57**: 115–121, 1978.

8

Tannins (Tannic Acid)

8.1 Occurrence, Chemistry and Use

The term "tannin" was applied in 1796 by Seguin to the constituents of oak gall, which are capable of converting animal skin to leather.[1] Tannin is not a single chemical compound, but a large group of phenolic compounds. Its structure varies depending upon the source vegetable from which it is extracted. Tannin is contained in wood, bark, fruit, twigs, leaves and roots of a large number of plants. The bark of oak (*Quercus*), eucalyptus, mangrove, hemlock, pine and willow, the wood of quebracho (*Schinopsis lorentzii*), chestnut (*Castanea sativa* Mill) and oak, the fruit of tara, myrobalans (*Terminalia chebula* Retz) and divi-divi, the leaves of sumac and gambier and the roots of canaigre and palmetto contain high amounts of tannin.[2] Early in the twentieth century, Fisher *et al.* disclosed the structure of tannic acid.[3] Further extensive studies on the chemistry of tannin were carried out by many groups of the chemists throughout the world and the vegetable tannins were divided into two groups — the hydrolyzable tannins and non-hydrolyzable, condensed tannins.[4] Hydrolyzable tannins are esters hydrolyzed by acids, alkalis and tannase such as gallic acid, ellagic acid and brevifolin. Gallotannins are usually contained in gall which is produced by the parasite, *Melaphis chinensis* Bell, living on *Rhus javanica* L and similar plants and is thus known as a pathological tannin. Extensive research on the structures of a variety of vegetable tannins has been carried out in recent years. Trapain, a novel hydrolyzable tannin, is one of the compounds newly isolated by the group of Nishioka[5] from the fruit shells of *Trapa japonica* Flerov (*Oenotherecease*) (Fig. 8–1). Condensed tannins, although they are polyphenolic substances similar to hydrolyzable ones, show the complexed structures of dimers, trimers, oligomers and polymers. The basic structures for this type of tannin reveal catechins, anthocyamis and flavones.[6]

161

Tannic acid (E. Fisher, 1912)

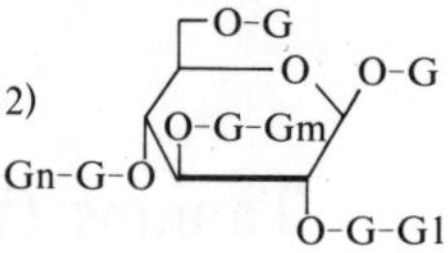

pentagalloylglucose	$:l+m+n=0$ 4%
hexa	$:l+m+n=1$ 12
hepta	$:l+m+n=2$ 19
octa	$:l+m+n=3$ 25
nona	$:l+m+n=4$ 20
deca-dodeca	: 21

G : galloyl

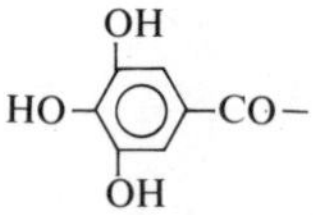

Trapain[5].

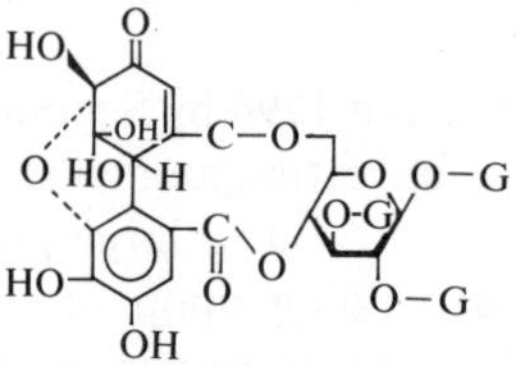

Fig. 8–1. Structures of tannic acid (Chinese gallotannin) and trapain.

Tannic acid (gallotannic acid, gallotannin, glycerite) is a principle of tannin, derived from Chinese nutgalls (*Gallae rhois*) belonging to *Anacardiaceae* and constitutes penta- to octa-galloylglucose (Fig. 8–1). However, the term tannin is ordinarily used as a synonym for tannic acid. Tannic acid is a colorless amorphous, bulky powder and very soluble in water, ethanol and aceton but almost insoluble in ether, chloroform and benzene. It is characteristic of astringent taste. One gram of tannic acid dissolves in 0.35 ml water, rendering an aqueous solution acidic. Applying its capacity to form insoluble precipitates with protein, gelatin, starch and heavy-metal ions, tannic acid is used largely by the textile industry as a treating agent. It is also used in pigment manufacture as an additive for inks and in medicinal products for humans, including those used for treatment of burns, diarrhea, chemical antidotes in poisoning and as local astringent. Many crude plant preparations, such as *Geranium* herb broth, are used for treatment of diarrhea by virtue of their tannin content, exerting a rather mild astringent effect on the mucous membrane of the gastrointestinal tract and causing constipation.

According to the IARC monograph[3] tannic acid is also added as a flavoring agent to foods and beverages and used as a clarifying agent in the brewing and wine industries.

8.2 Toxicology and Carcinogenicity

8.2.1 Human data

Local application of condensed tannin causes dryness and reduced taste of the oral mucosa by its astringent action. Tannic acid is known as a hepatotoxic agent causing centrolobular necrosis in the liver. Since a report of Wells *et al.* (1942)[7] on human burn cases, there have been several reported cases of acute hepatic injury probably caused by absorption in appreciable amounts of tannins with the use of tannin on burned skin surfaces or barium enemas containing tannic acid.[8,9] However, no case of human cancer caused by tannin or epidemiological information suggesting tannin as a causal factor for human cancer has been reported.[3]

8.2.2 Animal data.

Korpássy[10] observed the development of toxic hepatic damage with centrolobular necrosis in rats parenterally administered tannic acid. Administered orally, tannic acid produced similar necrosis in the liver.[11] A single dose of 250 mg/kg body weight tannic acid to rats caused centrolobular necrosis.[12] Histochemical and ultrastructural investigation on liver injury with tannic acid revealed a concentration of tannin acid in the nuclei of the liver cells as early as three hours following administration to rats. Sequential inhibition of nuclear RNA synthesis, nucleolar segregation, inhibition of protein synthesis and liver cell necrosis have been observed.[12-16]

Acute toxicity: oral LD_{50} of tannic acid is around 3.5 g/kg b.w. in mice[17] and 2.26 g/kg b.w. in rats.[18] S.c. LD_{50} of tannic acid in rats is 1.5 g/kg b.w.[19] Its i.v. LD_{50} in mice is 0.04 g/kg.[17]

Repeated parenteral administration of tannic acid to rats caused cirrhosis.[20] Subsequent study on white rats, subcutaneously administered for two months with tannic acid, generally every 5 days (altogether 49 injections) for 290 days (initial dose, 150 mg/kg b.w., later 200 mg/kg b.w. as a 1.5 to 2% aqueous solution) revealed development of liver tumors in 13 out of 23 rats (56%) which survived 100 days and died or were sacrificed between the 109th and 388th day of the experiment. Liver cirrhosis developed in 15 of 23 rats, mostly combined with liver tumor, while in 4 animals with liver tumors no cirrhosis was found (Table 8–1). The experiment was terminated after 388 days. Five out of 28 rats examined had

Table 8-1. Liver Tumors and Cirrhosis Produced by Parenteral Administration of Tannic Acid in Rats[21]

Days of experiment	Number of rats examined	Number of rats with liver cirrhosis	Number of rats with liver tumors				Cirrhosis in tumor rats
			Liver cell tumors (L)	Bile duct tumors (B)	L + B	Total	
11–64	5	—	—	—	—	—	—
109–185	11	8	1	3	1	5	4
215–295	7	5	2	2	—	4	4
320–388	5	2	2	1	1	4	1
Total	28	15	5	6	2	13	9

liver cell tumors and 6 out of 28 had bile duct tumors. From the histological description and photographic pictures of these tumors, some of the liver cell tumors look like liver cell adenomas and others liver cell carcinomas. Almost all of the bile duct tumors seem to be bile duct adenoma or choloangiofibrosis.[21] The sex of the animal did not seem to affect the incidence of induced liver tumors and cirrhosis.

No evident carcinogenic activity was observed in groups of 10 August strain rats, each injected with solutions of extracts from plant material (sulphited quebracho, mimosa and myrobalans) and tannic acid, though 2 out of 10 rats in each group of those injected with sulphited quebracho and mimosa extracts showed development of local sarcomas. No other tumors or hepatic lesions were observed in the rats in this experiment.[22]

When 5% aqueous solution of tannic acid was applied to the artificially burned and ulcerated skin of 20 white rats, no tumors or hepatic lesions were observed in 11 animals surviving 400 days.[21]

Tumors have been induced in mice by subcutaneous injections of various tannin extracts. Aqueous solutions of tannin extracts prepared from various plant materials (myrtan, quebracho, mimosa, myrobalans, chestnut and valonea) and tannic acid were injected subcutaneously at a dose of 0.25 ml in stock mice once weekly for 12 weeks. Myrtan, quebracho and mimosa tannins produced 5, 8 and 2 local sarcomas, respectively, and 7,5 and 9 liver tumors, respectively. Tannic acid, myrobalans, chestnut and valonea induced only liver tumors, 7, 4, 4 and 1, respectively. No histological description or photographic picture of these liver tumors was given in the report; no controls were reported, and there was no indication of the number of mice used in this experiment.[22]

Intramuscular injections of tannic acid, a complex of esters of D-glucose with gallo tannic acid and galloyl gallotannic acid, to young C3H/A mice, a group of 30 males and 30 females, every second week at a dose of 0.75 mg/kg b.w. for 12 months induced no local tumors after 18 months of experiment.[23]

8.3 Conclusion

At present, there are no significant animal data demonstrating carcinogenic activity of tannin. There is no published carcinogenicity study on
tannin by oral application. However, the early evidence obtained by
Korpássy's group on the hepatotoxic action of tannin causing centrolobular
necrosis and subsequent cirrhosis and/or liver tumors suggests the
presence of carcinogenic agents in vegetable tannins, when compared
with the carcinogenic property seen in similar centrolobular necro-
sis-inducing hepatotoxins including CCl_4 and $CHCl_3$.[24] Recent advances
in chemical isolation and structural determination of tannins will rapidly
increase the available information on toxicity and carcinogenicity of tannins in the near future. As noted by Nishioka in his review,[6] accumulation
of data on a variety of biological activities of tannins, including their
binding property with protein, effect on protease and its inhibitors, effect
on biosynthesis of prostaglandins and reducing effect on urea nitrogen
concentrations in serum and liver, will further the study of the chemistry
and biological effects of tannins.

REFERENCES

1. Haworth, R.D., Some problems in the chemistry of the gallotannins, *Proc. Chem. Soc.*, 1961, 401–412.
2. Flaherty, F., and Stubbings, R.L., Leather. In: *Encyclopedia of Chemical Techno- logy*, (R.E. Kirk and D.F. Othmer, eds.) vol. 12, John Wiley and Sons, pp. 314– 315, 1967 (Cited in Ref. 3).
3. *IARC Monographs on the Evaluation of Carcinogenic Risk of Chemicals to Man*, Tannic Acid and Tannins, vol. 10, pp. 253–262, Lyons, France, International Agency for Research on Cancer, 1976.
4. Haslam, E., Chemistry of Vegetable Tannins, Academic Press, London, New York, 1966.
5. Nonaka, G., Matsumoto, Y., Nishioka, I., Nishizawa, M., and Yamagishi, T., Trapain, a new hydrolyzable tannin from *Trapa japonica* Flerow, *Chem. Pharm. Bull.*, 29: 1184–1187, 1981.
6. Nishioka, I., Chemistry and biological activities of tannins *Yakugaku Zasshi*, 103: 125–142, 1983 (in Japanese).
7. Wells, D.B., Humphery, J.D., and Coll, J.S., The relation of tannic acid to the liver necrosis occurring in burns, *New Engl. J. Med.*, 226: 629–635, 1942.
8. Lucke, H.H., Hodge, K.E., and Patt, N.L., Fatal liver damage after barium enemas containing tannic acid, *Canad. Med. Ass. J.*, 89: 1111–1114, 1963.
9. McAlister, W.H., Anderson, M.S., Bloomberg, G.R. and Margulis, A.R., Lethal effects of tannic acid in the barium enema, *Radiology*, 80: 765–773, 1963.

10. Korpássy, B., Leber shädigung durch gerbsäure, *Schweiz Z. Path. Bakt.*, **12**: 13–23, 1949 (in German).
11. Korpássy, B., Koltay, N., and Hovai, R., Toxizität peroral verabreichter Gerbsäure, *Wien klin. Wschr.*, **62**: 270, 1950 (in German).
12. Horvath, E., Solyom, A., and Korpássy, B., Histochemical and biochemical studies in acute poisoning with tannic acid, *Brit. J. Exp. Path.*, **41**: 298–304, 1960.
13. Arhelger, R.B., Broom, J.S., and Boler, R.K., Ultrastructural hepatic alterations following tannic acid administration to rabbits, *Amer. J. Path.*, **46**: 409–434, 1965.
14. Badawy, A.A.B., White, A.E., and Lathe, G.H., The effect of tannic acid on the synthesis of protein and nucleic acid by rat liver, *Biochem. J.*, **113**: 307–313, 1969.
15. Reddy, J.K., and Svoboda, D., The relationship of nucleolar segregation to ribonucleic acid synthesis following the administration of selected hepatocarcinogens, *Lab. Invest.*, **19**: 132–145, 1968.
16. Reddy, J.K., Chiga, M., Hariss, C.C., and Svoboda, D.J., Polyribosome disaggregation in rat liver following administration of tannic acid. *Cancer Res.*, **30**: 58–65, 1970.
17. Robinson, H.J., and Graessle, O.E., Toxicity of tannic acid, *J. Pharmacol. Exp. Ther.*, **77**: 63–69, 1943.
18. Boyd, E.M., The acute toxicity of tannic acid administered intragastrically, *Canad. Med. Assoc. J.*, **92**: 1292–1297, 1965.
19. Cameron, G.R., Milton, R.F., and Allen, J.W., Toxicity of tannic acid, An experimental investigation. *Lancet*, **ii**: 179–186, 1943.
20. Korpássy, B., and Kovács, K., Experimental liver cirrhosis in rats produced by prolonged subcutaneous administration of solutions of tannic acid, *Brit. J. Exp. Path.*, **30**: 266–272, 1949.
21. Korpássy, B., and Mosonyi, M., The carcinogenic activity of tannic acid, Liver tumors induced in rats by prolonged subcutaneous administration of tannic acid solution, *Brit. J. Cancer*, **4**: 411–420, 1950.
22. Kirby, K.S., Induction of tumors by tannin extracts, *Brit. J. Cancer*, **14**: 147–150, 1960.
23. Bichel, J. and Bach, A., Investigation on the toxicity of small chronic doses of tannic acid with special reference to possible carcinogenicity, *Acta Pharmacol. Toxicol.*, **26**: 41–45, 1968.
24. Cohen, A.J., and Grasso, P., Review of the hepatic response to hypolipidaemic drugs in rodents and assessment of its toxicological significance to man, *Food Cosmet. Toxicol.*, **19**: 585–605, 1981.

9

Betel Nut

Betel nut is the fruit of the betel palm, *Areca catechu,* and is used as the quid for betel chewing. A high incidence of oral cancer in central and southeast Asian countries is considered to be related to the habit.

9.1 History of Betel Chewing

The chewing of betel is a widespread habit found in many countries of the Orient which goes back hundreds of years. The chewing of the betel nut is mentioned in the Sanskrit *Susrata Samhita* believed to have been written about 600 A.D. The Sanskrit for the leaf of the betel vine, "tambula," remains in the Hindi word "tambuli" and in the Arabic and Persian "tambula." Betel chewing is known to have reached the Zanzibar coast between 1200–1400 A.D. It is said that the betel leaf was imported from India to Malacca, and the habit spread to southeast Asian countries including Indonesia, Malaysia, the Philippines, New Guinea, Taiwan and other Pacific islands.[1,2]

9.2 Type, Method and Composition of the Quid

Basic constituents of the betel quid are betel nut, betel leaf and lime (Fig. 9–1).[1-7] Tobacco, liquefied catechu and other spicy ingredients are also frequently used with the above. The type of betel quid varies depending on location, socioeconomic level and individual preference.[7] Tobacco is usually mixed in India,[1,4] but not in New Guinea.[5,6] In general, flaked, cracked or sliced betel nut is used for the quid. Lime is prepared from stone (slaked) or shells.[1] The aboriginal Veddas of Sri Lanka use the slaked

Table 9-1. Habit of Chewing Betel Quids in Different Areas of Asia

Countries		Ingredients of betel quids and the methods
India	Calcutta	Cracked betel nuts, tobacco cut in a small piece and spices are wrapped in betel leaf smeared liquid gambir and lime (usually stone lime).
	Delhi	Basically the same as quids of Calcutta, but more spices are usually used.
	Agra	Four principal ingredients — betel leaf, liquid gambir, cracked betel nuts and lime. Usually, tobacco is not used.
	Mainpuri	Chewing is distributed as "Mainpuli tobacco" (A mixture of powdered tobacco, sliced betel nuts, lime, cloves, cardamon seed sandal-wood powder, nutmeg, camphor, peppermint, gambir and others is chewed.). Betel leaf is not used.
	Bombay	Betel leaf, liquid gambir, lime and sliced betel nuts are also used as ingredients. Various spices are also supplemented if tobacco is not used.
Sri Lanka		Betel leaf, cracked betel nuts, cut tobacco and shell lime are chewed together.
Taiwan		Fresh unripe fruit of betel nuts in toto with lime (stone lime) paste, a slice of long pepper and *Glycyrrhiza glabra* are the basic ingredients.
Thailand		Fresh wedge-shaped piece of unripe fruit with a clove and betel leaf smeared with lime (red paste of shell lime) are used. Cut tobacco is also used to wipe teeth.
Malaysia		Dry slices of betel nuts, nutmeg and *Foeniculum vulgare* are wrapped in betel leaf smeared with lime (usually stone lime) and gambir, and pinned with a clove. Cured tobacco is sometimes used together with the above.
Singapore		Dry slices of betel nuts, betel leaf smeared lime (stone lime in mountainous areas, shell lime in coastal areas) paste and cured tobacco are used.
Indonesia		Dry slices of betel nuts are wrapped in a piper leaf smeared with lime and gambir. Cut tobacco is also used to wipe teeth.
Philippines		A piper betel leaf smeared lime paste and a tipped nut belted with a piper betel leaf wrapping lime (mostly shell lime) powder are used. Chewing tobacco (half dry and seasoned) is used together with the above.

The table is based on the contents of references 9 and 10.

lime from the shells of snails, and coral is also used in the Pacific islands.[6] The purpose of the lime appears to be for its alkalinity since the betel nut has an acidic reaction, as well as its promoting effect for the appearance of a red dye.[1] The ingredients of the quid are wrapped in a leaf of the betel vine on which an aqueous extract of the heart of *Acasia catechu* or *Acasia suma* is often smeared. Spices such as cardamon, cloves and aniseed may be supplemented for additional flavor.[8] In Thailand, turmeric, the ground root of *Curma aromatica,* is usually added to the chew.[1] Variations of the ingredients of the quid are shown in Table 9–1. The quid is carried to the gingivo buccal fold, or between the lower teeth. A quid is chewed for hours and some sleep with the quid in the mouth. Chewing betel quid leaves the mouth rather numb and promotes intense salivation and mild

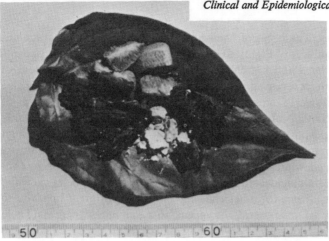

Fig. 9-1. A betel quid (unrolled) used in Sri Lanka. Cracked betel nuts, cut tobacco and lime on a betel leaf.

exhilaration. In countries where the habit is prevalent, the practice begins about 10–14 years of age. Chewing betel is currently being given up by increasingly large numbers of the younger generation, but it is still practiced especially among older people.[11]

9.3 Clinical and Epidemiological Evidence of Betel Chewing

The habit of betel chewing has been suggested to be related to high incidences of oral cancer.[3-20] Orr described 100 cases of oral cancer in betel/tobacco chewers in detail. Of these, 2 were not chewers, 9 chewed occasionally, 24 chewed from 3 to 5 quids a day, 40 chewed more, and 25 slept with a quid in the mouth. He stated that over two-thirds of the cancers involved the site directly. Sanghvi *et al.*[8] performed a statistical survey on 1,460 patients referred to the Tata Memorial Hospital, Bombay, in 1952–1954. Patients referred to this hospital in whom no cancer was detected formed a control group. The patients were asked whether they smoked "bids" or chewed betel. The survey showed that chewing betel/tobacco was associated with cancer of the oral cavity: chewing and smoking with tumors of the hypopharynx and the base of the tongue; smoking alone with cancers of the oropharynx, notably the tonsil, and the esophagus. Shanta and Krishnamurthi[12] reviewed 347 oral cancers seen in one year at the Cancer Institute, Madras. Seventy-one percent of all oral cancers arose from the buccal mucosa. The incidence of cheek cancer was higher in males. The habit of chewing tobacco, betel leaf and areca nut was highly significant. Eighty-five percent of cheek carcinoma patients were tobacco, betel and nut chewers as opposed to 12.5% in the control group. The authors reported that betel nut and botacco chewing were also important etiological factors for carcinomas of the anterior two-thirds of the tongue, although tobacco smoking appeared to play a dominant role in cancers of the posterior one third. Sanghvi et al.[8] attributed the high incidence of tumors at the base of tongue to the combined habit of smoking "bids" and chewing tobacco. Jussawalla and Deschpande[13] also conducted an epidemiological study to evaluate cancer risk in betel chewing. They showed evidence to indict chewing as a factor of great importance in the etiology of pharyngeal, laryngeal and esophageal cancer (Table 9–2). In particular, the risk of developing cancer in the buccal mucosa was found to be 7.7 times higher in chewers than in non-chewers and cancer of the buccal mucosa was moreover predominantly found in those with the habit of retaining the quid in the buccal groove. Similar epidemiological results were obtained by Wahi et al.,[4] who studied factors influencing oral and oropharyngeal cancers in 1,916 cases in India. Hirayama[14] conducted another epidemiological investigation on chewing habits in the three areas of Mainpuri (northern India), Neyyur (southern India), and Jaffna (Sri Lanka). A relative frequency of oral cancer and the risk of

Table 9–2. Relative Risk of Developing Oral Pharyngeal Laryngeal and Esophageal Cancers Among Chewers at Each Anatomical Site (after Jussawalla and Deschpande[13])

| Site-group | Chewing habit (assuming risk among non-chewers to be unity) | | | | Relative risk | χ^2 |
| | Cancer cases | | Control group | | | |
	Non-chewers	Chewers	Non-chewers	Chewers		
Cancer group	853	1152	1340	665	2.7	237.7***
Lip	8	6	1340	665	1.5	0.2 NS
Ant. 2/3 tongue	36	54	1340	665	3.0	26.3***
Floor mouth	10	4	1340	665	0.8	< 0.01 NS
Alveolus	26	44	1340	665	3.4	25.2***
Buccal mucosa	42	160	1340	665	7.7	164.2***
Hard palate	7	14	1340	665	4.0	9.0**
Oral cavity	129	282	1340	665	4.4	178.3***
Base tongue	175	187	1340	665	2.2	44.7***
Soft palate	35	18	1340	665	1.0	< 0.01 NS
Tonsils	99	128	1340	665	2.6	47.0***
Oropharynx	309	333	1340	665	2.2	71.6***
Nasopharynx	10	7	1340	665	1.4	0.2 NS
Hypopharynx	21	49	1340	665	4.7	39.0***
Larynx	246	314	1340	665	2.6	96.3***
Esophagus	138	167	1340	665	2.4	52.6***

The χ^2 values marked with single, double and triple asterisks were found to have $P < 0.05$, $P < 0.01$, and $P < 0.001$, while those marked "NS" were found to be not significant with $P < 0.05$.

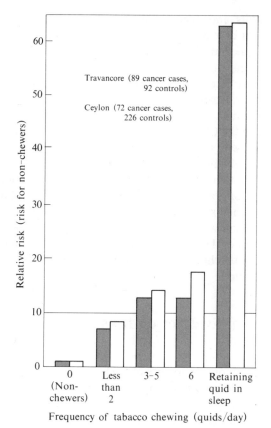

Travancore (89 cancer cases, 92 controls)

Ceylon (72 cancer cases, 226 controls)

Frequency of tabacco chewing (quids/day)

Fig. 9–2. Relative risk of developing oral cancer according to frequency of tobacco (betel) chewing in Travancore and Ceylon, 1964.[14]

developing oral cancer according to frequency of tobacco chewing in these areas with high prevalence of chewing was obtained (Fig. 9–2). Epidemiological study of precancerous conditions such as leukoplakia and the habit of betel or tobacco chewing has also been reported by several investigators. Mehta *et al.*[15] performed a study of oral cancer and precancerous conditions among 101,761 villagers in a district of India. In the house-to-house survey, precancerous conditions were established for leukoplakia (0.67%), preleukoplakia (0.86%) and submucosal fibrosis (0.03%) in addition to the detection of 12 oral cancers. About 54% of the study population had a habit of either chewing or smoking. The dominant habit of chewing tobacco with lime was found in 52% of males and 38.9% of females. Similar epidemiological studies have been conducted on the same group,[16–18] including a study of dose-response relationship between chewing habit and oral leukoplakia.[18] Dose-response relationship was significant for chewing habits and occurrence of leukoplakia, but the relationship was weaker than that between tobacco smoking and leukoplakia. Ramanathan and Lakshimi[11] carried out an epidemiological analysis of the incidence of oral cancer in peninsular Malaysia, especially in relation to racial variations among the Indians, Malays, Chinese and Caucasians. Of a total 898 oral cancer patients, 31.3% occurred in the Indian female, 29.1% in the Indian male, 10.6% in the Malay male, 11.1% in the Malay female, 14.1% in the Chinese male, and 4.0% in the Chinese female. In the Indian females, with the highest incidence of the oral cancer, the single habit of chewing betel quid was most popular. Similar epidemiological data on this area was obtained by Marsden.[19] Earlier, Friedell and Rosenthal[20] reported 8 cases of oral cancer in white American males who habitually chewed tobacco. They stated that widespread areas of leukoplakia surrounding the neoplasm were seen in these cases. Such evidence suggests that the occurrence of oral cancer is due mainly to environmental factors such as the habit of betel chewing more so than the genetic background of the human population.

9.4 Experimental Evidence on Betel Quid

Attempts to confirm the carcinogenic activity of the betel nut or the quid using experimental animals have been made by many investigators. Muir and Kirk[1] performed an experiment in which the ears of 53 Swiss white mice were painted daily with an aqueous extract of a typical Singaporean betel/tobacco quid for 2 years; two squamous cell carcinomas and a papilloma appeared in the painted area. Reddy and Anguli[21] conducted another study in which the mixed ingredients of betel quid were instilled daily into the vagina of 60 mice. In this experiment, papillomas appeared in three animals. A similar investigation was performed by Suli et al.[22] using hamster cheek pouches treated with dimethyl sulphoxide (DMSO) extract of betel nut alone or in combination with tobacco. Extract of betel nut induced 38% incidence of tumors in the mucosa of the pouches, and the mixture of extracts of tobacco and betel nut caused a 76% incidence of tumors. The authors suggested that tobacco contains materials which although not in themselves carcinogenic, can enhance the carcinogenic actions of substances present in betel nut. They also showed the time course of the appearance of leukoplakia and tumors during the application of the extracts. However, Dunham and Herrold[23] induced no tumors except a papilloma in the cheek pouches of 375 hamsters treated with the pellets that contained betel quid ingredients. Ranadive et al.[24] tested carcinogenicity of sun-dried Mangalore betel nut extracts in water and in DMSO, and sun-cured Vadakkan tobacco extract in DMSO in mice and hamsters. Sixty percent of Swiss mice developed transplantable fibrosarcomas at the site of injection, and hamster cheek pouches painted with DMSO extract of betel nut showed early malignant changes. Dunham *et al.*[25] examined the effect of calcium hydroxide (lime) by repeated applications in hamster cheek pouches and obtained a small number of cases of epithelial atypia associated with inflammatory and hyperplastic lesions. Kapadia *et al.*[26] reported that the uncured seed extract of betel nut caused tumors in all 30 NIH black rats at the injected subcutaneous sites. Shivapurkar *et al.*[27] performed subcutaneous injections of aqueous extracts of betel nut and betel quid in Swiss mice and obtained local malignancies in 30–50%. Furthermore, the polyphenolic fraction of betel nut induced 100% tumors at treated sites in the study. Experimental study for carcinogenic testing of the betel quid in animals other than rodents was done by Hamner and Reed.[28] Five baboons received the basic betel quid in a surgically-created buccal pouch and 7 had Indian tobacco added to the quid. Of the baboons given the betel/tobacco quid, 1 developed malignant lesion after 34 months of the treatment, although no malignant lesions occurred in the baboons which received the basic quid alone. Thus, carcinogenicity studies of betel quid have been carried out entirely by local administration of the extract and the results obtained were positive in some cases and negative in others. Mori *et al.*[29] examined the carcinogenicity of betel nut, betel leaf and lime, separately or in combination, by feeding to animals. Rats received diets containing dry powder of the test materials for 480 days. The concentration of betel nuts and leaves in the diet was 20% of the total, and that of calcium hydroxide used as slaked lime was 1%. Although malignant tumors were not induced in any group of this experiment, epidermal thickening was frequently observed in the tongue, esophagus, or stomach of rats in groups fed the betel nut diet mixed with calcium hydroxide and the betel leaves diet. It seems probable as stated by Jussawalla and Deschpande,[13] that the habit of chewing betel, in association with the pungent diet common in southeast Asia, malnutrition as well as poor oral hygiene, leads to the development of cancer in the oral cavity. The effect of vitamin A deficiency on the carcinogenicity of betel quid was also studied using long-term feeding of vitamin-A-deficient and vitamin-A-sufficient diets with and without betel nut and calcium hydroxide in rats.[30] A high incidence of focal epithelial hyperplasia was observed in the upper digestive tract of rats in the group given the vitamin-A-deficient diet mixed with betel nut and calcium hydroxide. The vitamin-A-deficient group also showed a high incidence of squamous papilloma in the tongue, buccal oral mucosa, and forestomach. The incidence of hyperplastic lesions of the tongue and buccal oral mucosa was significantly higher in this group than in the group receiving the vitamin-A-sufficient diet. Furthermore, a high incidence of altered liver cell foci was observed with a few cases of hepatocellular neoplasms in the groups given diets of betel quid ingredients in this study. Altered liver cell foci in rats have been recently regarded as one of the important precursor lesions for hepatocellular malignancies.[31-33] Therefore, the results suggest the possibility that betel quid ingredients have some carcinogenic or tumor-promoting activities in the liver as well as in the upper digestive tract. Bhide et al.[34] also reported that the aqueous extract and polyphenolic fraction of betel nut induced hepatomas in mice by oral administration. Very recently, Rao[35] reported some modifying effects of betel quid ingredients on carcinogenesis in hamster buccal pouches following short-term and long-term topical exposures to graded doses of benzo(a)pyrene either alone or in combination with extract of tobacco, betel nut or betel leaf. Short-term treatments with individual ingredients of betel quid did not produce any tumor while long-term treatments produced tumors only with tobacco and betel nut. When benzo-(a)pyrene and betel quid ingredients were painted concomitantly for 10-days, there was complete or partial suppression of tumor production. But there was a considerable increase in tumor incidence when benzo-(a)pyrene-plus-tobacco or benzo(a)pyrene-plus-betel nut treatments were given for 6 months. Betel leaf extract, in both short-term and long-term studies, expressed its inhibitory influence on benzo(a)pyrene-induced tumorigenesis.

9.5 Genotoxicity and Possible Carcinogens of the Betel Nut and Betel Quid Ingredients

Jussawalla and Deschpande,[13] stated, based on their epidemiological study, that betel chewers who do not include tobacco in the quid often swallow the juice which comes into direct contact with the oropharynx and esophagus thereby leading to a higher risk of cancer at these sites. Thus even without the tobacco content, the quid appears to contain some carcinogens or tumor-promoting agents. Atkinson et al.[5] reported that a high incidence of oral cancer in New Guinea is also due to the habit of chewing betel quid, even though the betel quid is never mixed with tobacco. Therefore, betel nut and lime, with or without piper betel leaf, seem to have some carcinogenic effect when chewed without tobacco. Regardless of the intensive studies on the carcinogenicity of betel quid, active principles clearly carcinogenic have not yet been isolated from betel nuts or other ingredients of the quid. Shirname *et al.*[36] examined the mutagenic activity of betel quid and its ingredients using 4 tester strains of *Salmonella typhimurium*. Aqueous extracts of betel quid, betel quid tobacco, and betel nut were mutagenic in one strain, but aqueous extract of betel leaf was not mutagenic in any of the 4 strains. Genotoxicities of several chemicals contained in the betel quid have been examined by many workers. Stich *et al.*[37] tested clastogenic effects of 5 compounds of the betel quid, *i.e.*, arecolin, euganol, quercetin, chlorogenic acid and Mn^{2+}. The clastogenic effects of the concurrent application of arecolin plus chlorogenic acid were greater than the sum of the action of each individual component. The combination of arecolin, chlorogenic acid and Mn^{2+} induced frequencies of chromosome aberrations which exceeded the sum of the clastogenic activities of individually applied compounds. Stich *et al.*[38] aslo reported that saliva of volunteers chewing betel quid, cured betel nut, betel leaves, a mixture of quid ingredients (dried betel nut flakes, catechu, lime, copra and menthol) and Indian tobacco demonstrated chromosome-damaging activity in Chinese hamster ovary (CHO) cells. In this study, after 5 min of chewing betel quid, betel nut, betel leaves, quid ingredients and Indian tobacco, the saliva smaples showed relatively potent clastogenic activities, and after removal of the betel quid or its components from the mouth, the clastogenic activity disappeared within 5 min. Furthermore, they applied a micronucleus test to the buccal mucosal cells of 2 population groups at high risk for oral cancer, who eat raw betel nuts together with betel leaves and lime, who chew betel quids consisting mainly of performed tobacco, dried betel nut, betel leaf, lime and several spices. All 17 raw betel nut eaters and all 20 chewers of betel quids had significantly elevated frequencies of micronucleated mucosal cells over non-chewing controls of comparable ethnic background and dietary habits.[39] They also reported that the frequencies of micronucleated exfoliated cells during a chewing period were reduced by the treatment of vitamin A and β-carotene administration.[40]

It is well known that the betel nut contains several pyridine alkaloids such as arecoline, arecaidine, guvacoline and guvacine (Fig. 9–3).[41] Arecoline is the pyridine alkaloid of importance. The dried nut contains about 1 %. The alkaloid is cholinergic, exerting a sialogogue and diaphoretic action.[1] Cell transformation capability of arecoline and arecaidine was proved by Ashby *et al.*[42] in the transformation assay of Styles.[43] Ashby *et al.* implicated arecaidine as a suspected human carcinogen. Panigrahi and Rao[44] examined chromosome-breaking ability of arecoline in mouse bone-marrow cells. They also clarified *in vivo* sister chromatid exchanges of arecaidine in mouse bone-marrow cells.[45] Mutagenicity of arecoline or arecaidine in *Salmonella typhimurium* strains is known,[36] but the carcinogenicity of these alkaloids has not yet been proved. Previously, Dunham

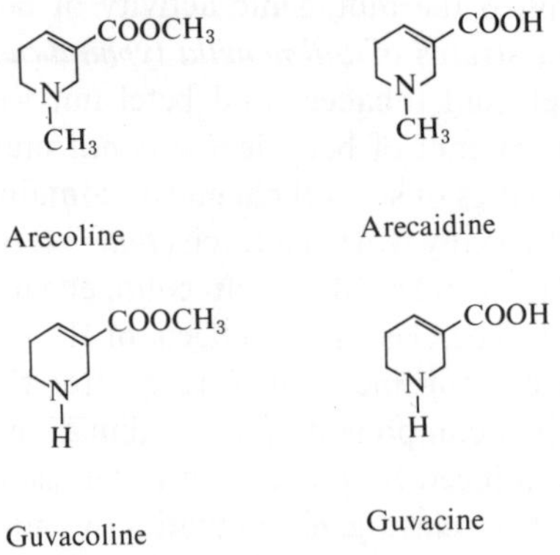

Arecoline

Arecaidine

Guvacoline

Guvacine

Fig. 9–3. Major pyridine alkaloids contained in the betel nut.

et al.[46] examined the carcinogenic activity of arecoline. Proliferative lesions developed in the esophagus of 2 animals in a group of 9 hamsters that received calcium hydroxide applied to the cheek pouch followed by painting with arecoline, but no tumors were found in animals that had their pouches with arecoline in DMSO and others that ingested arecoline solution or were fed the chemical in their food. Shivapurkar *et al.*[27] performed a carcinogenicity testing of arecoline by subcutaneous injection in Swiss mice; however, it induced no tumors in the injected sites. Bhide *et al.*[47] conducted another experiment on the carcinogenicity of arecoline. Arecoline was administered daily by gavage feeding to Swiss mice at a dose of 1 mg/day/mouse 5 times a week, either alone or in combination with KNO_3 or KNO_3 + lime. In the male mice receiving arecoline on a normal diet, tumors such as liver hemangiomas, lung adenocarcinomas and stomach squamous cell carcinomas developed in 40%, while no tumors were seen in females receiving the same. Arecoline tumorigenicity in females was evident only when they received a vitamin B-deficient diet. Futhermore, arecoline tumorigenicity was not evident in males when they were treated simultaneously with KNO_3 + lime, although the same treatment administered to male mice kept on a vitamin B complex-deficient diet induced tumors in 39%. The present authors examined the genotoxicity of both chemicals, arecoline and arecaidine, in the hepatocyte primary culture/DNA repair test,[48] which measures repairing unscheduled DNA synthesis and is considered to be sensitive for the screening of carcinogens, especially genotoxic carcinogens. The chemicals did not elicit DNA repair (unpublished data) suggesting that these chemicals are not carcinogens of genotoxic class.

Studies have also been conducted the effects of chewing betel quid on

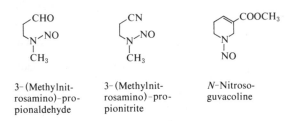

| 3- (Methylnit-
rosamino)-pro-
pionaldehyde | 3- (Methylnit-
rosamino)-pro-
pionitrite | *N*-Nitroso-
guvacoline |

Fig. 9-4. Nitrosamines derived from arecoline by *N*-nitrosation.

salivary levels of nitrite and other factors of importance in the formation of nitrosamines.[49] Wenke and Hoffman[50] recently clarified the fact that arecoline gives rise to *N*-nitrosamines such as 3-(methylnitrosamino)-propionitrite (MNPN) and 3-(methylnitrosamino)-propioaldehyde (Fig. 9-4). They also showed that MNPN is a potent carcinogen and suggested that MNPN is generated during betel quid chewing especially when tobacco is added to the quid.[51] Very recently, they stated that the saliva of chewers contains the areca-derived *N*-nitrosoguvacoline (Fig. 9-4), and other tobacco-specific *N*-nitrosamines when tobacco is added to the quid.[52] Stich *et al.*[53] on the other hand, reported an inhibitory effect of betel nut extracts on endogenous nitrosation in humans by measurement of urinary *N*-nitroso-L-proline following ingestion of sodium nitrate and L-proline, suggesting that phenolic-containing betel nut extracts affect the endogenous formation of carcinogenic nitrosamines.

REFERENCES

1. Muir, C.S., and Kirk, R., Betel, tobacco, and cancer of the mouth, *Br. J. Cancer.*, **14**: 597–608, 1960.
2. Burkhill, I.H., *A Dictionary of the Economic Products of the Malay Peninsula*, Crown Agents for the Colonies, London, **1935**.
3. Orr, I.M., Oral cancers in betel nut chewers in Travancore; its aetiology, pathology, and treatment, *Lancet*, **2**: 575–580, 1933.
4. Wahi, P.N., Kehar, U., and Lahiri, B. Factors influencing oral and oropharyngeal cancers in India, *Br. J. Cancer*, **19**: 642–662, 1965.
5. Atkinson, L., Chester, I.C., Smith, F.G., and Ten Seldam, R.E.J., Oral cancer in New Guinea, A study in demography and etiology, *Cancer*, **17**: 1289–1298, 1964.
6. Eisen, M.J., Betel chewing among natives of the south west Pacific islands; Lack of carcinogenic action, *Cancer Res.*, **6**: 139–141, 1946.
7. Hirono, I., Natural carcinogenic products of plant origin, *CRC Crit. Rev. Toxicol.*, **11**: 235–277, 1981.
8. Sanghvi, L.D., Rao, K.C.M., and Khanolkar, V.R., Smoking and chewing of tobacco in relation to cancer of the upper alimentary tract, *Br. Med. J.*, **1**: 1111–1114, 1955.

9. Hirono, I., 1974 report of the actual survey on cancer causation in southeast Asia. In: Annual Report of Mutagenicity and Carcinogenicity Testing Group of U.S.-Japan Cooperative Medical Sience Program (Japanese). Edited by T. Yamamoto. Tokyo, 1974: pp. 141–154.

10. Hirono, I., 1975 report of the actual survey on cancer causation in southeast Asia. In: Annual Report of Mutagenicity and Carcinogenicity Testing Group of U.S.-Japan Cooperative Medical Science Program (Japanese). Edited by T. Yamamoto. Tokyo, 1975, pp. 51–58.

11. Ramanathan, K., and Lakshimi, S., Oral carcinoma in peninsular Malaysia: racial variations in the Indians, Malays, Chinese, and Caucasians, Gann Monogr. Cancer Research, 18: 27–36, 1976.

12. Shanta, V., and Krishnamurthi, S., A study of aetiological factors in oral squamous cell carcinoma, Br. J. Cancer, 13: 381–388, 1959.

13. Jussawalla, D.J., Deschpande, V.A., Evaluation of cancer risk in tobacco chewers and smokers: an epidemiologic assessment, Cancer, 28: 244–252, 1971.

14. Hirayama, T., Epidemiological evaluation of the role of naturally occurring carcinogens and modulators of carcinogenesis, In: Naturally Occurring Carcinogens-Mutagens and Modulators of Carcinogenesis. Edited by E.C. Miller, J.A. Miller, I. Hirono, T. Sugimura, S. Takayama, University Park Press, Baltimore, 1979, pp. 359–380.

15. Mehta, F.S., Gupta, P.C., Daftary, D.K., Pindborg, J.J., and Choksi, S.K., An epidemiology study of oral cancer and precancerous conditions among 101, 761 villagers in Maharashtra, India. Int. J. Cancer, 10: 134–141, 1972.

16. Mehta, F.S., Shroff, B.C., Gupta, P.C., and Daftary, D.K., Oral leukoplakia in relation to tobacco habits, Oral Surgery, 34: 426–433, 1972.

17. Mehta, F.S., Gupta, P.C., and Pindborg, J.J. Chewing and smoking habits in relation to precancer and oral cancer. J. Cancer Res. Clin. Oncol., 99: 35–44, 1981.

18. Gupta, P.C., A study of dose-response relationship between tobacco habits and oral leukoplakia, Br. J. Cancer, 50: 527–531, 1984.

19. Marsden, A.T.H., Betel cancer in Malaya, Med. J. Malaya, 14: 162–165, 1960.

20. Friedell, H.L., and Rosenthal, L.M., The etiologic role of chewing tobacco in cancer of the mouth, J. Amer. Med. Assoc., 116: 2130–2135, 1941.

21. Reddy, D.G., and Anguli, V.C., Exerimental production of cancer with betel nut, tobacco and slaked lime mixture, J. Ind. Med. Assoc., 49: 315–318, 1967.

22. Suli, K., Goldman, H.M., and Wells, H., Carcinogenic effect of a dimethylsulphoxide extract of betel nut on the mucosa of the hamster buccal pouch, Nature (Lond.), 230: 383–384, 1971.

23. Dunham, L.J., Herrold, K.M., Failure to produce tumors in the hamster cheek pouch by exposure to ingredients of betel quid, histopathologic changes in the pouch and other organs by exposure to known carcinogens, J. Natl. Cancer Inst., 29: 1047–1067, 1962.

24. Ranadive, K.J., Gothoskar, S.V., Rao, A.R., Tezabwalla, B.U., and Ambaye, R.Y., Experimental studies on betel nut and tobacco carcinogenicity, Int. J. Cancer, 17: 469–476, 1976.

25. Dunham, L.J., Muir, C.S., and Hamner, J.E., Epithelial atypia in hamster cheek pouches treated repeatedly with calcium hydroxide, Br. J. Cancer., 20: 588–593, 1966.

26. Kapadia, G.J., Chung, E.B., Chosh, B., Shukla, Y.N., Basak, S.P., Morton, J.F., and Pradhan, S.N., Carcinogenicity of some folk medicinal herbs in rats, J. Natl. Cancer Inst., 60: 683–686, 1978.

27. Shivapurkar, N.M., Ranadive, S.N., Gothoskar, S.V., Bhide, S.V., and Ranadive, K.J., Tumorigenic effect of aquest & polyphenolic fractions of betel nut in Swiss strain mice, Ind. J. Exp. Biol., 18: 1159–1161, 1980.

28. Hamner, J.E., and Reed, O.M., Betel quid carcinogenesis in baboon, J. Med. Primatol., 1: 75–85, 1972.

29. Mori, H., Matsubara, N., Ushimaru, Y., and Hirono, I., Carcinogenicity examination of betel nuts and piper betel leaves, *Experientia,* **35**: 384–385, 1979.

30. Tanaka, T., Mori, H., Fujii, M., Takahashi, M., and Hirono, I., Carcinogenecity examination of betel quid, II Effects of vitamin A deficiency on rats fed semipurified diet containing betel nut and calcium hydroxide, *Nutr. Cancer,* **4**: 260–266, 1983.

31. Emmelot, P., Scherer, E., The first relevant cell stage in rat liver carcinogenesis: a quantitative approach. *Biochim. Biophys. Acta,* **605**: 247–304, 1980.

32. Farber, E., The sequential analysis of liver cancer induction, *Biochim. Biophys. Acta,* **605**: 149–166, 1980.

33. Williams, G.M., The pathogenesis of rat liver cancer caused by chemical carcinogenesis, *Biochim. Biophys. Acta.,* **605**: 167–189, 1980.

34. Bhide, S.V., Shivapurkar, N.M., Gothoskar, S.V., and Ranadive, K.J., Carcinogenicity of betel quid ingredients: feeding mice with aqueous extract and the polyphenol fraction of betel nut, *Br. J. Cancer.,* **40**: 922–926, 1979.

35. Rao, A.R., Modifying influences of betel quid ingredients on B(a)P-induced carcinogenesis in the buccal pouch of hamster, *Int. J. Cancer,* **33**: 581–586, 1984.

36. Shirname, L.P., Menon, M.M., Nair, J., and Bhide, S., Correlation of mutagenicity and tumorigenicity of betel quid and its ingedients, *Nutr. Cancer,* **5**: 87–91, 1983.

37. Stich, H.F., Stich, W., and Lam, P.P.S., Potentiation of genotoxicity by concurrent application of compounds found in betel quid: arecoline, eugenol, quercetin, chlorogenic acid and Mn^{2+}, *Mutat. Res.,* **90**: 355–363, 1981.

38. Stich, H.F., and Stich, W., Chromosome-damaging activity of saliva of betel nut and tobacco chewers, *Cancer Letters,* **15**: 193–202, 1982.

39. Stich H.F., Stich, W., and Prida, B.B., Elevated frequency of micronucleated cells in the buccal mucosa of individuals at high risk for oral cancer: betel quid chewers, *Cancer Letters,* **17**: 125–134, 1982.

40. Stich, H.F., Rosin, M.P., and Vallejera, M.O., Effect of vitamin A and β-carotene administration on the frequencies of micronucleated buccal mucosa cells of betel nut and tobacco chewers. *Proc. Amer. Assoc. Cancer Res.,* **25**: 125, 1984.

41. Henry, T.A., In: *The Plant Alkaloids,* 4, p.8, Churchill Press, London, **1949**,

42. Ashby, J., Styles, J.A., and Boyland, E., Betel nuts, arecoline, and oral cancer, *Lancet,* **1**: 112, 1979.

43. Styles, J.A., A method for detecting carcinogenic organic chemicals using mammalian cells in culture, *Br. J. Cancer,* **36**: 558–563, 1977.

44. Panigrahi, G.B., and Rao, A.R., Chromosome-breaking ability of arecoline, a major betel-nut alkaloid, in mouse bone-marrow cells *in vivo, Mutat. Res.,* **103**: 197–204, 1982.

45. Panigrahi, G.B., and Rao, A.R., Induction of *in vivo* sister chromatid exchanges by arecoline, a betel nut alkaloid, in mouse bone-marrow cells, *Cancer Letters* **23**: 189–192, 1984.

46. Dunham, L.J., Sheets, R.H., and Morton, J.F., Proliferative lesions in cheek pouch and esophagus of hamsters treated with plants from Curacao, Netherland Antilles, *J. Natl. Cancer Inst.,* **53**: 1259–1269, 1974.

47. Bhide, S.V., Gothoskar, S.V., and Shivapurkar, N.M., Arecoline tumorigenicity in Swiss strain mice on normal and vitamin B-deficient diet, *J. Cancer Res. Clin. Oncol.,* **107**: 169–171, 1984.

48. Williams, G.M., Detection of chemical carcinogens by unscheduled DNA synthesis in rat liver primary cell cultures, *Cancer Res.,* **37**: 1845–1851, 1977.

49. Shivapurkar, N.M., D'Souza, A.V., and Bhide, S.V., Effect of betel-quid chewing on nitrite levels in saliva, *Fd. Cosmet. Toxicol.,* **18**: 277–281, 1980.

50. Wenke, G., and Hoffman, D., A study of betel quid carcinogenesis. 1. On the *in vitro* N-nitrosation of arecoline, *Carcinogenesis* **4**: 169–172 1983.

51. Wenke, G., Rivenson, A., and Hoffman, D., A study of betel quid carcinogenesis. 3,3-(methylnitrosamino)-propionitrite, a powerful carcinogen in F344 rats, *Carcinogenesis,* **5**: 1137–1140, 1984.

52. Wenke G., Brunneman, K.D., Hoffman, D., and Bhide, S.V. A study of betel quid carcinogenesis. 4. Analysis of the saliva of chewers. A preliminary report. *J. Cancer Res. Clin. Oncol.*, **108**: 110–113 1984.

53. Stich, H.F., Ohshima H., Pignatelli, B., Michelon, J., and Bartsch, H., Inhibitory effect of betel nut extracts on endogenous nitrosation in humans. *J. Natl. Cancer Inst.*, **70**: 1047–1050, 1983.

10

The Active Principles of
the Euphorbiaceae and Thymelaeaceae

The plant family Euphorbiaceae consists of about 290 genera and includes about 8,000 species. One of these genera, Euphorbia itself, comprises 1,600 species.

Although the seeds of *Croton tiglium* (Croton genera indigenous to Africa) are known to be toxic and to cause skin inflammation, they have been used as a purgative, and studies on toxic principles have been conducted over a long period of time.

On the Caribbean island of Curaçao (Dutch Antilles), a very high rate of esophageal cancer has been observed among the black and creole people.

This phenomenon was found to be closely connected with the fact that they use the fresh aromatic leaves of the bush *Croton flavens* L. (Euphorbiaceae) to make a daily beverage. Another Euphorbiaceae, *Yatropha gossypifolia*, is habitually used in folk medicine. In these areas prevalence of esophageal cancer is extremely high. Etiologic investigation revealed that certain principles of Euphorbiaceae are closely related to esophageal cancer.

In 1941, Berenblum found that croton oil exhibited cocarcinogenesis[1] and that the oil, upon alkaline hydrolysis, was converted to a non-toxic diterpene phorbol.[2]

Hecker established a toxicity test for use with frogs, a method for producing inflammatory action on mouse-ear skin, and a bioassay for cocarcinogenesis.[3] By the application of the methods developed, he and his group succeeded in isolating eleven bioactive constituents by the combined use of chromatography and counter-current method.[4,5]

All these constituents were demonstrated to be phorobol-12,13-diesters of which either ester at 12 or 13 position is a long fatty acid and the other a short one.[6,48]

Evans and his co-workers began their study of toxic principles of Euphorbia in 1975.[57]

Hecker *et al.* successfully employed a variety of diterpene esters originating from Euphorbiaceae and Thymelaeaceae as model promoters in the three-stage mechanism of cancer generation, as shown in Fig. 10.1.

Initiation   *Promotion*

Normal cell ⟶ Potential tumor cell ⟶

Initiater   Promoter

DMBA*[1], urethane   Diterpene esters
TPA*[2]

Progression

Benign tumor ⟶ Malignant tumor

(papilloma)   Progressor   (carcinoma)

DMBA, urethane

*1 DMBA, (7,12-dimethylbenzeanthrathrene)
*2 TPA, (12–O–tetradecanolylphorbol-13-acetate)

Fig. 10.1. The three-stage protocol.

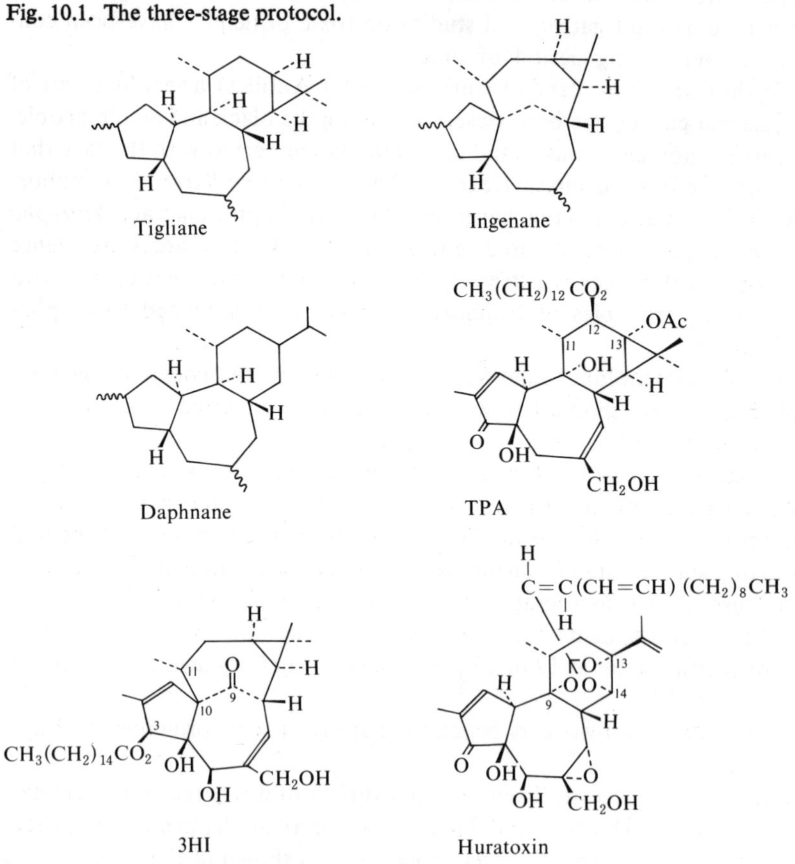

Tigliane

Ingenane

Daphnane

$CH_3(CH_2)_{12}CO_2$ .OAc .OH

TPA

CH_2OH

$CH_3(CH_2)_{14}CO_2$

3HI

H
$C=C(CH=CH)(CH_2)_8CH_3$
H

Huratoxin

Fig 10.2. The diterpene skeltons and their derivatiues

It was found that these diterpenes are biologically effective for such trace amounts as those found in hormones.[7,74]

As shown in Fig. 10.1, the three-stage model of carcinogenesis in mouse skin has proved to be one of the most advanced experimental models for studies of mechanisms of initiators and promoters.[74] It was found that irritant diterpenes include double bonds and oxygen functions in their parent skeltons, tigliane, ingenane, and daphnane, for example, 12-O-tetra–decanoylphorbol–13–acetate (TPA)[8], 3–O–hexadecanoyl ingenol (3HI),[9,10] or huratoxin (5β-hydroxy-6α,7α-epoxyresiniferonol-9,13,14-orthoester)[13] as shown.

Sakata *et al.* investigated piscicidal constituents of *Hura crepitans* (Euphorbiaceae) and isolated huratoxin.[13] Interestingly, a structurally similar compound, daphnetoxin, was obtained from the cortex of *Daphne mezereum* (Thymelaeaceae).[14] A biologically active component of the seed of the plant was isolated and chemically characterized as a new diterpene mezerein. This compound was demonstrated to exhibit inflammation activity (ID$_{50}$ 0.025 μg/mouse ear) and cocarcinogenesis.[15]

The active esters of these diterpenes also show ornithine decarboxylase-inducing activities[16,35,56] and Epstein-Barr Virus-activating effects.[17,73] Cocarcinogenesis of various kinds of constituents of Euphorbiaceae and Thymelaeaceae were also examined.

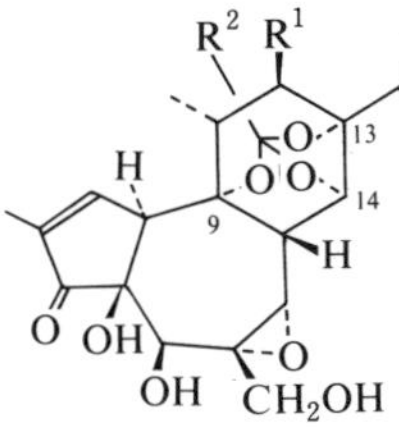

Huratoxin $R^1 = H$

$$R^2 = \underset{H}{\overset{H}{\underset{}{}}}C=C\overset{CH=CH-(CH)_8CH_3}{\underset{H}{}}$$

Daphnetoxin $R^1 = H$

$R^2 = C_6H_5-$

Mezerein $R^1 = C_6H_5(CH\,E\,CH)_2COO-$

$R^2 = C_6H_5-$

In Japan there exist a great number of plants of Euphorbiaceae, most of which have been recognized as toxic plants, but the nature of these toxic constituents were not clarified until around 1965. Therefore, in order to investigate toxic principles of Euphorbiaceae, we started with daphyniphyllum (alkaloids now Daphyniphyllaceae), at that time classified as a member of the Euphorbiaceae. in some books, because an existence of some alkaloids had bcen demonstrated.

Through intensive research, we had by 1975 isolated and chemically characterized twenty-seven new alkaloids with complex, novel skeletons that were classified into five skeleton types. (so far a total of thirty-seven diterpenes have been isolated, structurally determined, and classified into six skeleton types.) To our regret, while their toxicities have been determined,[18] cancer promoter tests have not yet been conducted. After finishing the studies of daphyniphyllum alkaloids, we were able to separate three new constituents from *Euphorbia milii*, milliamine A, B and C, all of which gave positive Dragendorf reagent tests.[18-20]

After we had determined the structures of the peptide moiety of the milliamines, Zechmeister *et al.* reported on the structure of ingenol determined by means of X-ray analysis technique.[21] Besides these milliamines, they isolated a few analogues and examined their cancer promoter activity.[22]

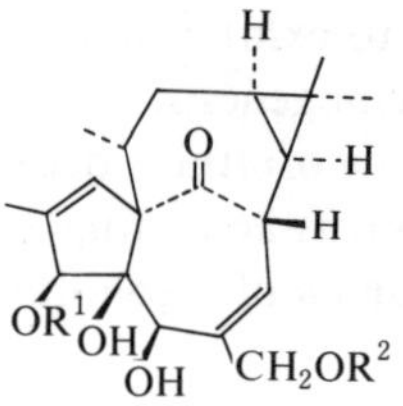

Milliamine A
$R^1 = X$ $R^2 = CH_3CO-$

Milliamine B
$R^1 = H$ $R^2 = X$

Milliamine C
$R^1 = X$ $R^2 = H$

$X =$

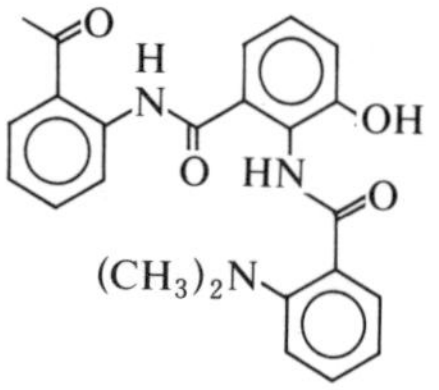

We also obtained a new toxic component of *Euphorbia jolkinii* Boiss, whose structure was assigned to be an ingenol ester of 2,4,6,8,10-tetra-decapentaenoic acid.[20] This acid is linked to the hydroxyl group at the 3-position of the ingenol forming the above ester. It has undergone test-ing for toxicity but not for cancer promoter activity.

In connection with the structures of milliamines, many phorbol amino acid or peptide derivatives were synthesized by condensation of phorbol with amino acids or peptides and examined with regard to their promoter activity.[23] To investigate structure/activity relationships, a large number of phorbol and ingenol derivatives have been synthesized so far.[8, 24]

Structurally analogous antileukemic diterpenes were obtained from *Euphorbia esula, Croton tiglium, Cunria spruceana*, and others.[25] *Euphorbia milii* Desmoul et Boiss is known as a wart remover.[26]

10.1 The Principal Parent Diterpene Skeletons

As described above, toxic and carcinogenic-related substances obtained from Euphorbiaceae and Thymlaeaceae have been proved hitherto to have the structures of diterpene esters with tigliane, ingenane or daphnane skeletons. Several are already known: TPA from *Croton tiglium* of the tigliane type, 3HI from *E. ingens* and *E. lathyris* of the ingenane type and huratoxin from *Hura crepitans* of the daphnane type. Carcinogenic-related substances isolated from naturally occurring products will be presented by classifying them into these three types. New substances will be explained in detail, with those which are already known indicated briefly in the tables.

10.1.1 Tigliane diterpenes

The diterpenes of this type are usually ester derivatives of diterpenoid alcohol involving a tetracyclic nucleus that consists of a five-membered ring (ring A), a seven-membered ring (ring B), a six-membered ring (ring C), and a three-membered ring (ring D). The representative example of this type of diterpene is phorbol ester. Phorbol itself carries alcoholic groups at the 4, 9, 12, 13, and 20 positions. In addition, there exist several parent alcohols such as 16-hydroxyphorbol, 12-deoxyphorbol, 5-hydroxyphorbol, 12-deoxy-16-hydroxy-phorbol, 4-deoxyphorbol and 12,20-dideoxyphorbol, most of which occur largely in the form of their ester derivatives.

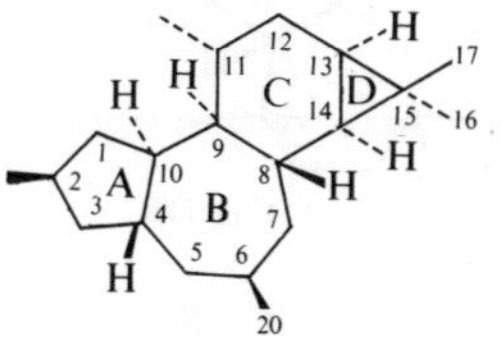

Tigliane nucleus

A. Phorbol esters

As presented above, phorbol esters, components of *Euphorbia tiglium*, were used for researching carcinogenic effect.[6,8,25] In particular, 12-*O*-tetradecanoylphorbol-13-acetate (TPA) was employed as a representative specimen which exhibited strong cocarcinogenesis.[33,74] The structure of phorbol was determined by a combination of chemical and X-ray analyses.[27]

Phorbol itself shows no biological activities such as toxicology. However, when either ester group of 12,13-diesters is constituted of medium or higher fatty acids, the ester derivatives of phorbol will demonstrate cocarcinogenesis.[6,73]

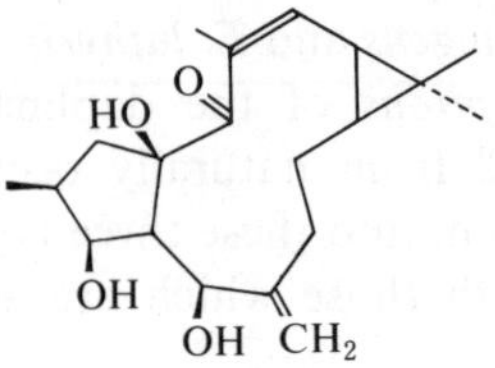

Lathyrol

Such large-ring diterpenoid alcohols as lathyrol were isolated from *E. lathyris* as esters. Since this alcohol has a skeleton with the same origin as that of phorbol, the former can be considered to have a biosynthetic relationship to the latter, but lathyrol does not exhibit significant cocarcinogenesis.[48] Some compounds of this type possess anti-cancer activity.[28]

Table 10.1   Phorbol Esters

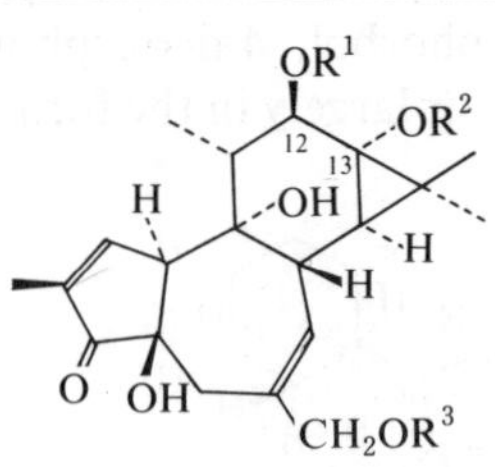

Phorbol (R^1=R^2=R^3=H)

Phorbol-12, 13-diesters (R^3 = H)

Many phorbol esters (R^3 = H)[6,8,25] were isolated from *Croton tiglium*. Either ester group (R^1 or R^2) of 12,13-diesters is constituted of a long fatty acid but the other is a short.

R^1 or $R^2 = CH_3CO-$, $CH_3 (CH_2)_nCO-$ ($n = 2$, 8, 10[†], 12 and 14);

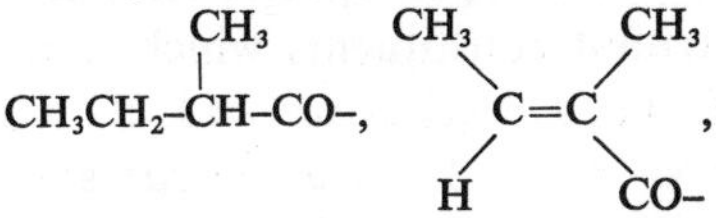

$$CH_3CH_2-\underset{\underset{CH_3}{|}}{CH}-CO-, \quad \underset{H}{\overset{CH_3}{\diagdown}}C=C\underset{CO-}{\overset{CH_3}{\diagup}} \quad , \text{octenoate}$$

The additional diesters shown below were obtained from other plants. Plant source is indicated in the parentheses.

$R^1 = CH_3(CH_2)_{10}CO-$, $R^2 = CH_3CO-$
   (*Croton sparciflorus*)[29]

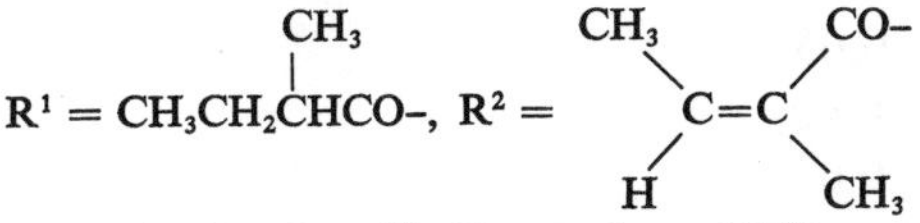

$$R^1 = CH_3CH_2\underset{\underset{CH_3}{|}}{C}HCO-, \quad R^2 = \quad \underset{H}{\overset{CH_3}{\diagdown}}C=C\underset{CH_3}{\overset{CO-}{\diagup}}$$

   (*E. franckiana*[30], *E. coerulescens*[30,31]);
$R^1 = CH_3(CH_2)_2(CH = CH)_3 CO-$, $R^2 = CH_3CO-$
   (*Sapium japonicum*[32])

Phorbol-12, 13, 20-triesters
   $R^1 = CH_3(CH_2)_{10}CO-$, $R^2 = CH_3CO-$, $R^3 =$ linolenate
      (*Croton sparciflorus*[29])

$$R^1 = (CH_3)_2CHCO-, \quad R^2 = CH_3CO-, \quad R^3 = \quad \underset{H}{\overset{CH_3}{\diagdown}}C=C\underset{CH_3}{\overset{CO-}{\diagup}}$$

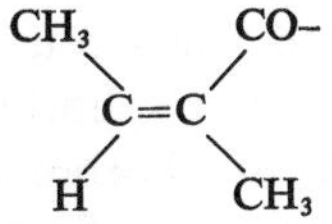

   (*E. franckiana*[30], *E. coerulescens*[30,31])

[†] This compound was isolated form *Sapium sebiferum*.[17]

B. 16-Hydroxyphorbol esters

A biologically active substance, 16-hydroxyphorbol ester, was isolated from *Aleurites fordii* (Euphorbiaceae).[34,35]

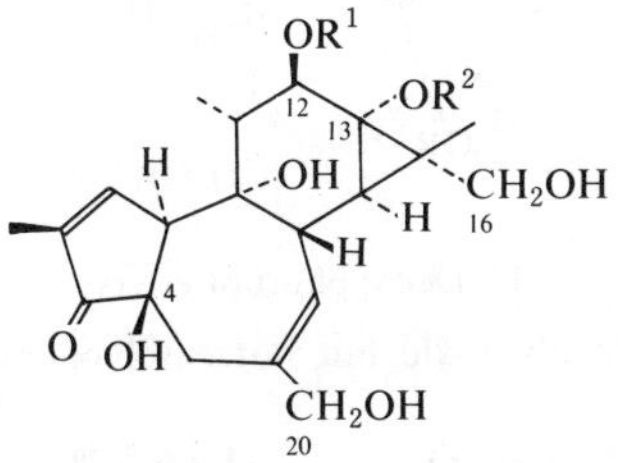

16-Hydroxyphorbol esters

Additional compounds, 12-O-palmitoyl-16-hydroxyphorbol-13-acetate and its 4-deoxy derivative, were also obtained from the same plant. The latter exists as a mixture of 4α- and 4β-isomers. In addition to these compounds, new skeleton compounds with carbon-carbon bonds between the 2- and 6-positions and between the 1- and 7-positions were isolated.[35]

The seed oil of four kinds of Jatropha species (Euphorbiaceae) used in folk medicine gave new irritant constituents which were assigned as 16-hydroxyphorbol esters from *J. podagrica* and *J. multifida* and as 12-deoxy-16-hydroxyphorbol esters from *J. curcas* and *J. gossypifolia*. The whole structures of these esters still remain unknown except for partial structures such as polyunsaturated esters. The strength of each irritant thus obtained is as follows.[36]

	ID_{50}^{24} (μg/ear)
J. podagrica	0.07
J. multifida	0.05
J. curcas	0.02
J. gossypifolia	0.02

C. 12-Deoxyphorbol esters

12-Deoxyphorbol esters are esters of phorbol derivatives lacking a hydroxyl group at the 12-position of phorbol. An active principle of *Croton tiglium* was proven to be a phorbol ester while that of *Euphorbia triangularis* was identified as a 12-deoxyphorbol ester.[37]

Evans and Soper found that many compounds of this type are distributed widely in Euphorbia.[57] The acids of the ester part are distinguished from those of phorbol because they consist of rather shorter carbon chains, i.e. four or five carbon acids.

TABLE 10.2.   12-Deoxyphorbol Esters

12-Deoxyphorbol esters ($R^1 = R^2 = H$)

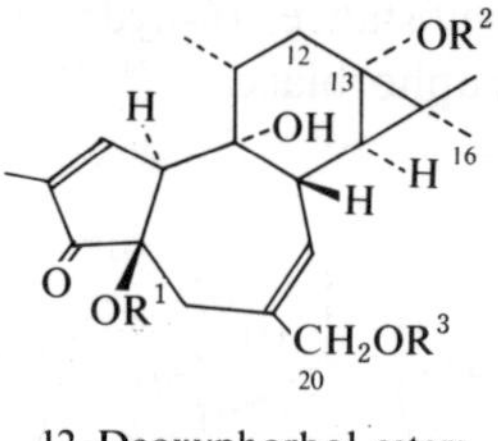

12-Deoxyphorbol esters

$R^2 = CH_3CO-$ (prostratin: highly toxic but not carcinogenic; *Pimelea prostrata*,[38] *Daphnopsis racemosa*[39]);

$R^2 = (CH_3)_2CHCO-$ $(1,2,6)^{37,40,41)}$

$$R^2 = CH_3CH_2\overset{\overset{\textstyle CH_3}{|}}{C}HCO- \qquad (1,4,6)^{31,37,40,43)}$$

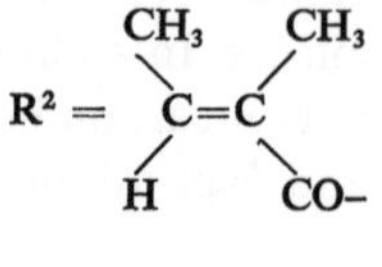

$$R^2 = \underset{H}{\overset{CH_3}{\diagdown}}C=C\underset{CO-}{\overset{CH_3}{\diagup}} \qquad (1,3,7)^{37,42,43}$$

$$R^2 = \quad \overset{CH_3}{\underset{H}{\diagdown}}C = C\overset{CO-}{\underset{CH^3}{\diagup}} \qquad (2,6)^{40,41)}$$

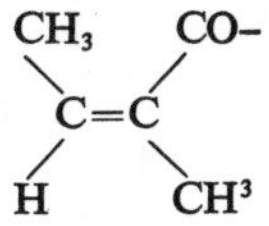

$R^2 = CH_3 (CH_2)_5CO-$ $(4)^{31,43)}$

$R^2 = $ Dodecenoate $(3)^{42)}$

$R^2 = CH_3(CH_2)_{10}CO-$ $(3,4)^{,31,42,43)}$

$R^2 = C_6H_5CH_2CO-$ $(2,6)^{,41,45,47)}$

12-Deoxyphorbol-20-acetate ($R^1 = H$, $R^3 = Ac$)

$R^2 = (CH_3)_2CHCO-$ $(1\dagger,2,3,6)^{37,40,41,42)}$

$$R^2 = \quad \overset{CH_3}{\underset{H}{\diagdown}}C = C\overset{CH_3}{\underset{CO-}{\diagup}} \qquad (1,3,4,7)^{37,42,43)}$$

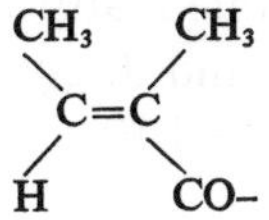

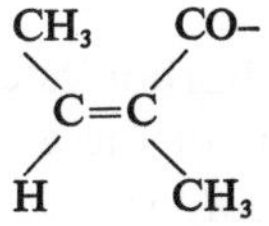

$$R^2 = \quad \overset{CH_3}{\underset{H}{\diagdown}}C = C\overset{CO-}{\underset{CH_3}{\diagup}} \qquad (2,6)^{40,41)}$$

$$R^2 = CH_3CH_2\overset{\overset{\textstyle CH_3}{|}}{C}HCO- \qquad (1,3,4,6)^{31,37,40,42,43)}$$

$R^2 = $ octenoate $(5)^{43,44)}$

$R^2 = $ decadienoate $(5)^{43)}$

$R^2 = CH_3 (CH_2)_{10} CO-$ $(4)^{31,43,44)}$

$R^2 = $ dodecenoate $(3,4)^{42,43,44)}$

$R^2 = $ dodecadienoate $(7)^{43)}$

$R^2 = C_6H_5CH_2CO-$ $(2,6)^{41,45,47)}$

$R^2 = $ *p*-OH-phenylacetate $(6)^{46)}$

---

† Figures in parentheses indicate the botanical source as shown below.
1. *E. triangularis*   2. *E. resinifera*   3. *E. fortissima*   4. *E. coerulescens*
5. *E. polyacantha*   6. *E. poisonii*   7. *E. pelioscopia*

12-Deoxy-16-hydroyxphorbol esters:

12-Deoxy-16-hydroxyphorbol esters have been found from two Euphorbia species as shown in Table 10.3.

TABLE 10.3 12–Deoxy-16-Hydroxyphorbol Esters

R^1	R^2	R^3	Plant source
angelate	isobutyrate	H	*E. cooperi*[50)]
angelate	isobutyrate	Ac	*E. cooperi*
Phenylacetate	α-methylbutyrate	Ac	*E. poisonii*[51)]
Phenylacetate	α-methylbutyrate	H	*E. poisonii*

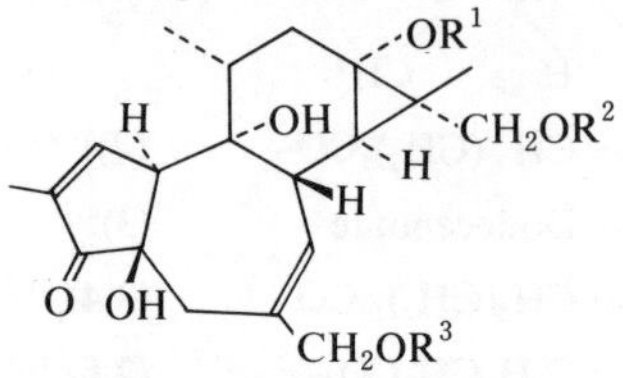

12-Deoxy-16-hydroxyphorbol esters

The occurrence of new highly unsaturated fatty acid esters of 12-deoxy-16-hydroxyphorbol in *Jatropha curcas* and *J. gossypifolia* was observed and described above.[36] (see section 10.1.1.B).

D. Other deoxyphorbol esters

4-Deoxyphorbol and 12,20-dideoxyphorbol esters have been isolated hitherto, although the number of kinds of these types of compounds is not as large as that of 12-deoxyphorbol esters.

4-Deoxyphorbol esters:

4-Deoxyphorbol-12,13-diesters were extracted from *E. tirucalli*; one ester group consists of acetic acid and the other one of the following acids.

acid residue: CH_3CO- or $CH_3(CH_2)_m(CH=CH)_n CO-$

$$m = 2, \quad n = 2, 3, 4, 5$$
$$m = 4, \quad n = 1, 2, 3, 4$$

Both kinds of compounds showed very strong biological activity (ID_{50} 0.003 μg/ear) compared with TPA (ID_{50} 0.01 μg/ear). Another 4α-epimer of 4-deoxyphorbol was found but proved to have no biological activity. This compound is apparently epimerized in alkaline solution.[33]

Isolation of 12-*O*-palmitoyl-4-deoxy-16-hydroxy-phorbol-13-acetate together with other constituents has been presented in a previous section (10.1.1.B).[34]

12,20-Dideoxyphorbol esters:

There occur 12,20-dideoxyphorbol-13-isobutyrate (*E. unispiria*) and 12,20-dideoxyphorbol-13-angelate (*E. resinifera*), both of which show no biological activity.[52]

E. Other tigliane type diterpene esters

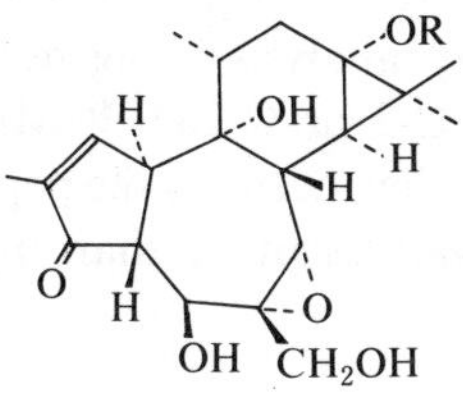

Pimelea factor P_5:
Pimelea prostrata
(Thymelaeaceae)[12,53]
$R = CH_3 (CH_2)_{12} CO-$

Mancinellin:
Hippomane mancinella
(Euphorbiaceae)[12,53]
$R = CH_3(CH = CH)_2CO-$

The two compounds below were isolated as Epstein-Barr Virus-activating principles from *Sapium sebiferum* (Euphorbiaceae).[17]

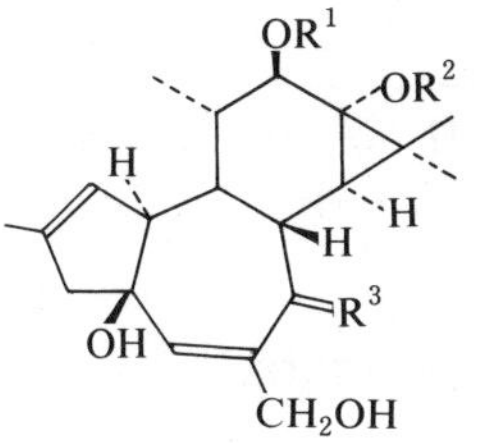

$$\begin{cases} R^1 = C_{15}H_{31} CO- \\ R^2 = Ac \\ R^3 = {}^{OOH}_{\cdots H} \end{cases}$$

$$\begin{cases} R^1 = C_{15} H_{31} CO- \\ R^2 = Ac \\ R^3 = =O \end{cases}$$

10.1.2 Ingenane diterpenes

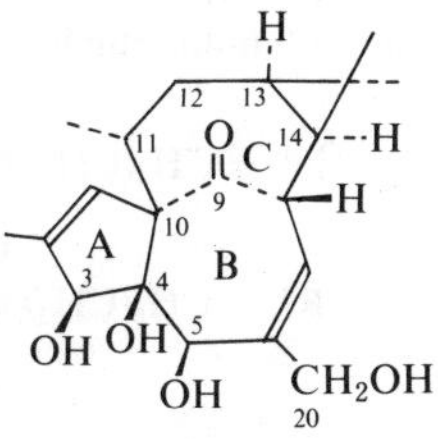

Ingenol

Ingenol is a tetracyclic diterpenoid alcohol which includes a parent ingenane skeleton. It has a seven-membered ring as ring C which can apparently be derived from phorbol by the shift of a C-9 and C-11 bond of phorbol to a C-10 and C-11 bond. Although phorbol holds one hydroxyl group each at C-12 and C-13 of its C ring, ingenol has no hydroxyl groups at C-12 and C-13. Instead, ingenol carries two hydroxyl functions at C-3 and C-5. Although phorbol has a carbonyl group at C-3 and a hydroxyl group at C-9, ingenol has a hydroxyl group at C-3 and a carbonyl group at C-9. Ingenol has been derived by hydrolysis of key constituents of certain Euphorbia families (*E. ingens, E. desomondi* and *E. lathyris*).

The whole structure of ingenol including the absolute structure was determined by X-ray crystallography analysis.[21] Ingenol esters contain at least one ester function at either C-3 or C-20.[6,33] Milliamines from *E. milii* attracted much attention since they occur as the peptide derivatives of ingenol. Ingenane diterpene derivatives other than ingenol also have been found.

A. Ingenol esters

A variety of esters derivatives of 3-OH in ingenol have been isolated from *E. resinifera* and *E. heloscopia*, as described below.

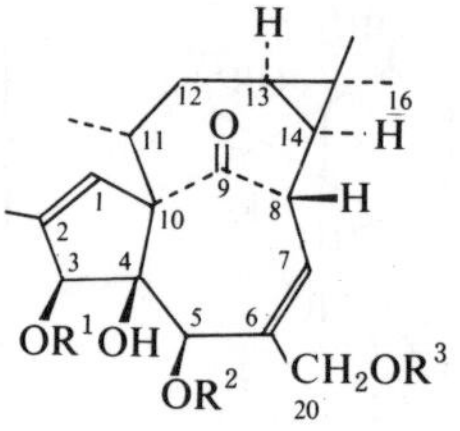

Ingenol esters

$$R^2 = R^3 = H,$$

E. resinifera[41]: R^1 = 2,6-dimethyloctenoate

R^1 = CH$_3$(CH$_2$)$_6$CHCO–
            |
            CH$_3$

R^1 = CH$_3$ (CH$_2$)$_7$ CHCO–
            |
            CH$_3$

R^1 = CH$_3$(CH$_2$)$_2$CH(CH$_2$)$_3$CHCO–
               | |
              CH$_3$ CH$_3$

R^1 = CH$_3$(CH$_2$)$_8$CHCO–
            |
            CH$_3$

E. heloscopia[55]: R^1 = 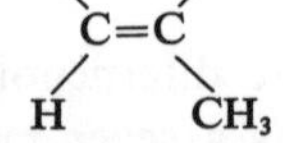
$$\underset{H}{\overset{CH_3}{\diagdown}} C = C \underset{CH_3}{\overset{CO-}{\diagup}}$$
(ID_{50}^{24} 0.12):

(This compound was also isolated from *E. antiquorum*.)

R^1 = CH$_3$(CH$_2$)$_2$(CH=CH)$_3$CO– (ID_{50}^{24} 0.22)

R^1 = CH$_3$ (CH$_2$)$_2$ (CH=CH)$_4$ CO–

R^1 = CH$_3$(CH$_2$)$_4$(CH=CH)$_2$ CO– (geometric isomers ID_{50}^{20} 0.06, 0.08)

20-*O*-Isobutyryl-ingenol and three kinds of 3,20-*O,O*-diacyl-ingenols were found in *E. cotinifolia* L.[56] by measuring both piscicidal activities and the induction of ornithine decarboxylase activity.

$$
\begin{aligned}
R^1 : R^2 &= H : (CH_3)_2CHCO- \\
&= CH_3CH_2CO- : (CH_3)_2CHCO- \\
&= (CH_3)_2\ CHCO- : (CH_3)_2CHCO- \\
&\qquad\qquad\qquad\qquad\qquad\overset{\textstyle S}{|} \\
&= CH_3CH_2CO- : CH_3CH_2\overset{|}{C}HCO- \\
&\qquad\qquad\qquad\qquad\qquad\underset{\textstyle CH_3}{|}
\end{aligned}
$$

In 1971, milliamines A, B and C were isolated from *E. milii* as toxic constituents by Uemura and Hirata.[19, 20] Marston and Hecker studied the other kinds of milliamines, which consist of the peptide derivatives of ingenol, and examined biological activities not only of the above milliamines but also other constituents.[22]

TABLE 10.4. Toxicity of Milliamines Isolated from *E. milii*

milliamines	R^1	R^2	R^3	ID_{50}^{24}
A	peptide X	H	Ac	0.04
B	H	H	X	3.0
C	X	H	H	0.0066
D	H	X	Ac	0.16
E	X	Ac	H	0.09
F	H	Y	Ac	0.14
G	Y	H	H	0.015

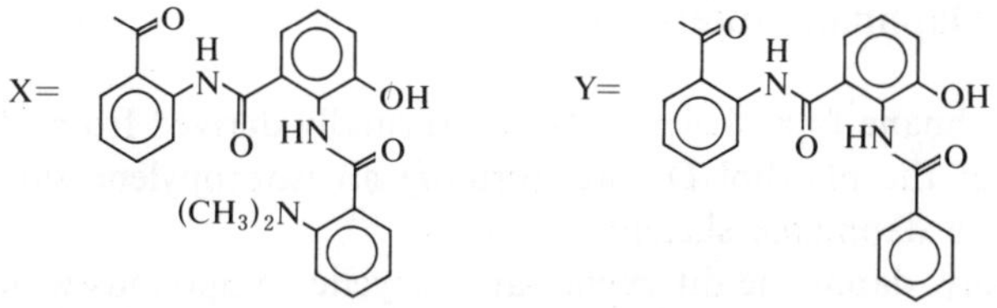

The compounds in Table 10.5 were obtained from various members of the Euphorbia family.[57]

TABLE 10.5. Compounds Obtained from Euphorbia

R^1	R^3	Plant source
$CH_3(CH_2)_4CO-$	H	(1), (2)
H	$CH_3(CH_2)_4\ CO-$	(1), (2)
$CH_3(CH_2)_2(CH=CH)_3CO-$	H	(2)
$CH_3(CH_2)_2(CH=CH)_5CO-$	H	(1), (2), (3)
$CH_3(CH_2)_4(CH=CH)_2CO-$	Ac	(4)
C_6H_5CO-	C_6H_5CO-	(5)
$CH_3\diagdownCO-$	Ac	(6)
$C=C$	$(ID_{50}^{24}\ 0.09)$	
$H\diagup\diagdown CH_3$		

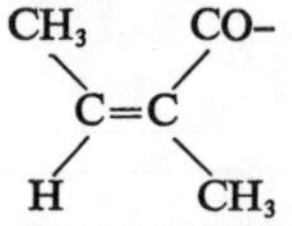

Figures in parentheses indicate the plant source as shown below.
1. *E. lathyris*   2. *E. ingens*   3. *E. jolkini*
4. *E. kansui*   5. *E. esula*   6. *E. peplus*

B.   Other ingenane derivative esters

The ester derivatives of the following parent ingenane diterpenes have been found so far. The plant source is noted in parentheses.
13-hydroxyingenol   (*E. kansui*[58])
16-hydroxyingenol   (*E. ingens*[59], *E. lactes*[59],
                             E. lathyris[9] and *E. esula*[60])
13,19-dihydroxyingenol (*E. cyparissis*[61])
4-deoxyingenol (*E. glandulosa*[62])
5-deoxyingenol (*E. myrsinites* and *E. biglandulas*[63])
12-deoxyingenol (*E. helioscopia*[64])
20-deoxyingenol (*E. kansui*[65])

10.1.3   Daphnane diterpenes

The daphnane type skeleton can be formally derived from phorbol by cleavage of the phorbol D ring, forming an isopropylene side chain at C-13 of the daphnane skeleton.

Accordingly, daphnane diterpenes are tricyclic compounds which consist of a five-membered ring (ring A), a seven-membered ring (ring B) and a six-membered ring (ring C). They contain two additional hydroxyl groups at C-5 and C-14, and an α-epoxy structure at C-6 and C-7. Among natural products, the daphnane diterpenes are characterized by their occurrence as the rare orthoester structure which is formed by condensation of carboxylic acid with three α-hydroxyl groups at C-9, C-13 and C-14 in ring C. The carboxylic acid of the orthoester is an aromatic acid or a fatty acid involving mostly unsaturated acid.

A number of new irritant factors were obtained from Thymelaeaceae.

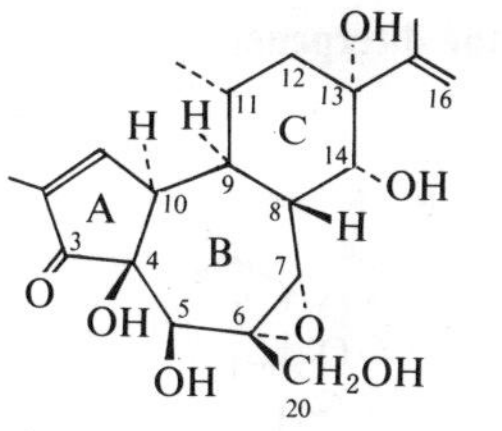

Daphnane diterpene

These structures contain 1α-alkyl-daphnane system where the end of the fatty acid is linked to C-1 in ring A.

A. Aromatic acid orthoester daphnane diterpenes

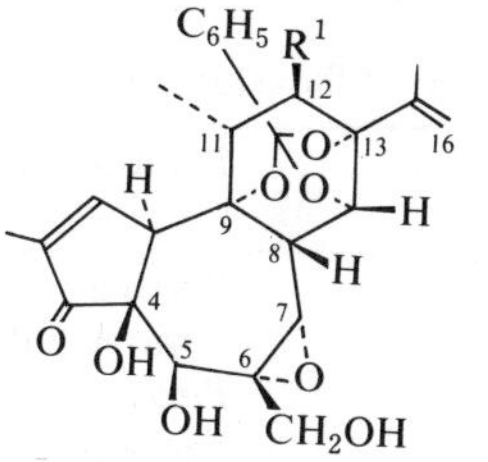

Daphnetoxin $(R^1=H)$[14]

TABLE 10. 6. Aromatic Acid Orthoester Daphnane Diterpenes

R^1 (compound)	Plant source
$C_6H_5(CH=CH)_2COO-$ (mezerein)[15,16,69]	*Daphne mezereum* *Daphne odora* *Lasiosiphon burchelli*
$CH_3(CH_2)_2(CH=CH)_3COO-$[16]	*Daphne odora*
H (daphnetoxin)[14]	*Daphne mezereum*
$CH_3(CH_2)_4(CH=CH)_2COO-$ (gnididin)	† *Daphne odora*[16,69] *Gnidia lamprantha*[66]
†$CH_3(CH_2)_2(CH=CH)_2COO-$ (gniditrin)	
$C_6H_5CH=CHCOO-$ (gnidicin)	

B. Fatty acid orthoester daphnane diterpenes

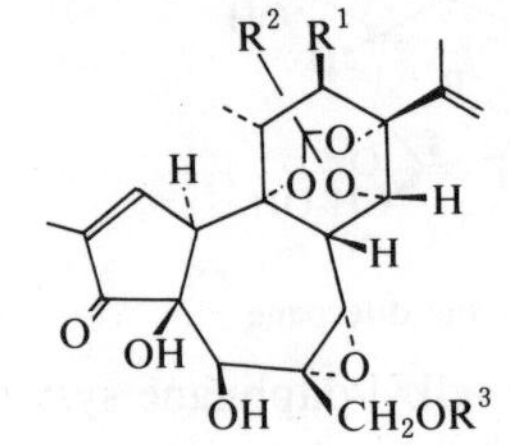

Orthoester daphna diterpene

TABLE 10. 7.   Fatty Acid Orthoester Daphnane Diterpenes

monoester R^2 ($R^1 = R^3 = H$)	Plant source
$CH_3(CH_2)_8-$	*Pimelea prostrata,*[53] *Daphnopsis racemosa*[39]
$CH_3(CH_2)_{12}-$	*Pimelea prostrata*[53]
$CH_3(CH_2)_4(CH=CH)_2-$ E	*Excoecaria agallocha*[68]
$CH_3(CH_2)_4(CH=CH)_2-$ E	*Daphne odora*[69]
$CH_3(CH_2)_8(CH=CH)_2-$	*Hura crepitans,*[13] *Hippomane mancinella*[49]
$CH_3(CH_2)_8(CH=CH)_3-$	*Hippomane mancinella*[49]
diester R^2 ($R^1 = C_6H_5CO_2-$, $R^3 = H$)	Plant source
$CH_3(CH_2)_8-$	*Gnidia latifolia* *Gnidia glaucus*[67]
$CH_3(CH_2)_8(CH=CH)-$	*Gnidia latifolia* *Gnidia glaucus*[67]
$CH_3(CH_2)_4(CH=CH)_2-$ E	*Daphne odora*[69]
$CH_3(CH=CH)_2(CH=CH)-$ E	*Daphne odora*[69]

E

R^2 ($R^1 = C_6H_5(CH=CH)CO_2-$, $R^3 = H$)

E $CH_3(CH_2)_4(CH=CH)_2-$ E	*Daphne odora*[69]
$CH_3(CH_2)_4(CH=CH)_2(CH=CH)-$ E	*Daphne odora*[69]
$CH_3(CH_2)_2(CH=CH)_2(CH=CH)-$	*Daphne odora*[69]

($R^1 = AcO-$, $R^3 = H$)

$R^2 = CH_3(CH_2)_8-$ *Gnidia latifolia*
                                         Gnidia glaucus[67]

$R^1 = H$
$R^2 = CH_3(CH_2)_8(CH=CH)_3-$ *Hippomane mancinella*[49]
$R^3 = CH_3(CH_2)_nCO-$
      $n = 14, 16, 18$

---

triester
$(R^1 = C_6H_5CO_2-, R^3 = CH_3(CH_2)_4 CO-)$
$R^2 = CH_3(CH_2)_8-$ *Gnidia latifolia*[67]
$R^2 = CH_3(CH_2)_4 (CH=CH)_2-$ *Gnidia glaucus*

C. 1α-Alkyldaphnane type

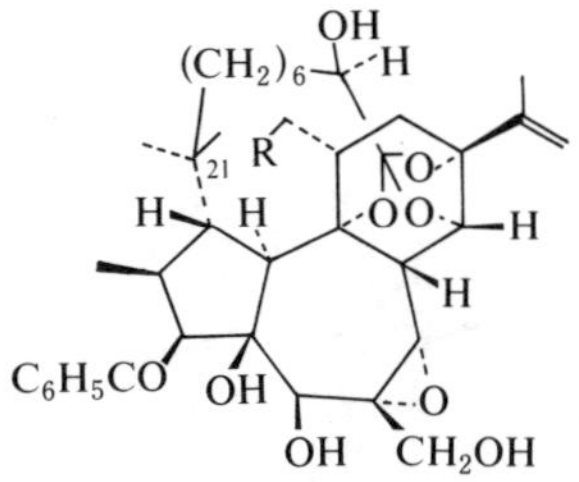

Gnidimacrin

In 1976, this type of compound gnidimacrin was isolated as the first antileukemic diterpenoid ester from *Gnidia subcordata* (Thymelaeaceae) by Kupchan *et al.*[70] Gnidimacrin-20-palmitate was also isolated.

Zayed *et al.* obtained strong irritant analogues from *Pimelea, Daphnopsis*, and *Synaptolepis* (Thymelaeaceae).[71] Recently, other compounds involving a structure similar to that of 1-alkyldaphnane diterpene were

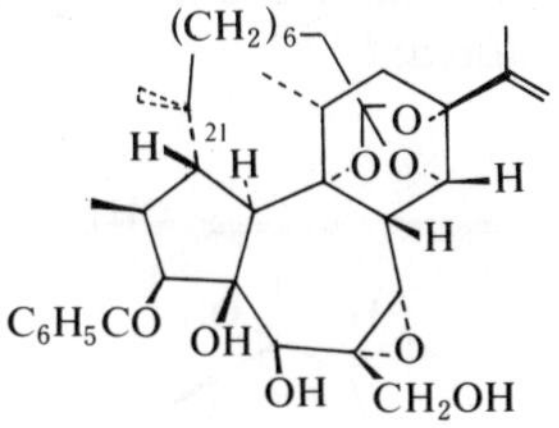

Pimelea factor P$_2$

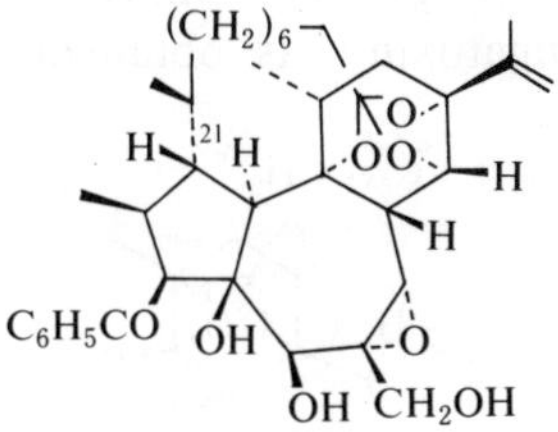

Pimelea factor P$_3$

isolated from *Daphnospsis, racemosa* and *Pimelea prostrata* and exhibited strong irritant and cocarcinogenic activity.[39,53] Pimelea factor P_2 and P_3 were shown to exhibit high cocarcinogenic activity (ID_{50} 0.006 and 0.02, respectively) compared with TPA (ID_{50} 0.016). Both are considered to be the C-21 epimers.

In addition to both these compounds, their 5-deoxy derivatives were isolated from *Daphnopsis racemosa*[39] and the 21α- and 21β-isomers showed almost the same biological activities (ID_{50} 0.04 and 0.09, respectively). Other 1-alkyldaphnane type derivatives shown below were also obtained from some plants.[53]

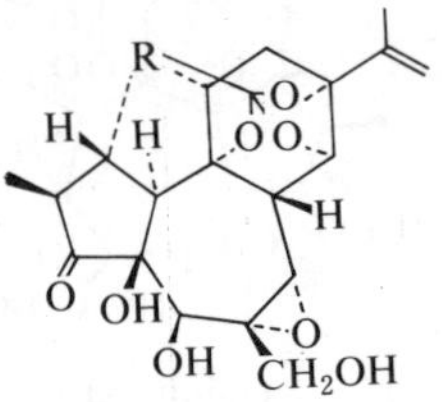

	Plant source
$\text{(C-1)-R} = \text{(C-1)-CH(CH}_3\text{)-(CH}_2)_6\text{-}\overset{\text{OCOC}_6\text{H}_5}{\overset{|}{\text{CH}}}\text{-}$	*Pimelea prostrata*
$\text{(C-1)-R} = \text{(C-1)CH(CH}_3\text{)-(CH}_2)_7\text{-}$	*P. simplex*
$\text{(C-1)-R} = \text{(C-1)-C}_{13}\text{H}_{26}\text{-CH=CH-}$	*Synaptolepis kirkii*

D. Other daphnane diterpene esters

Resiniferatoxin[45,52] and pro-resiniferatoxin[52] were found from three species of Euphorbia family, *E. resinifera, E. unispina* and *E. poisonii*, while tingatoxin was obtained from *E. poisonii*.[47]

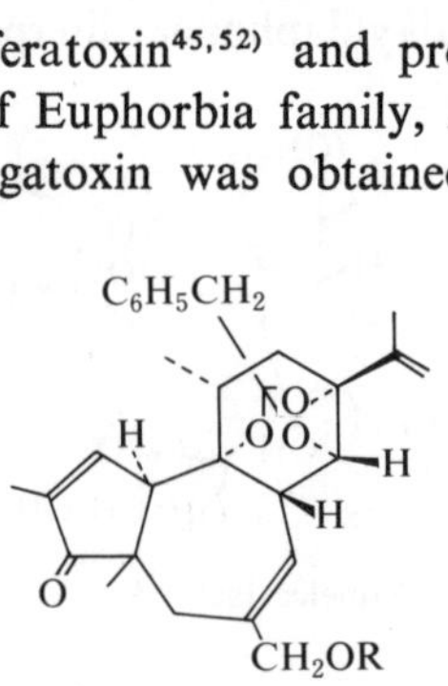

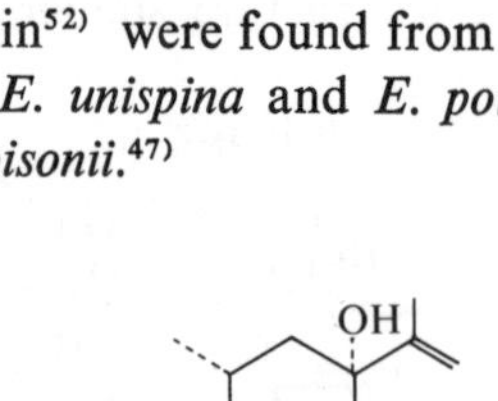

R =

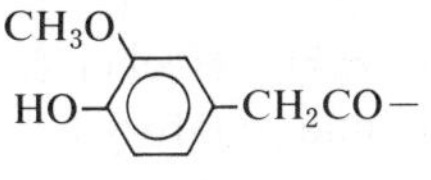

CH$_3$O, HO—⬡—CH$_2$CO—

R^1=C$_6$H$_5$CH$_2$CO—

Resiniferatoxin

R^2=

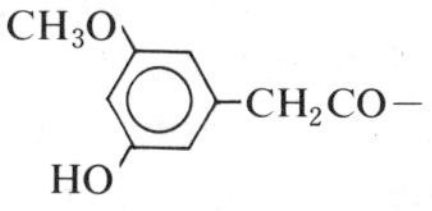

CH$_3$O, ⬡ —CH$_2$CO— HO

Pro-resiniferatoxin

R = HO—⬡—CH$_2$CO—

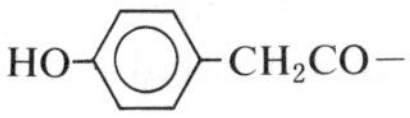

Tingatoxin

The following daphnane diterpenes were isolated from the same plant, *Daphne odorata*.[16]

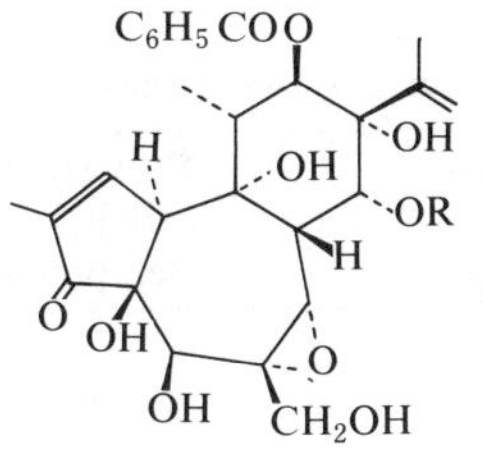

E

R=CH$_3$(CH$_2$)$_4$(CH=CH)$_2$CO—

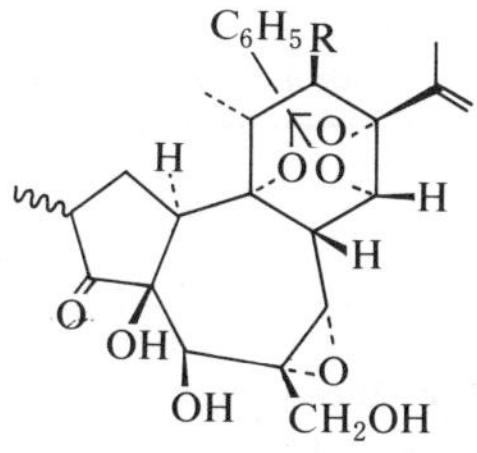

E

R=CH$_3$(CH=CH)$_2$(CH=CH)CO$_2$—

10.2 Irritation and Tumor Promotion

Phorbol diester itself exhibits carcinogenesis at a high dosage. However, phorbol ester shows cocarcinogenesis by administering it twice weekly after a dosage of a carcinogenic substance such as 7,12-dimethyl-benzanthracene (DMBA). Cocarcinogenesis is determined quantitatively by calculating the TD$_{50}$ (tumor dose) required to produce at least one manifestation of cancer per mouse for half the tested mice by administering a certain amount (0.1 ml) of DMBA followed by an ester twice a week.[5]

If animals are used for cocarcinogenesis testing, a long period of time is required to examine the activity as well as a great deal of expense. Thus a relatively easy first screening method is desirable. Hecker *et al.* employed inflammatory action. In order to examine inflammatory action a solution of the screening sample in a solvent was applied to mouse-ear skin and after 24 h, the action was determined by appearance of inflammation and indicated as the minimum amount of inflammatory dose (n mol ID_{50}^{24}) to produce inflammation.[72]

Inflammatory action is comparable to cocarcinogenesis as long as phorbal diesters and other constituents of Thymelaeaceae and Euphorbiaceae are involved.[5]

As described previously, Koshimizu, Ito and their coworkers perceived that some piscicidal diterpene esters of Euphorbiaceae and Thymeleaceae exhibit cocarcinogenesis. They investigated the first cocarcinogenesis screening of Euphorbiaceae and Thymelaeaceae using Epstein-Bar Virus-activation[17,73] and ornithine decarboxylase activity induction in mouse skin.

The results of biological activity on these diterpenes obtained by Hecker are summarized in Table 10.8[12,22,33,36,39,42,53,55,71,74]

TABLE 10.8   Biological Activities of Various Diterpenes

	Irritation ID_{50}^{24} (n mol)	Promotion activity (rel. potencies)
Tigliane types		
TPA (12–*O*-tetradecanoyl phorbol-13-acetate)	0.016	++++
4-OMe TPA	2.3	(+)
PDD (phorbol didecanoate)	0.01	+++
4α-PDD	> 150	0
12-Deoxyphorbol-13-decanoate	0.017	+++
RPA (synthetic 12–retinoic acid ester)	0.018	(+)
12–*O*–Acetylphorbol–13–decanoate	0.087	
12–*O*–Acetylphorbol–13–decadienoate	0.042	
Phorbol–12,13-didecanoate	0.01	
12-Decanoylphorbol–13–deca△²,⁴ dienoate	0.0007	
12-Deoxyphorobol–13–tigliate	0.045 (0.06)†	
12-Deoxyphorbol–13–dodecenoate	(0.006)	
12–Deoxyphorbol–13–isobutyrate–20–acetate	0.024 (0.1)	

TABLE 10.8—*Continued*

	Irritation ID_{50}^{24}(n mol)	Promotion activity (rel. potencies)
TPA–20–tetradecanoate	0.77	
Mancinellin	0.1	
Milliamine H	8.1	
Milliamine I	>10.0	
Phorbol	>270	0
Ingenane types		
Ingenol	>287	
3–*O*–Hexadecanoyl ingenol (3HI)	0.086	+++
3–*O*–Tetradecanoyl ingenol (3TI)	0.011	
3TI–20–tetradecanoate	0.05	
Ingenol–3–acetate	0.43	
Ingenol–3–butyrate	0.096	
Ingenol–3–hexanoate	0.025	
Ingenol–3–octanoate	0.042	
Ingenol–3–decanoate	0.030	
Ingenol–3–dodecanoate	0.027	
Milliamine A	0.040	
Milliamine C	0.007	(+)
Milliamine G	0.015	
Daphnane types		
Hippomane factor $M_1 + M_2$	0.02	+++
Pimelea factor P_1 (Simplexin)	0.01	
Pimelea factor P_4	0.03	
Daphnopsis factor R_3	0.02	
Daphnopsis factor R_4	0.1	
Mezerein	0.03	++
Resiniferatoxin	0.00001 (ID_{50}^2)	0
1-Alkyldaphnane types		
Synaptolepis factor K_7	0.02	
K_7–20–hexadecanoate	0.16	
Synaptolepis factor K_1	0.0015	
K_1–20–hexadecanoate	0.017	
Pimelea factor P_2 (Daphnopsis factor R_1)	0.006	+++
Pimelea factor P_3 (Daphnopsis factor R_5)	0.02	
Daphnopsis factor R_6	0.04	
Daphnopsis factor R_7	0.09	
Pimelea factor P_6	0.08	

† Figures in parentheses indicate $ID_{50}^3 \mu g \mu l^{-1}$ shown by F. J. Evans.[42]

REFERENCES

1. Berenblum, I., Cocarcinogenic action of croton resin, *Cancer Res.*, **1**: 44–48, 807 (1941).

2. Böhm, R., Flaschentrager, B., *Ber. ges. Phisiol. u. exp. Pharmakol.*, **42**: 585 (1927); Flaschentrager, B., and von Falkenhasen, F. Frhv., Über den giftstoff im Krontonöl II. Zur Konstitution von Krotophorfolon, *Ann.*, **514**: 252–257 (1934).

3. Hecker E., (Uber die Wirkstoffe des Crotonols I, Biologische Teste zur quantitativen Messung der entzundlichen, cocarcinogenen und toxischen wirkung, *Z. Krebsforsch*, **65**: 325 (1963).

4. Bartsch, H., Bresch, H., Gschwendt, M., Harle, E., Kreibich, G., Kubinyi, H., Schairer, H. U., Szczepanski, Ch. v., Thielman H. W., and Hecker, E., Kombination wirksamer Trennverfahren mit modernen analytischen Methoden in der Naturstoffchemie, *Z. Anal. Chem.*, **221**: 424–432 (1966).

5. Hecker, E., Schairer, H. U., Uber die Wirkstoffe des Crotonols VIII. Verbessertes Isotierungsverfahren fur die Wirkstoffgruppen A und B sowie Isolierung und Charakterisierung weiterer Wirkstoffe der Gruppe A, *Z. Krebsforsch*, **70**: 1–12 (1967)*Z. Krebsforsch*, 7, 1 (1967): Hecker, E. Phorbol Esters from Croton Oil Chemical Nature and Biological Activities, *Naturwiss.*, **54**: 282–284 (1967).

6. Hecker, E., Co-carcinogenic principles from the seed oil of *Croton tiglium* and from other Euphorbiaceae, *Cancer Res.*, **28**: 2338–2349 (1968).

7. Hecker E., and Bresch, H., Über die Wirkstoffe des Crotonöls, III. Reindarstellung und Charakterisierung eines toxisch, entzundlich und cocarcinogen hochaktiven Wirkstoffs, *Z. Naturforsch*, **20b**: 216–226 (1965).

8. Hecker E., and Schmidt, R., Phorbol esters-the irritants and cocarcinogens of *Croton tiglium* L., *Prog. Chem. Org. Natur. Prod.*, **31**: 377–467 (1974).

9. Adolf, W., and Hecker, E., On the active principles of the spurge family (Euphorbiaceae) III. Skin irritant and cocarcinogenic factors from the caper spurge, *Z. Krebsfor sch*, **84**: 325–344 (1975).

10. Opferkuch, H. J., and Hecker, E., On the active principles of the spruge family (Euphorbiaceae) IV. Skin irritant and tumor promoting diterpene esters from *Euphorbia ingens* E. May., *J. Cancer Res. Clin. Oncol.*, **103**: 255–268 (1982).

11. Roberts, H. B., Mc Clure, J. T., Ritchie, E., Taylor, W. C. and Freeman, P. W., The isolation and structure of the toxin of *Pimelea simplex*, responsible for St. George disease of cattle, *Aust. Vet. J.*, **51**: 325–326 (1975).

12. Zayed, S., Hafez, A., Adolf, W., and Hecker, E., New tigliane and daphnane derivatives from *Pimelea prostrata* and *Pimelea simplex.*, *Experientia*, **33**: 1554–1555 (1977).

13. Sakata, K., Kawazu, K., Mitsui, T., Structure and Stereochemistry of Huratoxin, a piscicidal constituent of *Hura crepitans*, *Tetrahedron Lett.*, 1141–1144 [(1971); Sakata, K., Kawazu, K., and Mitsui, T., Studies on a Piscicidal Constituent of *Hura crepitans* Part I. Isolation and Characterization of Huratoxin and its Piscicidal Activity, *Agr. Biol. Chem.*, **35**: 1084–1091, (1971).

14. Stout, G. H., Balkenhol, W. G., Poling, M., and Hickernell, G. L., The Isolation and Structure of Daphnetoxin, the Poisonous Principle of *Daphne* Species, *J. Am. Chem. Soc.*, **92**: 1070–1071 (1970).

15. Ronlan, A., and Wickberg, B., The Structure of Mezerein, A Major Toxic Principle of *Daphne Mezereum* L., *Tetrahedron Lett.*, 4261–4264 (1970); Ciezer J., and Pieterse, M. G., *J. van die Suid Afrikaanse Chem. Inst.* 24: 241 (1971).

16. Ohigashi, H., Hirota, M., Ohtsuka, T., Koshimizu, K., Fujiki, H., Suganuma, M., Yamaizumi, Z., and Sugimura, T., Resiniferonol-related Diterpene Esters from *Daphne odora* Thunb. and their Ornithine Decarboxylase-inducing Activity in Mouse Skin, *Agr. Biol. Chem.*, **46**: 2605–2608 (1982).

17. Ohigashi, H., Ohtsuka, T., Hirota, M., Koshimizu, K., Tokuda H., and Ito, Y.,

Tigliane Type Diterpene-esters with Epstein-Barr Virus-inducing Activity from *Sapium sebiferum, Agr. Biol. Chem.,* **47**: 1617–1622 (1983).

18. Hirata, Y., Toxic Substances of Euphorbiaceae, *Pure Apple. Chem.,* **41**: 175–199 (1975) and references cited therein.

19. Uemura, D., and Hirata, Y., The Isolation and Structures of Two New Alkaloids, Milliamines A and B, obtained from *Euphorbia milii, Tetrahedron Lett.,* 3673–3676 (1971); The Isolation and Structure of Toxic Principles, Milliamines A, B and C, from *Euphorbia milii, Bull. Chem. Soc. Japan,* **50**: 2005–2009 (1977).

20. Uemura D., and Hirata, Y., Isolation and Structures of Irritant Substances obtained from *Euphorbia* species *(Euphorbiaceae), Tetrahedron Lett.,* 881–884 (1973).

21. Zechmeister, K., Brandl, F., Hoppe, W., Hecker, E., Opferkuch, H. J., and Adolf, W., Structure Determination of the New Tetracyclic Diterpene Ingenoltriacetate with triple Product Methods, *Tetrahedron Lett.,* 4075–4078 (1970) and references cited therein.

22. Marston A., and Hecker, E., On the Active Principles of the Euphorbiaceae VI: Isolation and Biological Activities of Seven Milliamines from *Euphorbia milii, Planta Medica,* **47**: 141–147 (1983).

23. Marston, A., and Hecker, E., Structure-Activity Relationships of Polyfunctional Diterpenes of the Tigliane Type, V. Preparation and Irritant Activities of Amino Acid and Peptide Esters of Phorbol, *Z. Naturforsch,* **38b**: 1015–1021 (1983).

24. Theilmann, H. W., Jacovi P., and Hecker, E. photbol XVIII. Bromination of Phorbol pentaacetate, *Ann.,* **765**: 171–189 (1972); Sorg, B. and Hecker, E., On the Chemistry of Ingenor, III I Synthesis of3-Deoxy-3-oxoingenol, Some 5-Esters and of Ethers and Acetals of Ingenol, *Z. Naturforsch,* **37b**: 1640–1947 (1982).

25. Kupchan, S. M., Uchida, I., Braufman, A. R., Dailey, R. G., and Yu Fei, B., Antileukemic Principles Isolated from Euphorbiaceae Plants, *Science,* **191**: 571–572 (1976); Gunasekera, S. P., Cordell, G. A., and Farnsworth, N. R., Potential Anticancer Agents. XIV, Isolation of Spruceanol and Montanin from *Cunuria spruceana* (Euphorbiaceae), *J. Nat. Prod.,* **42**: 658–662 (1979).

26. Hartwell, J. L., Plants Used Against Cancer. A Survey, *Lloydia,* **32**: 153–205 (1969).

27. E. Hecker, H. Bartsch, G. Kreibich and C. v. Szczepanski, Chemistry of Phorbol X. Heavy-atom derivatives of Phorbol for X-ray structural analysis, *Ann.* **725**: 130–141 (1969); Crombie, L., Games, M. L. and Pointer, D. J., X-ray Structure Analysis of Neophorbol, Chemistry and Structure of Phorbol, the Diterpene Parent of the Cocarcinogenes of Croton oil, *J. Chem. Soc. (c),* 1347–1362 (1968).

28. Kupchan, S. M., Sigel, C. W., Matz, M. J., Renauld, J. A. S., Haltiwanger, R. C., and Bryan, R. F., Jatrophone, a Nobel Macrocyclic Diterpenoid Tumor Inhibtor from *Jatropha gossypiifolia, J. Am. Chem. Soc.,* **92**: 4476–4477 (1970).

29. Upadhyay, R. R. and Hecker, E., A new Cryptic Irritant and Cocarcinogen from seeds of *Croton sparciflarus, Phytochemistry,* **15**: 1070–1072 (1976).

30. Evans, F. J., A new Phorbol Triester from the Latices of *Euphorbia frankiana* and *E. coerulescens, Phytochemistry,* **16**: 395–396 (1977).

31. Evans, F. J., The Irritant Toxins of Blue *Euphorbia (Euphorbia coerulescens* Haw.), *Toxicon,* **16**: 51–57 (1978).

32. Ohigashi, H., Kawazu, K., Koshimizu, K., and Mitsui, T., A Piscicidal Constituent of *Sapium japonicum, Agr. Biol. Chem.,* **36**: 2529–2537 (1972).

33. Furstenberger, G., and Hecker, E., Zum Wirkungsmechanismus Cocarcinogener Pflanzeninhaltsstoffle, *Planta Medica,* **22**: 241–266 (1972).

34. Okuda, T., Yoshida, T., Koike, S. and Toh, N., The Toxic Constituents of the Fruits of the *Aleurites fordii, Chem. Pharm. Bull.,* **22**: 971–972 (1974); New Diterpene Esters from *Aleurites fordii* Fruits., *Phytochemistry,* **14**: 509–515 (1975).

35. Hirota, M., Ohigashi, H., and Koshimizu, K., Piscicidal Constituents and Related Diterpene Esters from *Aleurites fordii, Agr. Biol. Chem.,* **43**: 2523–2529 (1979); Fujiki, H., Mori, M., Sugimura, T., Hirota, M., Ohigashi, H., and Koshimizu, K., Relationship Between Ornithine Decarboxylase-inducing Activity and Configuration at C-4 in Phorbol Ester Derivatives, *J. Cancer Res. Clin. Oncol.,* **98**: 9–13 (1980).

36. Adolf, W., Opferkuch, H. J., and Hecker, E., Irritant phorbol derivatives from four *Jatropha* species, *Phytochemistry,* **23**: 129–132 (1984).
37. Geschwendt, M. G., and Hecker, E., Tumor Promoting Compounds from *Euphorbia Triangularis:* Mono- and Diesters of 12-Desoxy-phorbol, *Tetrahedron Lett.,* 3509–3512 (1969); M. Gschwendt und E. Hecker, Uber die Wirkstoffe der Euphorbiaceen II. Hautreizende und cocarcinogene Faktoren aus Euphorbia triangularis Desf. *Z. Krebsforsch,* **81**: 193–210 (1974). *Z. Krebsfprscj,* **81**: 193–210 (1974).
38. Cashmore, A. R., Seelye, R. N., Chain, B. F., Mack, H., Schimidt R., and Hecker, E., The Structure of Prostratin: A Toxic Tetracyclic Diterpene Ester from *Pimelea prostrata, Tetrahedron Lett.,* 1737–1738 (1976).
39. Adolf, W., and Hecker, E., On the Active Principles of the Thymelaeaceae II. Skin Irritant and Cocarcinogenic Diterpenoid Factors from *Daphnopsis racemosa, Planta Medica,* **45**: 177–182 (1982).
40. Schmidt R. J. and Evans, F. J., The Succulent *Euphorbias* of Nigeria. II. Aliphatic Diterpene Esters of the Latices of *E. poisonii* Pax. and *E. unispina* N. E. Br., *Lloydia,* **40**: 225–229 (1977).
41. Hergenhahn, M., Kusumoto S., and Hecker, E., Diterpene Esters from 'Euphorbium' and their Irritant and Cocarcinogenic Activity, *Experientia,* **30**: 1438–1440 (1974).
42. Kinghorn, A. D., and Evans, F. J., Skin irritants of *Euphorbia fortissima, J. Pharm. Pharmacol.,* **27**: 329–333 (1975).
43. Evans, F. J., Kinghorn, A. D. and Schmidt, R. J., Naturally occurring skin irritants, *Acta Pharmacol. et Toxicol.,* **37**: 250–256 (1975).
44. Evans, F. J., and Kinghorn, A. D., New Diesters of 12-Deoxy-phorbol, *Phytochemistry,* **14**: 1669–1670 (1975).
45. Evans, F. J., and Schmidt, R. J., Two New Toxins from The Latex of *Euphorbia poisonii, Phytochemistry,* **15**: 333–335 (1976).
46. Schmidt, R. J., and Evans, F. J., A new Aromatic Ester Diterpene from *Euphorbia poisonii, Phytochemistry,* **15**: 1778–1779 (1976).
47. Schmidt, R. J., and Evans, F. J., Structure and Potency of some 'Tinya' Toxins, *J. Pharm. Pharmacol.,* **27**: 50P (1975).
48. Hecker, E., New toxic, irritant and carcinogenic diterpene esters from Euphorbiaceae and from Thymelaeaceae, *Pure Appl. Chem.,* **49**: 1423–1431 (1977).
49. Adolf, W., and Hecker, E., On the Irritant and Cocarcinogenic Principles of *Hipponune mancinella, Tetrahedron Lett.,* 1587–1590 (1975).
50. Gschwendt, M., and Hecker, E., Biological active compounds of Euphorbiaceae, I. Skin irritant and cocarcinogenic factors from *Euphorbia cooperi, Z. Krebsforsch,* **8**: 335–350 (1973).
51. Schmidt, R. J., and Evans, F. J., Candletoxins A and B, 2 New Aromatic Esters of 12-deoxy-16-hydroxyphorbol, from the irritant latex of *Euphorbia poisonii* Pax., *Experientia,* **33**: 1197–1198 (1977).
52. Hergenhahn, M., Adolf, W. and Hecker, E., Resiniferatoxin and Other Esters of Novel Polyfunctional Diterpenes from *Euphorbia resinifera* and *unispinaa, Tetradron Lett.,* 1595–1598 (1975).
53. Zayed, S., Adolf, W. and Hecker, E., On the Active Principles of the Thymelaeceae, 1. The Irritants and Cocarcinogens of *Pimelea prostrata, Planta medica,* **45**: 67–77 (1982).
54. Kinghorn, A.D. and Evans, F. J., **26**: 150 (1967).
55. Gotta, H., Adolf, W., Opferkuch, H. J. and Hecker, E., On the Active Principles of the Euphorbiaceae, IX. Ingenane Type Diterpene Esters from Five Euphorbia Species, *Z. Naturforsch,* **39b**: 683–694 (1984).
56. Hirota, M., Ohigashi, H., Oki, Y. and Koshimizu, K., New Ingenol-Esters as Piscicidal Constituents of *Euphorbia cotinifolia* L., *Agr. Biol. Chem.,* **44**: 1351–1356 (1980); Fujiki, H., Sugimura, T., Ohigashi, H., Hirota, M., and Koshimizu, K., Relation Between the Structures of Ingenol Esters and Their Ornithine Decarboxylase-Inducing Activities in Mouse Skin *Carcinogenesis,* **7**: 65–67 (1982).

57. Evans, F. J. and Soper, C. J., The Tigliane, Daphnane and Ingenane Diterpenes, Their Chemistry, Distribution and Biological Activities. A Review, *Lloydia*, **41**: 193–233 (1977).

58. Uemura, D. and Hirata, Y., New Diterpene, 13-Oxyingenol, Derivative Isolated from *Euphorbia kansui* Lion, *Tetrahedron Lett.*, 2529–2532 (1974).

59. Opferkuch, H. J. and Hecker, E., New Diterpenoid Irritants from Euphorbia ingens, *Tetrahedron Lett.*, 261–264 (1974); Upadhyay, R. R. and Hecker, E., Diterpene Esters of the Irritant and Cocarcinogenic Latex of *Euphorbia lactea, Phytochemistry*, **14**: 2514–2516 (1975).

60. Seip, E. and Hecker, E., Skin Irritant Ingenol Esters from *Euphorbia esula, Planta medica*, **46**: 215–218 (1982).

61. Ott, H. H. and Hecker, E., Highly irritant ingenane type diterpene esters from *Euphorbia cyparissias* L., *Experientia*, **37**: 88–91 (1981).

62. Falsone, G., Crea, A. E. G. and Noack, A. E., Über Inhaltsstoffe von Euphorbiaceae, 7. Mitt. 20-Desox yingenolmonoester und Ingenoldiester aus *Euphorbia bigglandulosa* Desf. *Arch. Pharm.*, **315**: 1026–1032 (1982).

63. Evans, F. J. and Kinghorn, A. D., A New Ingenol Type Diterpene from the Irritant Factors of *Euphorbia myrsinites* and *Euphorbia biglandulosa, Phytochemistry*, **13**: 2324–2325 (1974).

64. Schmidt R. J., and Evans, F. J., Skin irritants of the sun spurge (Euphorbia helioscopia L.) *Contact Dermatitis*, **6**: 204–210 (1980).

65. Uemura, D., Ohwaki, D. and Hirata, Y., Isolation and Structure of 20-Deoxyingenol New Diterpene Derivatives and Ingenol Derivative Obtained from "Kansui", *Tetrahedron Lett.*, 2527–2528 (1974).

66. Kupchan, S. M., Sweeny, J. G., Baxter, R. L., Murae, T., Zimmerly, V. A. and Sickles, B. R., Gnididin, Gniditrin, and Gnidicin, Novel Potent Antileukemic Diterpenoid Esters from *Gnidia lamprantha, J. Am. Chem. Soc.*, **97**: 672–673 (1975).

67. Kupchan, S. M., Shizuri, Y., Sumner, W. C., Haynes, H. R., Leighton, A. P., Sickles, B. R., Isolation and Structual Elucidation of New Potent Antileukemic Diterpenoid Esters from *Gnidia* Species, *J. Org. Chem.*, **41**: 3850–3853 (1976).

68. Ohigashi, H., Katsumata, H., Kawazu, K., Koshimizu, K. and Mitsui, T., A Piscicidal Constituent of *Excoecaria agallocha, Agr. Biol. Chem.*, **38**: 1093–1095 (1974).

69. Kogiso, S., Wada, K. and Munakata, K., Odoracin, a Nematicidal Constituent from *Daphne odora, Agr. Biol. Chem.*, **40**: 2119–2120 (1976).

70. Kupchan, S. M., Shizuri, Y., Murae, T., Sweeny, J. G., Haynes, H. R., Shen, M. S., Barrick, J. C., Bryan, R. F., van der Helm, D., and Wu, K. K., Gnidimacrin and Gnidimacrin 20-Palmitate, Novel Macrocyclic Antileukemic Diterpenoid Esters from *Gnidia subcordata, J. Am. Chem. Soc.*, **98**: 5719–5720 (1976).

71. Zayed, S., Adolf, W., Hafez, A., and Hecker, E., New Highly Irritant 1-Alkyldaphnane Derivatives from Several Species of Thymelaeceae, *Tetrahedron Lett.*, 3481–3486 (1977).

72. Hecker, E., Immich, H., Bresch, H. and Schairer, H. U., Uber die Wirkstoffe des Crotonols VI. Entzungsteste am Mauseohr, *Z. Krebsforsch.*, **68**: 366–374 (1966).

73. Ito, Y., Yanase, S., Tokuda, H., Kishita, M., Ohigashi, H., Hirota, M. nad Koshimizu, K., Epstein-Barr Virus Activation by Tung Oil, Extracts of Aleurites Fordii and Its Diterpene Ester 12-*O*-Hexadecanoyl-16-Hydroxphorbol-13-acetate, *Cancer Lett.*, **18**: 87–95 (1983); Ito, Y., Ohigashi, H., Koshimizu, K., and Yi, Z., Epstein-Barr Virus-Activating Principle in the Ether Extracts of Soils Collected from Under Plants Which Contain Active Diterpene Esters, *Cander Lett.*, **19**: 113–117 (1983).

74. Fujiki, H., Hecker, E., Moore, R. E., Sugimura, T. and Weinstein I. B., (ed.), *Cellular Interactions by Environmental Tumor Promoters*, pp. 3–36, Japan Scientific Societies Press, VNU Science Press BV. (1984).

11
Noncarcinogenic Plants and Plant Materials of Japan

In Japan, especially in rural and mountainous areas, it is long established custom that various kinds of uncultivated wild plants are used as seasonal delicacies, famine relief, and/or folk remedies. Furthermore, many vegetables indigenous to Japan, such as bamboo shoots, roots of burdock ,and rhizomes of lotus, are also consumed. As described elsewhere in this volume, several wild plants, such as cycads, bracken and others, consumed by humans, have been shown to be carcinogenic to experimental animals, and powerful carcinogens have been isolated from these plants and their carcinogenicity proven.

Carcinogenicity of wild esculent plants, indigenous vegetables and herbal medicines traditionally consumed in Japan have been investigated in long-term feeding experiments[1-3] from the viewpoint of food safety.

Among the wild esculent plants, kernels of ginkgo nuts (*Ginkgo biloba,* "*ginnan*" in Japanese), fertile stems of common horsetail (*Equisetum arvense,* "tsukushi"), young furled fronds of osmund (*Osmunda japonica,* "zemmai"), and young ostrich-fern (*Matteuccia struthiopteris,* "kusasotetsu") were investigated. Ginkgo, like the cycads, is a gymnosperm and common horsetail, osmund and ostrich-fern, like bracken, are pteridophytes.

Other wild esculent plants investigated include young shoots of aralia *(Aralia cordata,* "udo"), cacalia (*Cacalia hastata,* "yobusumasou"), mugwort (*Artemisia princeps,* "yomogi") and vicia (*Vicia unijuga,* "nantenhagi").

Among vegetables indigenous to Japan, young shoots of bamboo *(Phyllostachys heterocyclia,* "take-no-ko"), roots of burdock *(Arctium lappa,* "gobou") and rhizomes of lotus (*Nelmbo nucifera,* "renkon") have been studied for carcinogenicity.

Of plants used as herbal medicine, dandelion roots *(Taraxacum platycarpum,* "hokouei-kon"), rhizomes of galangal *(Alpinia officinarum,* "kou-ryoukyou-kon"), terrestrial parts of lathyrus (*Lathyrus palustris,* "ezo-no-renrisou"), and leaves of lycium (*Lycium chinense,* "kuko") have been examined.

Caffeic acid and prunasin were investigated as plant constituents. Caffeic acid is widely distributed throughout the vegetable kingdom, and prunasin, a cyanogenetic glucoside, is found in poisonous plants and bracken.[4]

The following is the description of a long-term experiment conducted by the present author on carcinogenicity testing of various kinds of plants and plant materials found in Japan.

Animals and diets

Inbred strain ACI rats of both sexes were used in the study outlined in Table 11–1. The age and number of rats in each group, concentration of plant materials in diet and administration periods are summarized in the table. To prepare the diet containing plant materials, fresh plants in the same stage of growth as when used as human food or herbal remedies were dried in a dryer equipped with blower. The material was then milled and mixed with rat basal diet CE-2 (CLEA Japan Inc., Tokyo) in varying concentrations and made into pellets. Composition of basal diet CE-2 and preparation of pellets were the dame as described previously.[5] Upon termination of feeding with the diet containing plant materials, rats were returned to a normal diet. Water was given ad libitum. All animals were autopsied at death, i.e. when sacrificed due to a moribound condition or at the termination of the experiment. Tissues were fixed in 10% formalin, sectioned and stained with hematoxylin and eosin.

Plant Materials

Ginkgo nuts ("ginnan" in Japanese), seeds of maidenhair tree *(Ginkgo biloba* L., "ichou" in Japanese), were harvested in Aichi Prefecture in October. The young fronds of osmund *(Osmunda japonica* Thunb., "zemmai") in the fiddlehead or crosier stage of growth were collected in mountainous areas of Gifu Prefecture in April. Dried osmund as a foodstuff was purchased from a grocer. The young furled fronds of ostrichfern *(Matteuccia struthiopteris* (L.) Todaro, "kusasotetsu") were collected in Iwate Prefecture in May. The fertile stems ("tsukushi") of common horsetail *(Equisetum arvense* L., "sugina") were collected in Gifu Prefecture and Hokkaido in March and May, respectively. The young terrestrial parts of aralia *(Aralia cordata* Thunb., "yama-udo") were collected in a mountainous area of Gifu Prefecture in May. The young terrestrial parts of cacalia *(Cacalia hastata* L. var. *orientalis* (Kitam.), "yobusumasou") were collected in Iwate Prefecture in June. The young leaves of mugwort *(Artemisia princeps* Pampan., "yomogi") were collected in Gifu City in April and May. The young terrestrial parts of vicia *(Vicia unijuga* A. Br., "nanten-hagi" or "azukina") were collected in Gifu Prefecture in June.

The young shoots ("take-no-ko" in Japanese) of bamboo *(Phyllosta-*

Table 11–1. Experimental Design[†]

	ACI Rats		Treatment		
Group	Age (Months)	Number and Sex	Plant Materials	Concentration of Plant Materials in Diet	Period of Administration
I-1	1.0	15 (M7, F8)	Unprocessed ginkgo kernels	33%	337 days
I-2	1.0	15 (M8, F7)	Autoclaved (30 min at 1 atm) ginkgo kernels	33%	310 days
II-1	1.5	16 (M8, F8)	Curled top part of the young osmund frond in the fiddlehead or crosier stage	33%	113 days
II-2	1.5	25 (M13, F12)	Young osmund fern without curled top parts	33%	126 days
II-3	1.5	18 (M9, F9)	Young terrestrial part of osmund fern	33%	177 days including an interval of 45 days fed with normal diet
III-1	1.5	24 (M12, F12)	Young furled frond of ostrich-fern	33% 3 weeks, 20% for 3 days, basal diet for 10 days, 4% for 3 weeks, and finally 4% until the termination of experiment	480 days
III-2	1.5	26 (M13, F13)	Young furled frond of ostrich-fern	4%	480 days
IV	1.0–1.5	11 (M4, F7)	Fertile stems of common horsetail	33%	76 days
V	1.5	26 (M13, F13)	Young terrestrial part of Aralia	33%	230 days
VI	1.0	20 (M9, F11)	Rhizomes of lotus	33%	150 days
VII	1.5	24 (M12, F12)	Young terrestrial part of Cacalia	4%	480 days
VIII	1.5	25 (M11, F14)	Young terrestrial part of mugwort	33%	86 days
IX	1.5	12 (M6, F6)	Roots of burdock	33%	120 days
X	1.0–1.5	20 (M10, F10)	Roots of dandelion	32%	209 days
XI	1.5	16 (M8, F8)	Bambooshoots	33%	131 days
XII	1.5	18 (M9, F9)	Terrestrial part of Lathyrus	33%	180 days
XIII	1.5	24 (M12, F12)	Young terrestrial part of Vicia	16%	285 days
XIV	1.5–2.0	30 (M15, F15)	Galangal	16%	397 days (M4 and F4 33% for 5 days and 16% for 385 days)
XV	1.0	20 (M10, F10)	Leaves of Lycium	33%	540 days
XVI	1.0	14 (M7, F7)	Caffeic acid	0.5%	180 days
XVII	1.5	20 (M10, F10)	Prunasin	0.03%	480 days
Control	1.0	151 (M80, F71)		None	

[†] The experiment was terminated after 480 days, except Group XV in which the experiment was terminated after 540 days.

chys heterocyclia (Carr.) Mitf. var. *Pubescens* (Mazel) Ohwi, "mousou-chiku") cultivated in Gifu Prefecture were harvested in April. The roots of burdock *(Arctum Lappa* L., "gobou") cultivated in Gifu Prefecture were harvested in May. Rhizomes ("renkon") of lotus *(Nelumbo nucifera* Gaert., "hasu" cultivated in Aichi Prefecture were harvested in October.

The roots ("hokouei-kon") of dandelion *(Taraxacum platycarpum* Dahlst., "tampopo") which were collected in Kagawa Prefecture in October and dried, were purchased from pharmacy specializing in herb medicine. The terrestrial parts of lathyrus *(Lathyrus palustris* L. var. *pilosus* Ledeb., "ezo-no-renrisou") were collected in Hokkaido in August. Dried galangal *(Alpinia officinarum* Hance, "kou-ryoukyou-kon") and dried leaves of matrimony vine *(Lycium chinense* Mill., "kuko") were purchased from a pharmacy specializing in herb medicine.

Caffeic acid used in the study was purchased from Nakarai Chemical Co. (Kyoto, Japan). Prunasin was synthesized according to the method described by Fischer and Bergmann.[6]

Group I

Neither the group fed for 337 days with pellets containing unprocessed kernels (Subgroup I-1) nor the group fed for 310 days with kernels treated in an autoclave (Subgroup I-2), developed tumors.

Group II

Glioma of the cerebellum was observed in one rat of Subgroup II–1, which died 451 days after the start of feeding. No tumor was observed in rats of Subgroup II-2. As for Subgroup II-3, only one rat had a tumor, fibroadenoma of breast. Since the animals in this subgroup II-3 were frequently reluctant to eat and lost weight, the concentration of the young osmund fern in the diet had to be reduced at times.

Group III

In Subgroup III-1, two out of 24 rats dies within 45 days, and another two died 306 and 411 days after the start of the experiment. The remaining 20 rats survived until the termination of the experiment. No tumors were observed in this group. All animals in Subgroup III-2 survived beyond 400 days after the start of the experiment, and 19 animals survived until the termination. None of the animals had tumors.

Group IV

Of 11 rats fed a diet containing common horsetail, 10 survived until the termination of the experiment, with no tumors indeuced.

Group V

Twenty-two out of 26 rats survived until the termination of the experiment. In these 22, and in another three which died between 218 and 300 days after the start of the feeding, no tumors were detected except a papilloma of the urinary bladder in one rat.

Group VI

Five out of the 20 rats in this group died or were sacrificed in a moribound condition between 172 and 435 days after the start of the experiment. One of the five had oligodendoroglioma of the cerebrum. The remaining 15 rats survived until the termination of the experiment and no tumors were observed.

Group VII

Two out of 24 rats died 184 and 245 days after the start of the experiment; the latter had subcutaneous fibrosarcoma in the back. Another four died between 329 and 443 days; one of them showed reticulum cell sarcoma in the mesentery. The remaining 18 rats, which were sacrificed 480 days after the start of the experiment, had no tumors.

Group VIII

All the animals except one which died of pneumonia survived beyond 390 days after the start of the experiment. Pituitary adenoma was observed in one rat, but the others did not develop any tumors.

Group IX

All the animals survived beyond one year after the start of the experiment, and ten rats survived until the termination. Tumors were not detected in any of the animals.

Group X

One of the 20 rats in this group died after 20 days, and another six rats dies 207, 259, 304, 367, 391, and 416 days after the start of the pexeriment. The remaining 13 rats survived until the termination of the experiment. However, no tumors were observed in this group.

Group XI

All the animals in this group survived beyond 414 days. No tumors were observed.

Group XII

Sixteen out of 18 rats (two rats died of pneumonia 125 and 247 days after the start of the feeding) survived beyond 440 days, and 14 rats were sacrificed at the termination of the experiment. Of three rats, one had urinary bladder papilloma, another adrenal cortical adenoma and a third testicular interstitial cell tumor.

Group XIII

All 24 rats in this group survived beyond 352 days after the start of the feeding. Two (one male and one female) out of 19 rats which were sacrificed at the termination of the experiment had adrenal cortical adenooma.

Group XIV

Animals in this group were frequently reluctant to feed on the diet and lost weight, necessitating reduction of the concentration of galangal in the diet. Five male and 6 female rats died of hunger within 8 days, being reluctant to eat the diet. Fifteen rats were sacrificed at the termination of the experiment, of which three had testicular interstitial cell tumor.

Group XV

Seventeen out of the 20 rats survived beyond about 500 days, and 14 of them were sacrificed at the termination of the experiment. Pituitary adenoma and hemangioma of the lung were observed in each of two rats. Testicular interstitial cell tumors were observed in two rats.

Group XVI

All rats survived beyond 233 days after the start of feeding the 0.5% caffeic acid diet. Nine of them survived until termination of the experiment. No tumors were observed.

Group XVII

Nineteen rats in this group (one rat died after 26 days) survived beyond 394 days; six died 394 to 453 days after the start of the feeding, and the remaining 13 were sacrificed at the termination of the experiment. One female rat which died after 451 days had leukemia, and one male had testicular interstitial cell tumor.

Control

Tumors observed in 151 rats of the control group were as follows: testicular interstitial cell tumor, 7 rats; adrenal cortical adenoma, 3; pituitary adenoma, 2; adrenal pheochromocytoma, 1; cecal adenoma, 1; urinary bladder carcinoma, 1 and papilloma, 1; pancreatic exocrine adenoma, 1; and reticulum cell sarcoma of the mesentery, 1.

The proportion by weight of each plant material and basal diet in pellets used in most studies was 1:2, the same as in the pellets used in the bracken experiment.[5,7]

Ginkgo is a gymnosperm and, like cycads, it is the most primitive among the living spermatophytes. It is well known that cycasin from cycads was hydrolyzed to its active aglycone by β-glucosidase in the kernel when the nut was crushed without pretreatment.[8,9] Taking this into account, ginkgo nuts treated in an autoclave before crushing were also tested in this study. No tumors were observed in any groups fed pellets containing ginkgo nuts for more than 300 days.

Osmund, ostrich-fern, and common horsetail, like bracken, are pteridophytes. In rats fed pellets containing osmund, no significant results suggesting its carcinogenicity were obtained. The young frond of ostrich-fern is used as human food in Japan as well as in Canada and the United States.[10,11] Carcinogenicity of ostrich-fern was not observed in either receiving group. Newberne[11] also reported that the young frond of ostrich-fern was not toxic of carcinogenic in Sprague-Dawley weanling rats. The feeding period for Group IV was 76 days, relatively short compared with the other groups. However, since a high incidence of tumor was observed in rats fed for only 60 days with bracken pellets,[12] it may be assumed that common horsetail does not possess carcinogenic activity.

Although rats received diets containing wild aralia and cultivated lotus for 230 and 150 days respectively, no tumors were observed except urinary bladder papilloma and oligodendoroglioma in one rat each of Group V and Group VI. Maekawa and Odashima[13] reported that urinary bladder papilloma was observed in 10 animals and oligodendoroglioma in one in their study on spontaneous tumors using 264 ACI rats. No histological finding to suggest the role of these plants materials as a cause of these tumors was detected. Therefore, these tumors were considered to have been induced spontaneously.

Hayashi *et al.*[14] reported that integerrimine, a pyrrolizidine alkaloid, is contained in the terrestrial part of *Cacalia hastata* L. In rats of Group VII fed a diet containing 4% cacalia, subcutaneous fibrosarcoma in the back was observed in one rat and reticulum cell sarcoma in the mesentery in another. The remaining 22 rats showed neither tumors nor morphological changes suggesting hepatotoxicity or the possibility of occurrence of tumors. Thus carcinogenic activity of cacalia could not be demonstrated as the result of a 4% cacalia diet.

In rats of Groups XIII and XIV fed diets containing vicia and galangal respectively, adrenal cortical adenoma was encountered in two rats and testicular interstitial cell tumor in three. Adrenal and testicular tumors were freuqnely observed in control ACI rats, so these tumors in the rats of Groups XIII and SIV were considered to be spontaneous. Thus carcinogenic activity of the young terrestrial part of vicia and galangal could not be detected under these experimental conditions.

Although one rat in Group XII fed a diet containing lathyrus developed urinary bladder papilloma, it was considered to be spontaneous because control animals occasionally developed the same type of tumor, as noted above in the case of aralia. Since rats in this group received the diet containing lathyrus in high concentration for 180 days, it is reasonable to assume that lathyrus is not carcinogenic.

It is known that galangal and lathyrus contain flavonoids, such as galangin[15] and kaempherol.[16] Recently, mutagenic activity of flavonoids was reported by Sugiura et al.[17] and Bjeldanes et al.[18] attracting a great deal of attention to the carcinogenicity testing of pure mutagenic flavonoids.

A diet containing matrimony vine was given to rats for 540 days in Group XV. However, all tumors observed in this group were spontaneous benign tumors, and carcinogenicity of matrimony vine was not be detected in the present study.

Caffeic acid is widely distributed as a plant constituent. Rats fed the diet containing caffeic acid in Group XVI had neither tumors nor morphological changes suggesting the possibility of cocurrence of tumors.

Prunasin (mandelonitril glucoside) is a toxic cyanogenetic glucoside and contained in bracken.[4] The LD_{50} of prunasin given by stomach tube was 790 mg/kg body weight in male rats of ACI strain. The concentration of prunasin used in the present study was determined based on the LD_{50}. However, prunasin was found to have no carcinogenic activity under the experimental conditions employed.

REFERENCES

1. Hirono, I., Shibuya, C., Shimizu, M., Fushimi, K., Mori, H., and Miwa, T., Carcinogenicity examination of some edible plants. *Gann.* **63**: 383–386 1972.
2. Hirono, I., Mori, H., Kato, K., Ushimaru, Y., Kato, T., and Haga, M., Safety examination of some edible plants, Part 2. *J. Environ Path. Toxicol.*, **1**: 71–74, 1977.
3. Hirono, I., Hosaka, S., Uchida, E., Takanashi, H., Haga, M., Sakata, M., Mori, H., Tanaka, T., and Hikino, H., Safety examination of some edible or medicinal plants and plant constituents, Part 3, *J. Food Safety*, **2**: 205–211, 1980.
4. Bennett, W.D., Isolation of the cyanogenetic glucoside prunasin from bracken fern. *Phytochemistry*, **7**: 151–152, 1968.
5. Hirono, I., Shibuya, C., Fushimi, K., and Haga, M., Studies on carcinogenic properties of bracken, *Pteridium aquilinum. J. Natl. Cancer Inst.*, **45**: 179–188, 1970.

6. Fischer, E. and Bergmann, M., Synthese des Mandelnitril-glucosids, Sambunigrins und ähnlicher Stoffs. *Ber. Dtsch. Chem. Ges.*, **50**: 1047–1069, 1917 (in German).
7. Hirono, I., Fushimi, K., Mori, H., Miwa, T., and Haga, M., Comparative study of carcinogenic activity in each part of bracken. *J. Natl. Cancer Inst.*, **50**: 1367–1371, 1973.
8. Kobayashi, A., Biochemical studies on cycasin. Part 1. Purification and properties of cycad β-glucosidase. *Agr. Biol. Chem.* (Tokyo) **26**: 203–207, 1962.
9. Laqueur, G.L., Mickelson, O., Whiting, M.G., and Kurland, L.T., Carcinogenic properties of nuts from *Cycas circinalis* L. indigenous to Guam. *J. Natl. Cancer Inst.*, **31**: 919–951, 1963.
10. Robert-Pichette, P., *Fiddleheads in New Brunswick.* Mimeograph, New Brunswick Department of Agriculture and Rural Development, Fredericton, 1971.
11. Newberne, P.M., Biologic effects of plant toxins and aflatoxins in rats. *J. Natl. Cancer Inst.*, **56**: 551–555, 1976.
12. Hirono, I., Mori, H., Miwa, T., and Haga, M., Unpublished results.
13. Maekawa, A. and Odashima, S. Spontaneous tumors in ACI/N rats. *J. Natl. Cancer Inst.*, **55**: 1437–1445, 1974.
14. Hayashi, K., Natorigawa, A., and Mitsuhashi, H., Integerrimine from *Cacalia hastata* L. *subsp. orientalis* Kitamura. *Chem. Pharm. Bull.*, **20**: 201–202, 1972.
15. Kariyone, T. and Kimura, K., *Hirokawa Yakuyo Shokubutsu Dai Jiten*, Hirokawa Publishing Co., Tokyo, **1970** (in Japanese).
16. Harborne, J.B., Distribution of flavonoids in leguminosae. In: *Chemotaxonomy of the Leguminosae*, (Harborne, J.B., Boutler, D., and Turner, B.L. eds.), p. 31, Academic Press, London and New York, 1971.
17. Sugimura, T., Nagao, M., Matsushima, T., Yahagi, T., Seino, Y., Shirai, A., Sawamura, M., Natori, S., Yoshihira, K., Fukuoka, M., and Kuroyanagi, M., Mutagenicity of flavone derivatives. *Proc. Jpn. Acad.*, Ser. B, **53**: 194–197, 1977.
18. Bjeldanes, L.F. and Chang, G.W., Mutagenic activity of quercetin and related compounds. *Science*, **197**: 577–578, 1977.

12

Plant Secondary Metabolites as Chemical Carcinogens

12.1 Biosynthesis and Functions of Plant Secondary Metabolites

More than one million species of all living things on earth grow, propagate, and evolve utilizing chemical substances. Recent advances in the field of biochemistry have greatly clarified the molecular basis of life and the common biosynthetic pathways of energy and anabolic metabolism of the compounds called primary metabolites such as sugars, amino acids, fatty acids, and of the biopolymers such as polysaccharides, lipids, peptides and proteins, and nucleic acids, which are both essential and ubiquitous. In contrast, so-called plant products and antibiotics belong to the category of secondary metabolites produced by specific organisms. Due to the development of separation methods and of physical methods for structure elucidation, the numbers of such secondary metabolites being characterized are ever increasing, but the roles they play in host organisms is generally not clear and they have been considered to be waste products of the metabolic processes.

The enormous numbers of secondary metabolites exhibit a variety of structural modifications but, since the 1930s, it has been pointed out that there exists some regularity in these structures to suggest their biogenetic origin. The application of the isotopical labeled precursors subsequently clarified the relationship of these compounds to primary metabolites and they are now systematically classified according to their biosynthetic pathways as shown in Fig. 12.1.[1] They are classified into i) acetogenins (polyketides) formed from the condensation of one mole of acetyl–Co A and several moles of malonyl–Co A, ii) phenylpropanoids (C_6–C_3) and related compounds formed from shikimic acid, derived from triose and tetrose, iii) isoprenoids such as terpenes, steroids, and carotenoids, formed from mevalonic acid, and iv) alkaloids formed from amino acids such as phenylalanine, tyrosine, tryptophan, lysine and

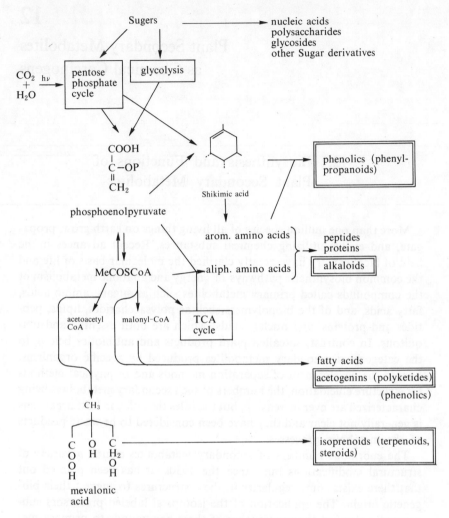

Fig. 12.1. Biosynthetic pathways of secondary metabolites.

ornithine. Some secondary metabolites are formed by the combination of the above units; e.g. flavonoids are formed from the C_6–C_3 unit and three malonates. Besides these, some secondary metabolites are assumed to be direct derivatives of primary metabolites, while some others are formed by the combination of the secondary metabolites formed from the above units with primary metabolites such as sugars (glycosides) and fatty acids (esters). As a whole, though the structural features of the secondary metabolites appear complicated, they are biosynthesized from the definite building blocks noted above with further modifications occurring by oxidation, reduction, condensation, migration, and other reactions including attachment of C_1-units (5-deoxyadenylmethionine).

The acute toxicities of some secondary metabolites, such as the principles of toxic plants, have been known for centuries and utilized as arrow poisons and fish poisons. Alkaloids and cardiotonic glycosides are examples of compounds later used for medicines. Recent developments in natural products chemistry have revealed that many secondary metabolites exhibit a diversity of biological activities to other organisms. The discovery of a variety of ecochemicals[2] is one example. As a result, secondary metabolites are now assumed to be products which do not directly influence the functions of the producers but play roles as ecochemicals in their existence. Thus the naturally occurring plant carcinogens may be assumed to be a kind of allomone for mammals.[2] However, the majority of the secondary metabolites remains to be isolated, characterized, and tested for further understanding of the chemical bases of the biological phenomena.

12.2 Naturally Occurring Carcinogens as Secondary Metabolites[3-6]

The numbers of natural products (secondary metabolites) are increasing rapidly. However, naturally occurring carcinogenic compounds which have been proved experimentally, number not more than forty. This is not an indication that only a few natural products among the vast numbers of compounds are carcinogenic but rather that compounds tested by adequate experimental methods are quite small compared with synthetic chemicals.

Cycacin in cycad, aflatoxins from *Aspergillus flavus*, and bracken carcinogens were first recognized as acutely toxic substances and then found to be carcinogenic in the course of studies using detailed animal experiments. Safrole is an exception; feeding experiments using large amounts of the material led to the discovery of its carcinogenicity. Feeding experiments for carcinogenicity testing require long periods of time and large amounts of material; sufficient amounts of materials for such tests are generally not available in the case of natural products. In this respect, relatively inexpensive and rapid mutagenicity tests, especially the *Salmonella*/microsome test (Ames' test), are suited to screening large numbers of compounds and they are now frequently used to test naturally occurring compounds. As a result, mutagenicity of flavonoids (*see* Chapter 3) and other phenolics has been reported. However, none of these compounds has so far been proved to be carcinogenic in animal experiments.

12.3 Chemical Structures of Naturally Occurring Carcinogens

Our knowledge of naturally occurring carcinogens is very limited at the moment by the chronic toxicity data available for the chemicals. It is within such limitations that the chemical structures of the carcinogenic compounds will be overviewed.

Our attention to natural products was stimulated by the discovery of the mycotoxins, aflatoxins. In 1960 an outbreak of "Turkey-X-disease," causing death of turkeys in the United Kingdom, attracted much attention and the cause was found to be contamination of *Aspergillus flavus* in the peanut meal used for feed. Further work revealed that the main metabolites of the mold aflatoxin B_1 (1), and congeners (2–4) were strongly carcinogenic: addition of 15 ppb of aflatoxin B_1 to the feed significantly induced hepatocarcinoma in rats. The presence of a bisfuran ring was noted in the chemical structures of the aflatoxins clarified.

This discovery stimulated work on mycotoxins. The carcinogenic compounds (5–12) thus far clarified are shown in Fig. 12.2.[7–10]

All these compounds except cyclochlorotin (8) belong to the polyketides (acetogenins) according to the biosynthetic classification shown in Fig. 12.1. Since acetogenins are most common in the mold secondary metabolites, it is impossible to correlate the carcinogenicity with the biosynthetic pathways. Among these, 1–4, 10 and 11 contain an α,β-unsaturated lactone moiety. A number of simple α,β-unsaturated lactones have been proved to induce subcutaneous sarcomas in rats and mice at the site of injection.

Several antibiotics (13–19) from various Streptomyces (Fig. 12.3) have been found to induce neoplasia in rats and mice by parenteral administration.

Carcinogens from higher plants, the subject of this volume, will now be reviewed according to their chemical structures and biosynthetic classification.

Carageenan (Chapter 5) consists mainly of varying amounts of the metal salts of sulphate esters of galactose and 3,6-anhydrogalactose copolymers and is classified as a polysaccharide belonging to the primary metabolites. Since they generally appear as mixtures, the exact chemical characteristics of the carcinogenicity is not known.

Cycasin (Chapter 1) is a glucoside of an aliphatic alcohol containing an azoxy group, which is quite rare among natural products. The biosynthesis of the compounds has not been proved experimentally, but the compound is assumed to be a derivative of an aliphatic amino acid.

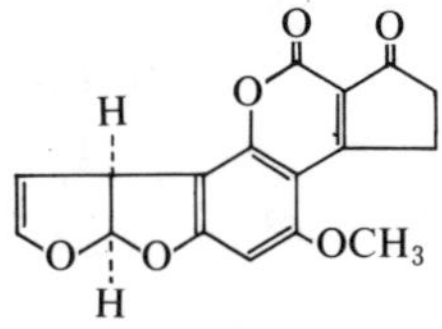

aflatoxin A₁ (1)   aflatoxin A₂ (2)   aflatoxin B₁ (3)   aflatoxin B₂ (4)

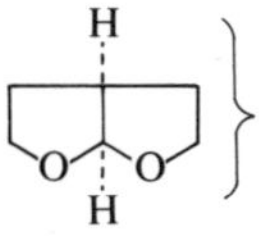

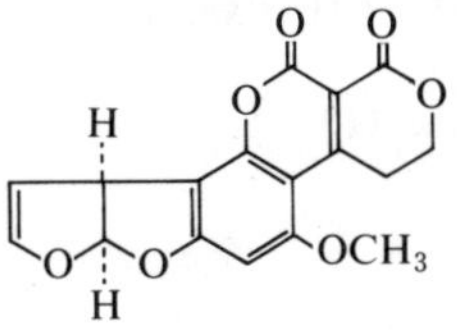

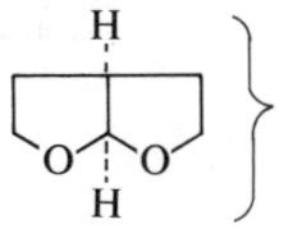

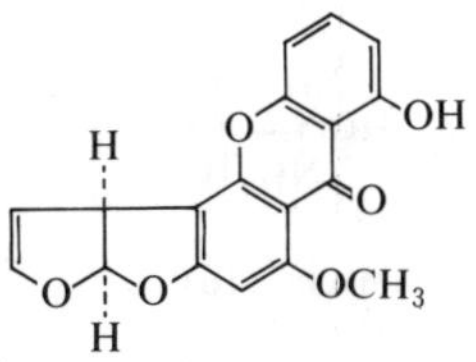

sterigmatocystin (5) 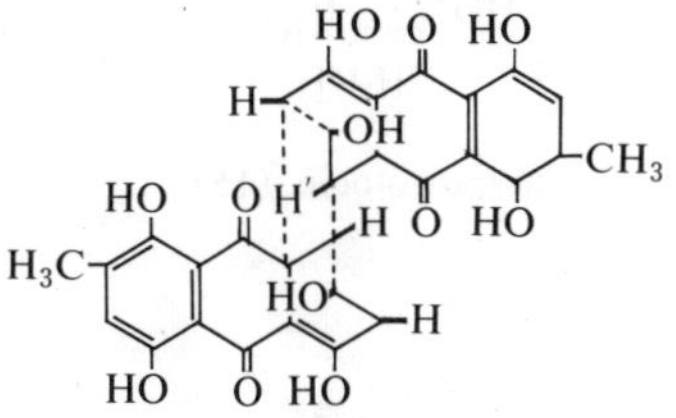   luteoskyrin (6)

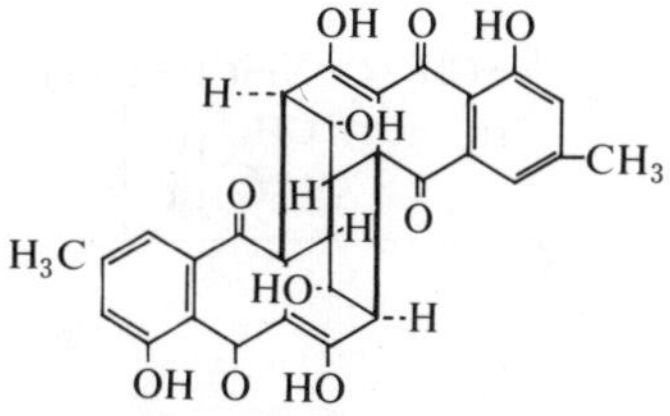

rugulosin (7)

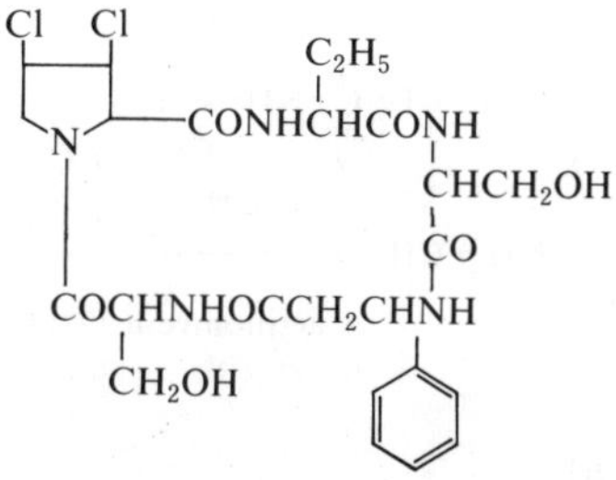

cyclochlorotin (8)

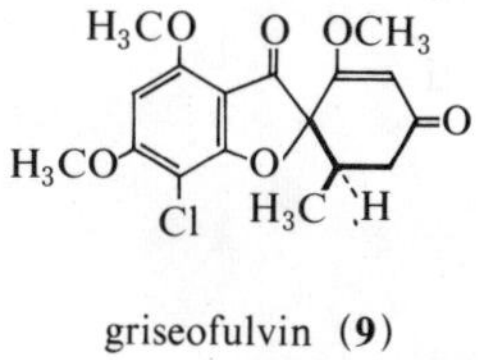

griseofulvin (9) 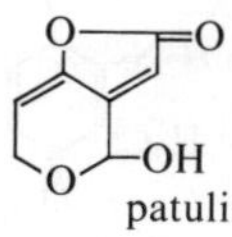   patulin (10) 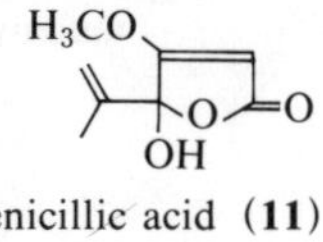   penicillic acid (11) 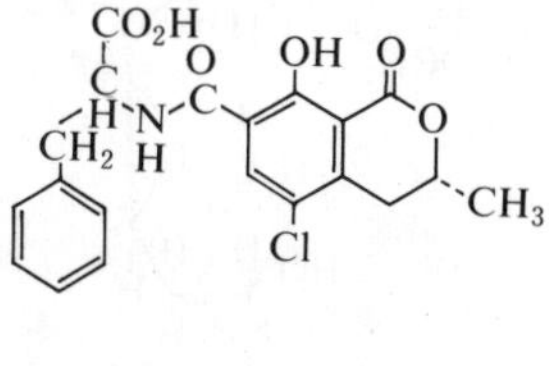   ochratoxin A (12)

Fig. 12.2. Carcinogenic mycotoxins.

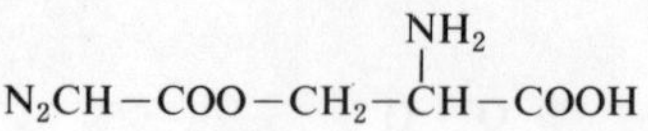

azaserine (13)

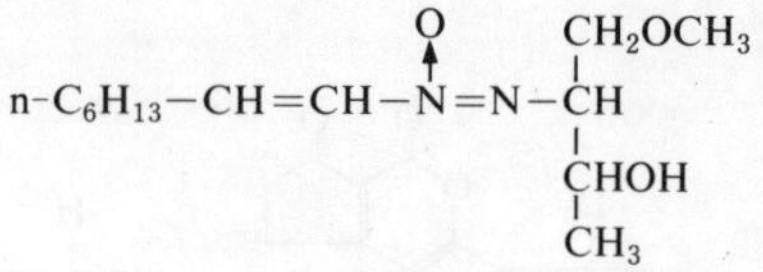

elaiomycin (14)

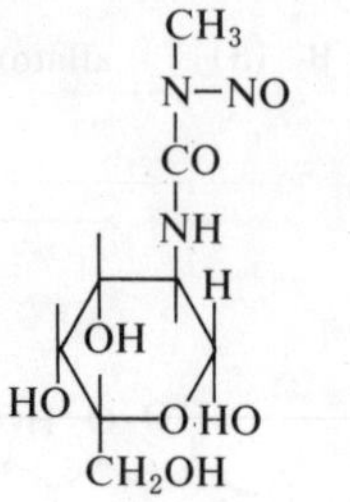

streptozotocin (15)

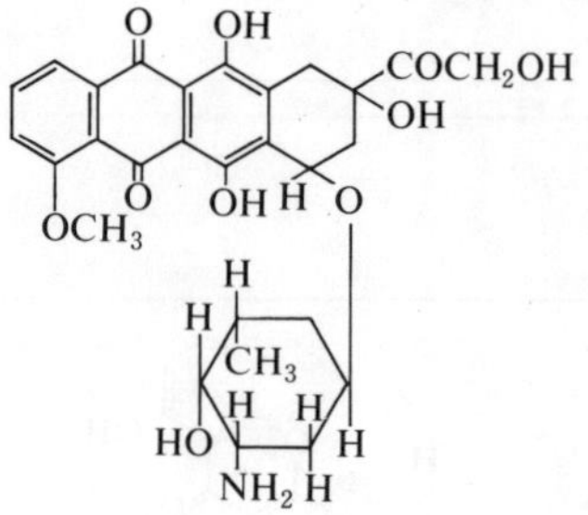

adriamycin (16)

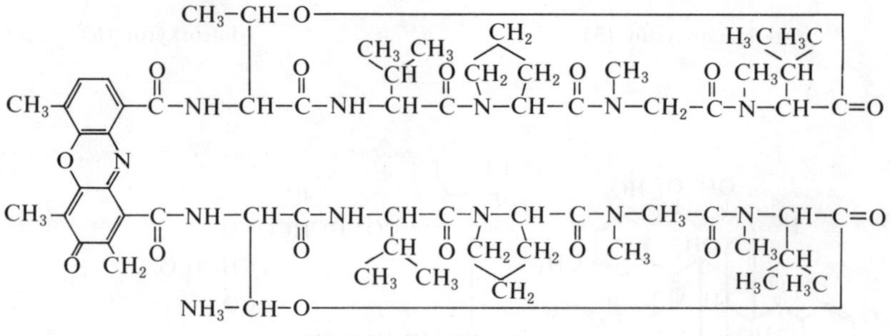

actinomycin D (17)

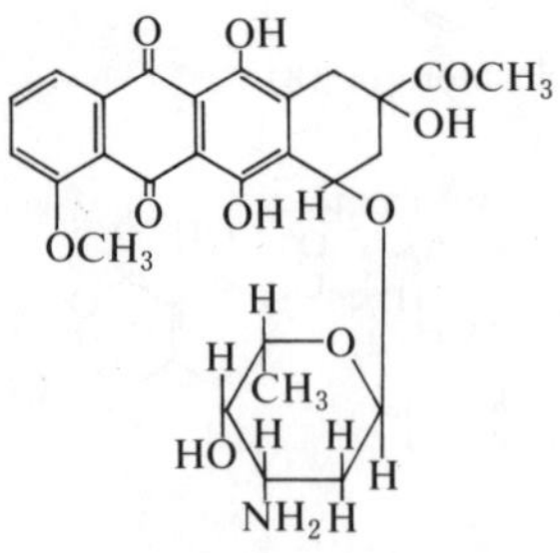

daunomycin (18)

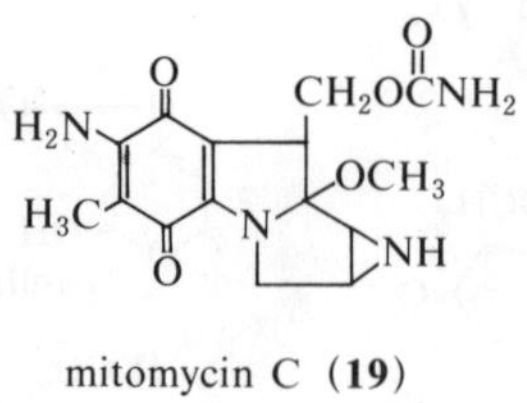

mitomycin C (19)

Fig. 12.3. Carcinogenic metabolites from *Streptomyces*.

Alkaloids are one of the most important groups of plant products and are formed from amino acids. Most of the alkaloids exhibit a variety of biological activities and have been widely used as medicines such as morphine and strychinine. Most are nitrogen-heterocyclic compounds and are usually classified by heterocyclic rings such as pyridine, isoquinoline, and indole. Although many alkaloids are acutely toxic, only those bearing the pyrrolizidine ring (Chapter 2) have been proved to be carcinogenic. The pyrrolizidine ring has been shown to come from an amino acid, ornithine, by the pathway shown in Fig. 12.4. The majority of the other alkaloids are not known to be carcinogenic.

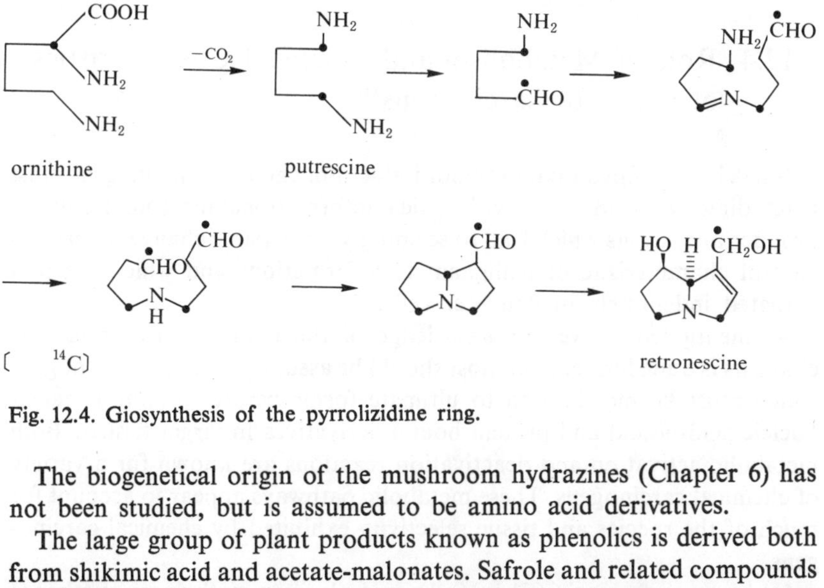

Fig. 12.4. Giosynthesis of the pyrrolizidine ring.

The biogenetical origin of the mushroom hydrazines (Chapter 6) has not been studied, but is assumed to be amino acid derivatives.

The large group of plant products known as phenolics is derived both from shikimic acid and acetate-malonates. Safrole and related compounds (Chapter 7) are examples of former origin. The mutagenic flavonoids (Chapter 3) are formed from both precursors as shown in section 3.1. Tannins (Chapter 8) are divided into two groups, hydrolyzable and non-hydrolyzable (condensed) tannins. The former is a group of compounds in which sugar residues are esterified with phenolic acids of shikimic acid origin, while the latter is a group of compounds formed by polymerization of catechins or leucoanthocyanidins belonging to the flavonoids (cf. p. 54 of Chapter 3). They appear naturally as mixtures and the chemical characteristics of the carcinogenic tannins have not been clarified.

Isoprenoids are compounds formed by the condensation of two to eight prenyl units derived from mevalonic acid. The recently unveiled carcinogenic principle of bracken, ptaquiloside (Chapter 4), is a glycoside of a norsesquiterpene, formed from three prenyl units. The structural characteristics of the compound are discussed in Chapter 4. In contrast, phorbol esters, tumor promoters (Chapter 10), are fatty acid esters of diterpenes formed from four prenyl units. In the diversity of the structural modifications of isoprenoids, these two may be unique in the instability to form an active form after hydrolysis in the former and in the specific physical properties originating from long fatty acid residues in the latter.

As a whole, naturally occurring carcinogens of plant origin are very diverse in their structural modifications, and no common structural features, functional groups, or biogenetical origins, are evident. In other words, we cannot predict *a priori* carcinogenicity from the chemical structure.

12.4 Role of Metabolism and Chemical Characteristics of Ultimate Carcinogens[11]

It has been defined that, in tumor induction, chemical carcinogens must react, directly or indirectly, with critical informational macromolecules to produce alterations which lead to seemingly irreversible changes in growth control characteristic of malignant transformations and which are perpetuated indefinitely in daughter cells.

As mentioned above our knowledge of the naturally occurring carcinogens is quite limited, but most should be assumed to be precarcinogens which must be metabolized to ultimate forms before forming covalent nucleic acid-bound and protein-bound derivatives in target tissues. Both metabolic activation and deactivation reactions are known for a variety of chemical carcinogens. These metabolic pathways appear to account for much of the species and tissue selectivity exhibited by chemical carcinogens.

In the case of cycasin (Chapter 1), hydrolysis to methylazoxymethanol by β-glycosidase of gut flora is prerequisite for carcinogenicity. Spontaneous loss of formaldehyde then gives rise the ultimate form, CH_3N_2OH, which reacts as an alkylating agent.[12]

In the case of pyrrolizidine alkaloids (Chapter 2), the metabolism to highly reactive pyrrol derivatives, which react as electrophiles bearing an allyl alcohol group to nucleophiles such as DNA, is an essential stage of the carcinogenic activity (*see* Chapter 2, Fig. 2.13).

Safrole (Chapter 7) also must be oxidized at the α-position to a benzylic and allylic alcohol type compound, 1'-hydroxysafrole, as the proximate carcinogen. The acyl esters of the alcohol, from which acyloxy groups tend to separate, act as ultimate carcinogens.

Such metabolism to form the reactive ultimate form has been more precisely demonstrated in the case of the mycotoxins, aflatoxin B_1 and sterigmatocystin. The furan ring in both compounds are metabolized to the epoxides by phenobarbital-induced rat liver microsomes *in vitro* and, in the presence of calf thymus DNA, transformed into carcinogen-modified DNAs, acid hydrolysis of which liberates major guanine-containing adducts, **20** and **21** (Fig. 12.5). These are examples of the isolation and characterization of the DNA adducts by chemical means *in vitro*.[13]

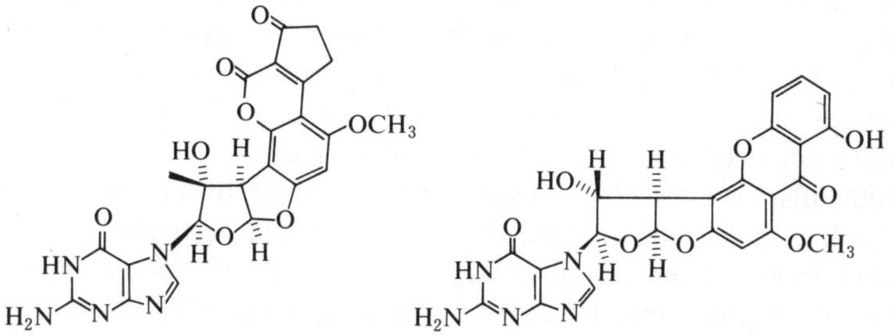

(20)   (21)

Fig.12.5. Structures of guanine-containing adducts of aflatoxin B and sterigmatocystin.

The recently established carcinogenic principle of bracken (Chapter 4), ptaquiloside, is a unique compound among the chemical carcinogens so far known. Most carcinogens must be *oxidatively* metabolized to the reactive and carcinogenic electrophiles. Ptaquiloside, a glycoside, itself is quite unstable both in acids and bases and an unstable conjugated dienone, an ultimate form, is formed spontaneously by hydrolysis. The quite unstable intermediate easily forms non-toxic indanone derivatives, pterosins, isolated earlier by the conventional methods of extraction and isolation.

Compounds such as ptaquiloside, which cannot be isolated by ordinary methods, should also be the subject of future studies on environmental carcinogens of natural origin.

From these results, we can conclude that metabolisis to potentially electrophilic compounds is usually, if not always, necessary for carcinogenesis. Furthermore, absorption, excretion and distribution to target organs must be considered to be accompanied by metabolic changes. Little is known regarding these points.

12.5 Effects of Naturally Occurring Carcinogens on Human Health

Human beings select harmless and tasty animals and plants as food-stuff, harmless here meaning not acutely toxic. The geographical pathology of cancer in humans suggests that a large percentage perhaps as high as 80%, of human cancer is of environmental origin. Thus, the chemical carcinogens in the total environment may rank as a major cause of human cancer. All plants and microorganisms produce secondary metabolites, which may exhibit some physiological activities. Thus the safety of foods and feeds should be examined, taking into consideration a wider view of toxicity including carcinogenicity. Recent surveys have revealed that compounds like the flavonoids, commonly distributed among the plant kingdom, exhibit a kind of genotoxicity, though carcinogenicity has fortunately not been proved for these compounds.

In foodstuffs we must also consider contamination by environmental factors such as polycyclic aromatic hydrocarbons and pesticide residues. The recent trend of increasing use of highly processed foodstuffs has given rise to new problems such as the use of many kinds of food additives including "natural food additives." The recent discovery of the strong mutagenicity of protein pyrolysates is another case in point. Generally speaking, cooking acts as a detoxification process but here it is an example of toxification. Formation of carcinogenic nitrosamines from naturally occurring secondary amines and nitrite ion present naturally or formed from nitrate, is another problem in which the secondary formation of carcinogens from natural products in foods occurs. The safety of foodstuffs must thus be considered from all these aspects.[14]

Recent progress described in this volume has demonstrated the occurrence of natural carcinogens of higher plants origin. Stimulated by the discovery of aflatoxins, general surveys on natural carcinogens have been extensively conducted over the past twenty years. Recently, mutagenicity testing has been applied to many natural resources. Contrary to our expectation, many new carcinogens have fortunately not been discovered, though many compounds have been shown to exhibit some mutagenicity or genotoxicity. This fact may indicate that genotoxic compounds exist widely in nature and may play a role as ecochemicals, but whether or not they are chemical hazardous to humans must be considered from a multidisciplinary standpoint. In any case, the reduction of the total amounts of carcinogenic natural products in the diet or intestinal content of humans may eventually constitute an important weapon in the prevention of cancer. Further work in this direction will contribute to the improvement of human health.

REFERENCES

1. Natori, S., Classification of natural products. In: *Natural Products Chemistry* vol. 1. (eds. K. Nakanishi, T. Goto, S. Ito, S. Natori, S. Nozoe) pp. 4–10, Kodansha, Tokyo, and Academic Press, New York, 1974.
2. Whittaker, R.H. and Feeny, P.P., Allelochemics: Chemical interaction between species, *Science,* **171**: 757–770 (1971).
3. Miller, J.M., Naturally occurring substances that can induce tumors. In: *Toxicants Occurring Naturally in Foods*, pp. 508–549, National Academy of Sciences, Washington, D.C., 1973.
4. Schoental, R., Carcinogens in plants and microorganisms. In: *Chemical Carcinogens* (ed. C.E. Searle) pp. 626–689, American Chemical Society, Washington, D.C., 1976.
5. IARC: *IARC Monographs on the Evaluation of Carcinogenic Risk of Chemicals to Humans,* vol. 10, 1976; vol. 31, 1983, IARC, Lyon.
6. Kinghorn, A. D., Carcinogenic and cocarcinogenic toxins from plants. In: *Plant and Fungal Toxins* (ed. R. F. Keeler, A. T. Tu), pp. 239–298, Marcel Dekker, New York, 1983.
7. Ciegler, A., Kadis, S., Ajl, S.J. (eds.) *Microbial Toxins,* vol. VI-VIII, Academic Press, New York, 1971–1972.
8. Purchase, I.F.H. (ed.), Mycotoxins, Elsevier, Amsterdam, 1974.
9. Rodricks, J.V., Hesseltine, C.W., and Mehlman, M.A. (eds.), *Mycotoxins in Human and Animal Health,* Pathotox Publishers, Ill., 1977.
10. Uraguchi, K., and Yamazaki, M. (eds.), *Toxicology, Biochemistry and Pathology of Mycotoxins,* Kodansha, Tokyo, 1978.
11. Miller, E.C., and Miller J.A., The metabolism of chemical carcinogens to reactive electrophiles and their possible mechanisms of action in carcinogenesis. In: *Chemical Carcinogens.* (ed. C.E. Searle), pp. 732–762, American Chemical Society, Washington, D.C., 1976.
12. Zedeck, M.S., Hydrazine derivatives, azo and azoxy compounds, and methylazoxymethanol. In: *Chemical Carcinogens,* Second Edition, vol. 2, (ed. C.E. Searle) pp. 915–944, American Chemical Society, Washington, D.C., 1984.
13. Essigmann, J.M., Croy, R.G., Nadzan, A.M., Busby, W.F. Jr, Reinhold, V.N., Büchi, G., and Wogan, G.N., *Proc. Natl. Acad. Sci. U.S.A.,* **74**: 1870–1874, 1977; Lin, J-K., Miller, J.A., and Miller, E.C., *Cancer Res.,* **37**: 4430–4438, 1977; Essigmann, J.M., Barker, L.J., Fowler, K.W., Francisco, M.A., Reinhold, V.N., Wogan, G.N., *Proc. Natl. Acad. Sci. U.S.A.,* **76**: 179-183, 1979.
14. Grasso, P., Carcinogens in food. In: *Chemical Carcinogens.* Second Edition, vol. 2. (ed. C.E. Searle) pp. 1205–1239, American Chemical Society, Washington, D.C., 1984.

Index

OF GREENWICH LIBRARY